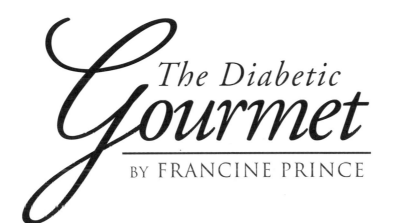

The Diabetic
Gourmet

BY FRANCINE PRINCE

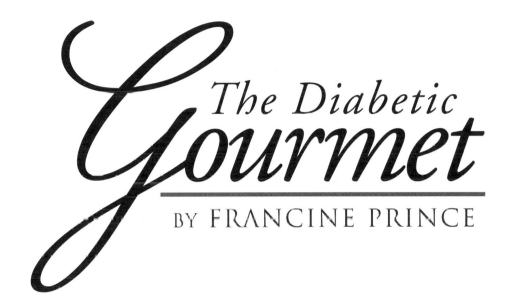

The Diabetic
Gourmet

BY FRANCINE PRINCE

A DIABETES SELF-MANAGEMENT COOKBOOK

Exchange Lists for Meal Planning in the Appendix copyright © 1989 American Diabetes Association and The American Dietetic Association. Reprinted with permission.

Library of Congress Cataloging-in-Publication Data
Prince, Francine.
   The diabetic gourmet / by Francine Prince.
    p. cm.
   Includes index.
   ISBN 0-9631701-3-9
   1. Diabetes—Diet therapy—Recipes.   I. Title
   RC662.P739 1994
   641.5´6314—dc20   94-5368
                           CIP

Editor: James Hazlett

Project Director: Maryanne Schott Turner

Design: Edward Noriega

Photography: Michael Grand

Food Stylist: Hillary Davis-Tonken

Prop Stylist: Michele Michael

The four-color separations for this book were done by Applied Graphics Technologies.

Printed and bound in the United States by Quebecor Printing Book Group.

10 9 8 7 6 5 4 3 2

Diabetes Self-Management Books is an imprint of R.A. Rapaport Publishing, Inc., 150 West 22nd Street, New York, NY 10011.

ABOUT THE AUTHOR

~

*F*rancine Prince is one of the nation's leading authorities on good cooking for better health. She is well known for creating innovative cookbooks that show people on special diets how to create nutritious, delicious dishes.

Her cooking methods and her recipes have been endorsed by leading medical experts and acclaimed by food critics. All the recipes she has written for this book are easy to prepare—even if you've never cooked before—and use ingredients readily available in the supermarket.

ACKNOWLEDGEMENTS

~

*O*ur boundless gratitude to Nancy Cooper, R.D., C.D.E., who spent many thoughtful hours writing the highly instructive Chef's Notes chapter of this book. Nancy also put her heart and soul (and many more hours) into creating the mouth-watering menus beginning on page 17. Her expertise, particularly in diabetic nutrition, was invaluable in helping to put this book together.

We are also deeply grateful to Nancy C. Patterson, M.S., R.D., C.D.E. for her painstaking and thoughtful nutrition analyses and exchange calculations. Her analyses will help you keep track of what you eat as you enjoy each scrumptious recipe in this book.

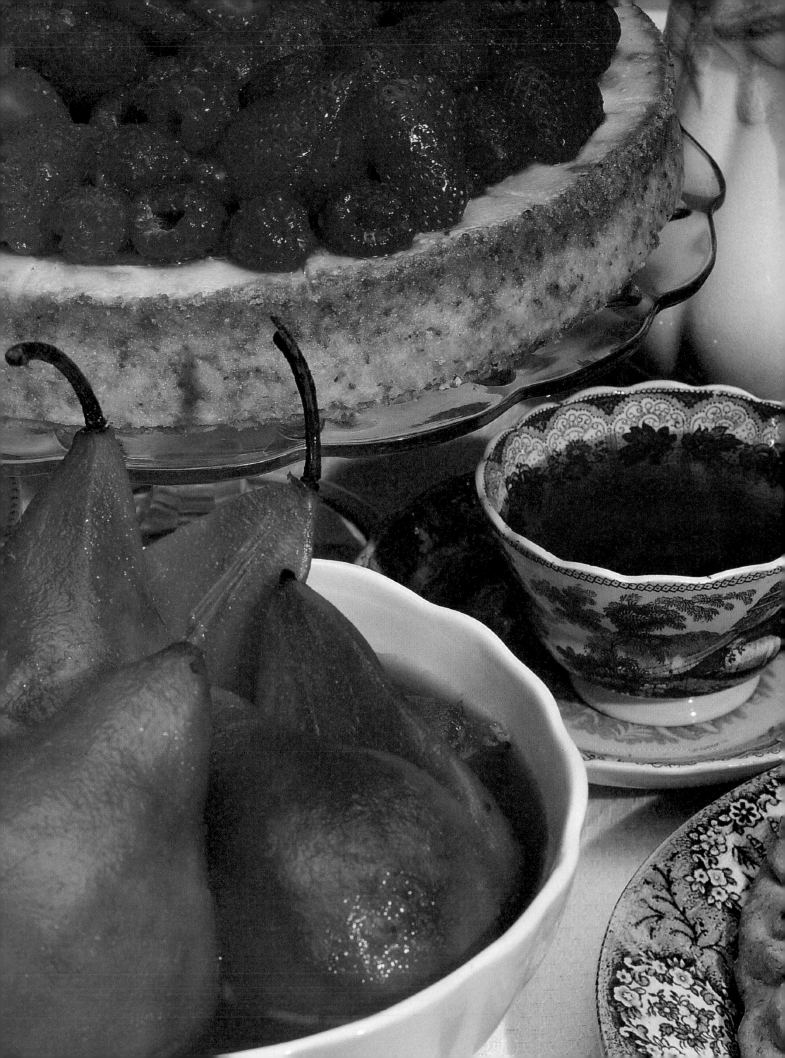

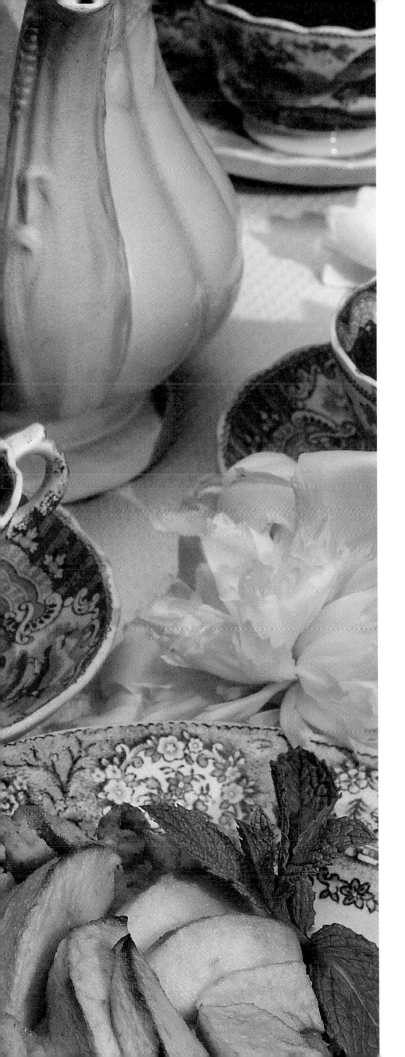

Table of Contents

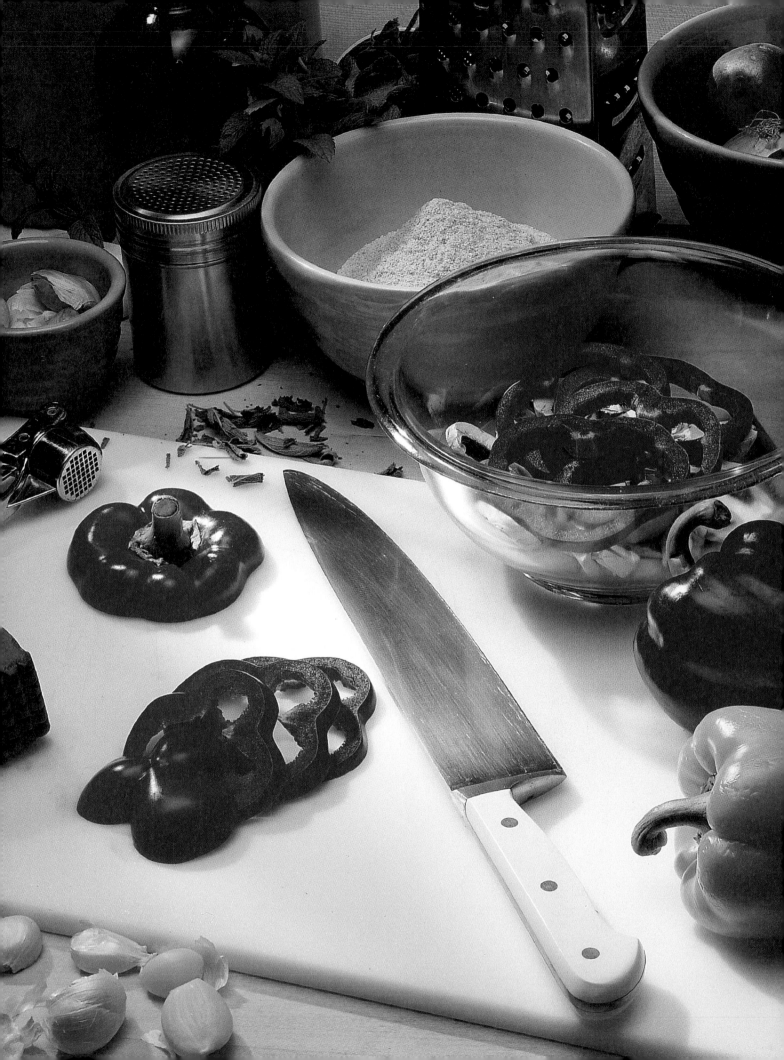

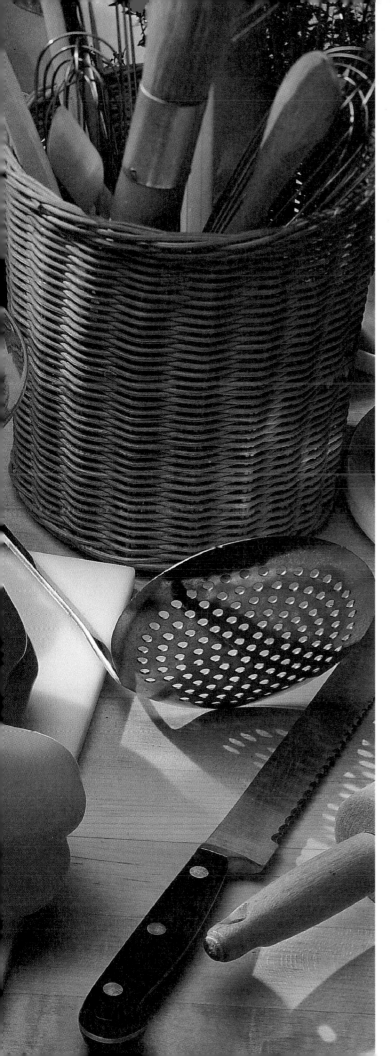

Chef's Notes

Whether you're an old pro or just beginning to cook, a fundamental understanding of cooking techniques brings added pleasure to your time in the kitchen. This section covers some basic knowledge picked up over many enjoyable years of cooking and can show you how to prepare great-tasting, healthier foods quickly and efficiently—and bring out your best as a cook.

CUTTING AND PREPARING INGREDIENTS

Cutting ingredients and preparing them correctly before cooking is an important step to success in the kitchen. Ingredients that are properly cut and prepared are more likely to cook within the time specified in the recipe and produce the desired texture, consistency and eye-appeal. To make easier work of the cutting and preparation techniques described below, start with a set of freshly sharpened knives and a cutting board.

CHOP: To cut food into irregular-shaped pieces, which can range from small (finely chopped) to large (coarsely chopped) in size.

CRUSH: To press, often with a garlic press, mallet, or the side of knife blade to extract juice.

CUBE: To cut food into equal-size cube-shaped pieces that are ½ inch or larger.

DICE: To cut food into equal-size small cubes that are less than ½ inch.

FILLET: To cut or slice meat, chicken, or fish from the bones.

GRATE: To change a solid food into tiny particles by rubbing it across a grating surface that has very small, round cutting holes. Grating can also be done using a food processor.

GRIND: To use a food processor, meat grinder, or mortar and pestle to change a solid piece of food into fine pieces.

JULIENNE: To cut food into thin matchstick-size strips of uniform length.

MINCE: To cut or chop food into very fine, irregular-shaped pieces no larger than ⅛ inch square.

PARE: To remove the skin or rind from fruits and vegetables with a thin, small knife or parer.

PEEL: To use a knife or vegetable peeler to strip the rind or peel from a fruit or vegetable.

SHRED: To cut food into long, thin strips with a knife or by pushing food over the oval-shaped, large cutting holes of a hand shredder or grater.

SLICE: To cut foods into pieces of uniform thickness with a knife. To slice *diagonally*, cut the food by holding the knife at a 45-degree angle to the food; slicing food diagonally exposes more surface area, allowing the food to cook quickly.

SLIVER: To cut food into long, thin pieces, as with almonds.

SNIP: To cut into very small pieces with a scissors before measuring, as with herbs.

LOW-FAT COOKING
METHODS

Keeping nutrients in and calories out takes a light touch in cooking. You can cut fat by stir-frying or sautéing instead of deep-frying, and rack-roasting instead of cooking in fatty drippings. Meats, poultry and fish will taste tender and juicy without heavy fat-laden sauces and gravies, and vegetables will retain their beautiful color and crunch. The cooking methods used in this book aim for the fullest flavor possible while keeping the fat content in check. Try the cooking methods outlined below. As you master them, your favorite meals and recipes will take on new character.

BAKE: To cook in an oven thereby cooking with free-circulating dry heat. It is very important to preheat the oven before putting in the food. Do not crowd food in an oven; give it room to cook evenly. Use low oven temperatures for foods that require slow cooking and little or no browning, such as meringue shells. Lean meats, poultry, and fish that are baked are generally covered. To prevent meats from drying out, a low-fat marinade is added.

BARBECUE: To cook food over a charcoal or hardwood fire on a grill, in open pits, or on a spit over intense heat. To prevent food from drying out, use a low-fat marinade before cooking and baste during cooking with a low-fat liquid.

BLANCH: To plunge vegetables, seafood, or fruit into boiling water for a very short time, then into cold water to stop the cooking process. Blanching is used to bring out the color, loosen skins for peeling, and/or mellow flavors.

BOIL: To cook food in a large amount of boiling water or other liquid. Large bubbles should rise continuously and break on the surface of the liquid. This method is often used for vegetables, seafood, and pasta.

BRAISE: A method of browning food in fat over high heat, then tightly covering and cooking slowly in a small amount of liquid on top of the stove or in the oven. Braising is a slow-cooking method used to develop flavors and tenderize tough foods. It is ideal for tougher cuts of meat, firm fish, and some vegetables. Oven-cooking bags are useful for braising foods in the oven. If possible, refrigerate braised dishes overnight to allow the fat to congeal on top; skim off and discard the hardened fat before reheating. Braising is also known as *stewing*. Stewing usually involves more liquid than braising and uses smaller pieces of meat.

BROIL: To cook food directly over or under intense direct heat. This is usually done in an oven under a broiler. Thick foods or foods that need to be cooked longer should be placed on a lower rack so they cook through without burning the outside, and thinner foods are broiled closer to the heat source for maximum browning. Meats, poultry, and fish that are broiled should be placed on a rack in the broiler pan to allow the fat to drip away from the food.

EN PAPILLOTE: A method of baking food inside a wrapping of parchment paper. As the food cooks and releases steam, the parchment puffs up into a dome. Using this method, food cooks in its own juices, thereby reducing the need for added fat. This is an excellent method for tender and delicate cuts of meat, fish, seafood, and boned poultry.

GRILL: To cook food on a rack over very hot coals to seal in juices. When using a grill, spray the grill rack with a nonstick cooking spray before placing the grill over the coals to prevent the food from sticking to the rack.

MICROWAVE: To cook food in a microwave oven. Microwaves are high-frequency electromagnetic waves that penetrate food and cause the molecules to vibrate, creating friction, which in turn creates heat and cooks the food. Microwaves cook food from the outside in to a depth of about $1\frac{1}{2}$ inches; the rest is cooked as heat is transferred from the outside of the food to the inside. Food prepared in the microwave cooks in its natural juices so there is no need to add any fat. In addition, foods with a high moisture content, such as fruits and vegetables, require little or no water for cooking, so nutrients that are usually leached out by cooking in boiling water are retained. Other high-moisture foods ideal for the microwave include fish and sauces.

OVEN-FRY: To bake foods in the oven at high temperatures. The food is often dipped in lemon juice, water, or milk and breaded. This results in food that is crispy on the outside and tender and juicy on the inside, similar to deep-fat fried foods. This method is ideal for chicken, fish, and pork chops.

PAN-BROIL: To cook meats, poultry, or fish on top of the stove in a preheated heavy skillet over high heat, pouring off the fat or liquid as it accumulates.

PARBOIL: To partially cook in boiling water, broth or other liquid. Dense vegetables such as carrots are often parboiled, added at the last minute to quicker-cooking ingredients, and finished in the oven or in a skillet.

POACH: To cook food in a simmering liquid that does not boil. Food should be started in warm water and slowly brought to a simmer for best results. No added fat is required and the poaching liquid may be strained through cheesecloth and used as a broth in soups or as a base for a sauce. Eggs, fish, poultry, and firm fruits such as apples, pears, and peaches are well suited for poaching.

PRESSURE COOK: To cook food with steam under pressure. The tightly sealed pots called pressure cookers are safe to use and have a valve release system for excess steam that controls the amount of pressure in the container. This method of cooking does not require the addition of fat in preparation and is useful in tenderizing tough cuts of meat, often reducing the cooking time by one-third to one-half.

ROAST: To oven-cook large cuts of meat or whole poultry on a rack set in an uncovered pan. Food is cooked without added fat or liquid until the outside is browned and the inside is tender and moist. Roasting requires fairly tender cuts. To prevent meats from drying out, use a low-fat marinade before roasting or baste with broth, water, juice, or other low-fat liquid during cooking. A meat thermometer is the best guide to doneness.

SAUTÉ OR STIR-FRY: To cook food quickly in a skillet (sauté) or wok (stir-fry) over medium-high heat with a very small amount of oil, water, broth, juice, wine, or other liquid. Foods to be sautéed or stir-fried should be thinly sliced, and stirred or tossed constantly to promote even cooking. Stir-frying is done with smaller pieces of food. Meats, poultry, seafood, and vegetables are delicious prepared in this way.

STEAM: To cook food over, rather than in, boiling water. Place food on a rack or in a perforated steamer basket, colander, or strainer in a saucepan or skillet. Add about one inch of water to the pan (water must be below the basket). Bring water to a boil over high heat and cover tightly. Reduce heat to medium and cook until tender. No fat is required and steaming is an excellent way to retain the natural flavor and texture of poultry, fish, seafood, and vegetables.

STEW: *See* Braise.

TOOLS OF THE TRADE

Certain equipment is especially well suited to low-fat cooking. The following items are not necessarily "must haves," since resourceful cooks can usually modify equipment and/or recipes to fit their needs. However, these items will offer valuable assistance when it comes to preparing dishes that are trimmed of extra calories and fat. You can add pieces of equipment as you try new recipes and learn more about your own cooking needs. Missing pieces may be added to a holiday or birthday wish list!

BLENDER: Use to puree, chop, and mix foods, and to blend beverages, sauces, soups, and dressings. A hand-held immersion blender is useful because it can be brought to the container of food, eliminating the need to transfer the food to the blender container.

BROILER PAN WITH RACK: The rack holds food out of the pan so the fat can drip away. Using the rack and pan also allows oven-fried foods to be exposed to free-circulating dry heat while cooking, preventing them from becoming soggy on the bottom.

COLANDER: A large, stainless steel mesh colander or strainer works well for draining pasta and other foods, and for draining fat from cooked ground meat. A smaller-mesh strainer or colander is useful for separating the pulp and seeds from fresh-squeezed fruit juice and for making yogurt cheese.

FAT-OFF LADLE: This ladle has slots around the edge that allow fat to be collected when lowered into soups, stews, or gravies. The fat runs into the ladle bowl through the slots and can then be poured off the other side and discarded.

FOOD PROCESSOR: Food processors vary in size and power, but whether you use a compact miniprocessor or a full-size model, it will make quick work out of food preparation. Food processors can chop, puree, mince, slice, grind, shred, knead, and mix a variety of foods very quickly and easily.

GARLIC PRESS: Garlic can be an important flavor in low-fat recipes and a press can be used to crush whole cloves of garlic while keeping the taste and aroma off your hands. Many cooks do not use a press, choosing instead to mince and sauté the garlic, which gives it a more pleasing flavor.

GRATER: Use a grater for grating cheese, fresh ginger root, citrus peel, and other foods. A four-sided upright stainless steel grater with a handle on top is recommended. Choose one that has several different sizes of grating holes.

GRAVY STRAINER: A gravy strainer is used to separate excess fat from gravy. It looks like a measuring cup with a spout attached near the bottom. As liquid is poured out of the spout on the bottom, the fat remains at the top and can be discarded.

KITCHEN SHEARS: Use shears to snip or mince herbs, cut dried fruit, chop canned tomatoes, trim fat and skin from meat and poultry, cut pita bread into wedges for tortillas, cut phyllo, and a variety of other kitchen tasks.

KNIVES: These are your most essential cooking tools. Invest in high-quality knives and keep the edges sharp and protected during storage. Knives perform many important tasks in healthy cooking such as trimming fat and skin from meats and poultry and cutting foods in specified sizes. Most professionals recommend high-carbon stainless steel knives for their durability, sharpness, and ease of care. A basic set of knives that can perform most kitchen tasks include a 3- or 4-inch paring knife, a 6-inch cook's knife, an 8-inch chef's knife, a 10-inch slicing or carving knife, and a serrated bread knife. A sharpening steel is also a wise investment to keep your knives in good cutting condition.

LOAF PAN, 2 PIECE: Ideal for baking meat loaves, this pan has an inner piece with draining holes so the fat drips away while the meat cooks.

MALLET: This hammerlike device has two different surfaces: one that is smooth for flattening delicate foods, such as chicken, and one that is covered with small spikes for tenderizing tougher foods, like red meats. Use a mallet to tenderize meats, flatten boneless chicken breasts, and crush ice for blenderized drinks.

MEAT THERMOMETER: Using a meat thermometer ensures that meats are done but not overcooked. Choose one that has a large dial for easy viewing.

MICROWAVE COOKWARE: There are a variety of containers developed especially for use in the microwave. Their advantage is they will not get hot during cooking and they allow maximum penetration of microwaves into the food to promote even cooking. Another advantage of using microwave cookware is that you can prepare, serve, and store food all in the same container so there are fewer dirty dishes to clean. Choose cookware with lids in a variety of sizes.

NONSTICK COOKWARE: Heavy-duty nonstick cookware lets you cook with virtually no fat. It usually heats evenly and does not warp. A vegetable cooking spray can be used on nonstick cookware to help prevent sticking of foods prepared without fat. A set of cookware that would cover most of your needs would include a large and small skillet with lids, 1-, 2-, and 3-quart saucepans with lids, a loaf pan, baking pans, baking sheets, and muffin tins.

PASTA PORTIONER: Used to measure the correct amount of pasta for a recipe, a pasta portioner is usually a flat disc with different size holes that correspond to different amounts of pasta. Place the pasta in the designated opening for the desired amount until the pasta fills the opening completely.

ROASTING RACK: A roasting rack is a collapsible V-shaped rack that fits into a shallow roasting pan. Meat is placed on the rack and the fat drips away during cooking. Meats brown evenly on all sides because the shape of the rack allows heat to circulate around all surfaces of the food.

RUBBER SPATULAS: Choose an assortment of wide and narrow rubber spatulas to use on nonstick cookware (the rubber variety will not scratch the surface).

SALAD SPINNER: Use a salad spinner to wash and dry salad greens in minutes. Salad dressing adheres better to drier greens, so you can get by with using a smaller quantity of dressing on a salad.

SCALE: A kitchen scale takes the guesswork out of measuring ingredients by weight. It is also helpful for accurately measuring food portions. Look for a scale that measures in ounces, can be reset to zero, and is easy to read and clean.

SKEWERS: A skewer is a very inexpensive gadget for low-fat cooking. Use skewers for cooking and serving cubes of lean meat and poultry, fruits, and vegetables. Kabobs are a favorite skewer dish: cubes of lean meat marinated in a low-fat sauce, then arranged on skewers with onions, mushrooms, and other bite-sized vegetables, and grilled or broiled.

SPOONS: Wood and plastic spoons will not scratch nonstick cookware or heat up and burn your hands. A large stirring spoon can be used for skimming fat off the top of soups, stews, gravies, and broths, and a slotted or perforated spoon can be used to lift foods out of liquids.

STEAMER BASKET: Collapsible steamer baskets can fit any size pan. Choose one that has legs at least one inch high, so it stands above the boiling water, and a handle that allows you to lift it easily. Many steamer baskets or inserts are stainless steel;

others may be made from porcelain or bamboo. Electric steamers with a see-through top are available for a much greater cost than the baskets or inserts (which do the job just as well).

WIRE GRILLING BASKET: These flat baskets with handles are used in grilling fish, tender meats, and vegetables over a barbecue and prevent them from falling through the grill rack. Be sure to spray the basket with cooking spray before using to prevent sticking and simplify cleaning.

WIRE WHISK: Stainless steel wire whisks in assorted sizes are ideal for beating eggs and egg whites, blending salad dressings, sauces, low-fat gravies, and other foods.

WOK: This traditional cooking vessel is a favorite for stir-frying because its sloping sides allow food to be cooked very quickly and evenly with a minimum amount of oil. Nonstick woks are also available that eliminate the need for any added fat. The round-bottom wok is ideal for cooking over a gas burner, while flat-bottom woks work well on an electric stove.

YOGURT CHEESE FUNNEL: This handy device is used to filter out the whey from yogurt, leaving a thick and low-fat cheese substitute to use in dressings, dips, and spreads. Place the funnel over a container, spoon in low-fat or nonfat yogurt, and place in the refrigerator. After 8–12 hours, gravity will force the whey through the funnel to the container below. Be sure to choose a yogurt that is free of gelatin or the whey will not drain properly.

MAKING YOUR FAVORITE RECIPES HEALTHIER

When most people consider a reduced-calorie and reduced-fat diet, they think of cutting back on fried chicken, French fries, and chocolate cake. What they may not realize is that a number of foods contain large amounts of "hidden fat" that cannot be seen, cut off, or trimmed away from the food. Did you know, for instance, that one-half cup of potato salad contains, on average, three teaspoons of added fat? That is equivalent to about 135 calories from fat. And one cup of macaroni and cheese has an average of 150 calories from fat, the equivalent of about three and a half teaspoons of fat.

There are many ways to lower the fat content in recipes without making a dent in the way the food tastes. One obvious way is to cut away the visible fat. If you have to add fat or oil, do it sparingly. Try reduced-fat or nonfat dressings on salads, and look for the words "low-fat" or "nonfat" when you buy condiments and dairy products. One of the best ways to jazz up your dishes is to flavor them with spices and herbs instead of using fatty sauces and gravies. Consider these and some other options for lowering fat and calories:

MEATS / POULTRY / FISH

- Buy lean cuts of meat and extra-lean ground beef. Trim all visible fat.

- Skin all poultry and trim visible fat.

- Choose water-packed canned fish instead of oil-packed.

- When roasting, use a rack so the meat does not sit in the drippings during cooking.

- Drain the extra fat after browning ground meat for spaghetti or casseroles. Rinsing the meat in a colander under water will remove even more fat.

- Baste meat with wine, fruit juice, or broth instead of fat drippings. Enhance the flavor of meats by placing them in a low-fat marinade and refrigerating several hours before cooking.

- Try ground turkey or chicken instead of ground beef in recipes. Or mix half ground beef with half ground turkey or chicken.

- When browning meat, spray a non-stick pan with cooking spray to avoid having to add any fat to the pan.

- Avoid high-fat meats such as bacon, sausage, hot dogs, luncheon meats, salami, bologna, organ meats, duck, and goose.

OILS/FATS

❧ Use a nonstick cooking spray when a recipe calls for a "greased pan."

❧ If a recipe calls for margarine or butter, try using less than is called for (except when preparing baked foods).

❧ Sauté vegetables or other foods in broth or water instead of oil.

❧ Use crushed cereal as a coating for meat, poultry, or fish instead of buttered bread crumbs.

❧ Choose reduced-fat or reduced-calorie spreads for table use.

❧ Use reduced-fat or fat-free salad dressings, or make dressings with nonfat or low-fat yogurt or buttermilk instead of oil.

EGGS

❧ Use two egg whites in place of a whole egg when preparing scrambled eggs and other egg dishes.

❧ Use a liquid egg substitute or beaten egg whites to coat chicken, fish, or other meats before breading.

DAIRY

❧ Use reduced-fat or skim milk cheeses such as mozzarella, farmer, string, ricotta, or cottage cheese in place of regular cheese.

❧ Substitute plain nonfat or low-fat yogurt for mayonnaise or sour cream in salad dressings, dips, and spreads.

❧ Make "cream" soups with skim or 1% milk instead of cream or whole milk.

❧ Use evaporated skim milk in place of cream in coffee or tea, or in recipes for quiche or cream sauces for pasta. Evaporated skim milk can also be whipped and used in place of whipped cream or whipped topping mixtures. To prepare, chill a mixing bowl, beaters, and a can of evaporated skim milk in the freezer for 30 minutes. Remove and beat the milk on high speed until soft peaks form. Use immediately as a nonfat topping.

❧ Substitute buttermilk for whole milk in biscuits, cakes, and pancakes. You'll add flavor with a minimum of fat.

❧ For drinking, use skim or 1% milk.

OTHER TIPS

~ When making soup, skim off the fat layer that floats on top. If possible, chill the soup before serving and remove the hardened layer of fat that forms on the surface.

~ Chicken or beef bouillon granules can be added to water and used as a lower-fat substitute for canned broths.

~ Thicken sauces with cornstarch or flour mixed with liquid rather than fat. Whisk the thickening agent into cold milk or water, using one tablespoon cornstarch or two tablespoons flour to one cup of liquid.

Everyone has favorite recipes. Not everyone, however, has favorite lower-fat recipes. But it's easy to modify your old favorite, cut fat and calories and enjoy a healthier eating style. As you modify a recipe of your own, try to determine these things:

~ Are all the ingredients that contain fat necessary to the recipe? Can any ingredients be omitted?

~ Is there a reduced-fat or no-fat version of an ingredient that can be substituted?

~ Can the cooking method be changed to reduce fat? For instance, can you broil or bake instead of fry?

Compare these two versions of a recipe as an example of
how to modify your own recipes:

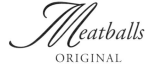

Meatballs
ORIGINAL

2   pounds ground beef

½   cup chopped onions

2   eggs

¼   cup milk

½   cup bread crumbs

¼   teaspoon pepper

½   teaspoon allspice

2   tablespoons butter for frying

Mix all ingredients except butter in a
large bowl. Form meatballs using a heaping tablespoon of mixture for each. Fry
in butter until browned. Serves 6.

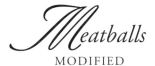

Meatballs
MODIFIED

1 ½ pounds extra-lean ground beef

½   cup chopped onions

2   egg whites or ½ cup egg substitute

¼   cup skim milk

½   cup bread crumbs

¼   teaspoon pepper

½   teaspoon allspice

Mix all ingredients in a large bowl. Form
meatballs using a heaping tablespoon of
mixture for each. Fry in a nonstick pan
with cooking spray or bake the meatballs
on a broiler pan in the oven. Serves 6.

The following changes were made in
this recipe:

∼ Ground beef: Extra-lean ground beef
  was used instead of regular, and the
  amount of meat was reduced.

∼ Eggs: Egg whites or egg substitute
  were used to omit the fat from the
  egg yolk.

∼ Milk: Skim milk was used instead of
  whole milk.

∼ Butter: The need for any fat was omitted by using a nonstick pan with
  cooking spray, or by changing the
  cooking method and broiling instead
  of frying.

How do these changes add up? One serving
of the original meatballs contains 450 calories and 32 grams of fat while one serving of
the modified version provides 260 calories
and 14 grams of fat—a savings of almost
200 calories and 18 grams of fat! As you can
see, what might seem to be minor or small
changes or substitutions really do make a
difference in nutrition.

RECIPE SUBSTITUTIONS

The following chart summarizes suggestions for modifying recipes to reduce calories, fat, sugar, and sodium, some of which were reviewed in other sections:

INSTEAD OF THIS	TRY THIS
bacon	Canadian bacon, lean ham, turkey bacon
baking chocolate	3 tablespoons powdered unsweetened cocoa plus 1 tablespoon oil
butter	margarine, reduced-calorie margarine
canned broth	dry bouillon granules or cubes, low-sodium bouillon granules or cubes
canned fruit, syrup-packed	canned fruit, juice-packed
cheese, regular	skim-milk cheese, reduced-fat cheese, or fat-free cheese; look for 5 grams fat or less per ounce on label
cream	evaporated skim milk
cream cheese	light or fat-free cream cheese product
cream soup	fat-free condensed cream soups or homemade white sauce made from 1 cup skim milk plus 2 tablespoons flour plus 1–2 tablespoons margarine; add chopped celery, mushrooms, or chicken bouillon for flavor
egg, whole	2 egg whites or ¼ cup egg substitute
gelatin, regular	sugar-free gelatin
ground beef, regular	extra-lean ground beef, ground turkey or chicken
ice cream	nonfat or low-fat frozen yogurt or dairy dessert, ice milk, sherbet, sorbet, fruit ice

INSTEAD OF THIS	TRY THIS
lard	oil, reduced in quantity by one-fourth to one-third
margarine	reduced-calorie margarine
mayonnaise	reduced-calorie or fat-free mayonnaise, plain nonfat or low-fat yogurt
milk, whole or 2%	skim or 1% milk, evaporated skim milk
nuts	reduce quantity or eliminate if possible
oil	reduce quantity or eliminate if possible
salad dressing	reduced-calorie or fat-free dressings
salt	reduce quantity or eliminate if possible
salt, flavored	powdered garlic, onion, or celery
shortening	oil, reduced in quantity by one-fourth to one-third
sour cream	light or nonfat sour cream alternative, nonfat or low-fat plain yogurt, 1 cup nonfat or low-fat cottage cheese blended with 2 tablespoons lemon juice until smooth
sugar	reduce quantity or eliminate if possible
tuna and salmon, packed in oil	water-packed tuna and salmon
whipped cream	evaporated skim milk, chilled and whipped

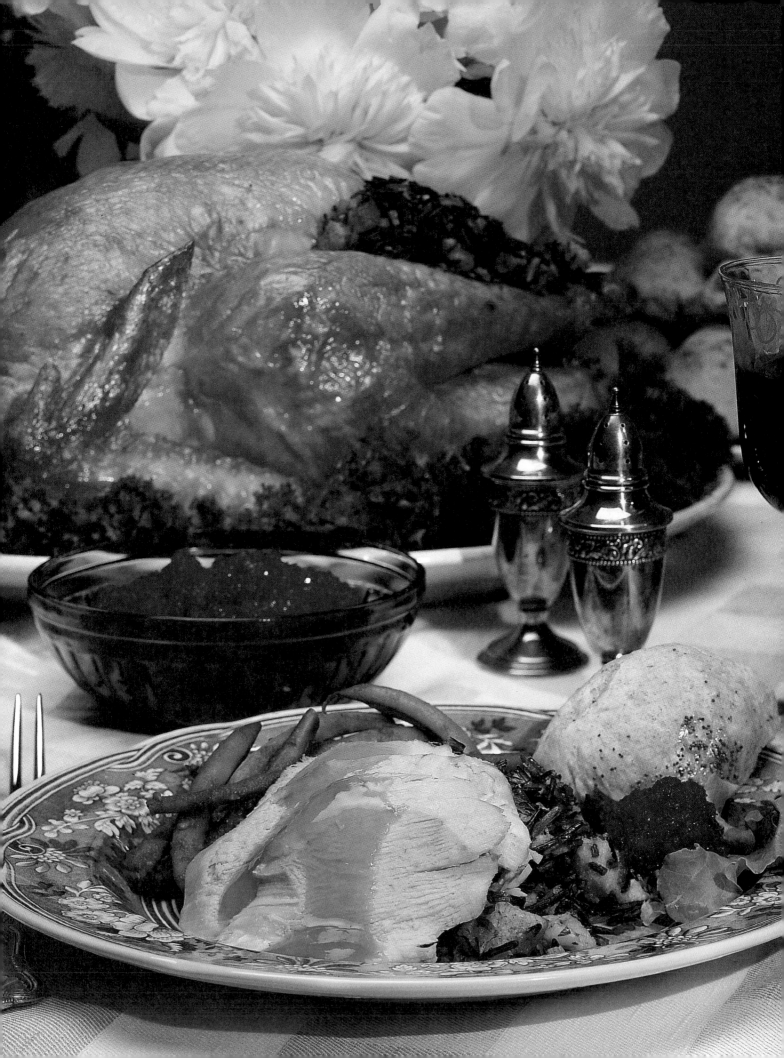

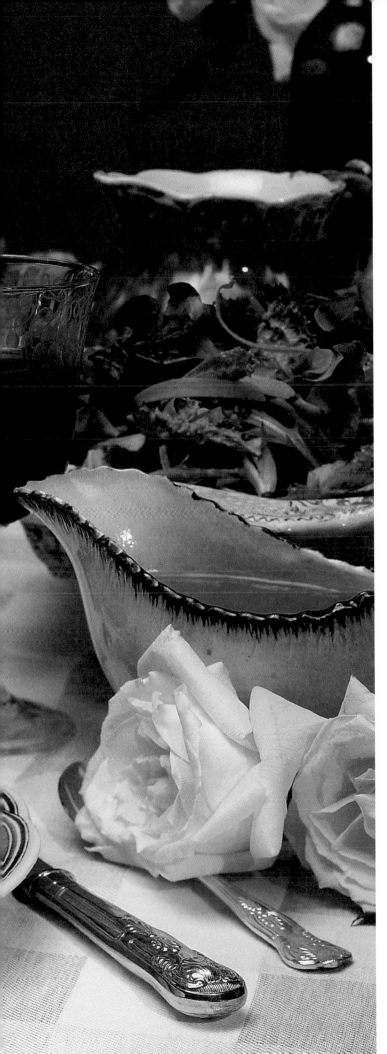

Menus for Healthy Meals

The menus that follow were developed for your enjoyment, using recipes from every chapter in this cookbook. Each menu lists the total calories per serving (rounded to the nearest 5 calories) and fits into the recommendations for low-fat, healthy eating.

You may want to follow each menu exactly as it is presented. Or you may want to use these menus simply as suggestions to get started in planning balanced meals, adding your own experience, creativity, and family preferences to the meal. When you want to make a substitution in a menu, draw from the many other flavorful dishes in this book or one of your own favorite recipes. To keep the calories similar for the total menu, substitute a recipe that is comparable in caloric content.

The menus in this section cover almost any occasion. Whether preparing a simple breakfast or brunch, a quick and easy lunch or supper for the family, or an elegant dinner for company, you're sure to find the perfect menu for your meal!

WEEKEND BREAKFAST

≈

After your next Saturday or Sunday morning walk or tennis game, revive yourself with this delicious breakfast. The menu calories reflect a serving of two pancakes, two ounces of broiled Canadian bacon, and one serving of apricots. Leftover pancakes can be easily frozen and used another day.

SPICED BRAN GRIDDLE CAKES
page 36

CANADIAN BACON

STEWED APRICOTS
page 38

SERVES 5
340 calories

COUNTRY MORNING BREAKFAST

≈

The homemade aroma of this meal will remind you of breakfast in the country. Serve each person one slice of whole wheat toast with one teaspoon margarine along with a serving of cream of wheat and one baked apple.

SMOOTH AND SATISFYING CREAM OF WHEAT
page 42

WHOLE WHEAT TOAST

NEW BAKED APPLES
page 39

SERVES 3
360 calories

BREAKFAST ON THE GO

≈

In a hurry? Here is a quick breakfast to eat in a jiffy. The muffins can be made ahead of time and frozen—simply take one out of the freezer the night before or pop in the microwave in the morning. The prunes can also be made ahead and stored in a jar in the refrigerator. They are delicious mixed with the cottage cheese. The menu calories are based on one muffin, three spiced prunes, and one-quarter cup low-fat cottage cheese.

SPICED BLUEBERRY-BRAN MUFFINS
page 45

SPICED PRUNES
page 38

COTTAGE CHEESE

SERVES 8

230 calories

DOWN-HOME DELICIOUS BREAKFAST

≈

Fond memories from childhood often include favorite family foods, like bowls of oatmeal swimming in butter and cream and fresh blueberry muffins baking in the oven. Here are the 1990's versions of these breakfast favorites, without all the fat. Add one cup of cut-up mixed fresh fruit to a serving of oatmeal and one muffin.

SWEET AND CHUNKY OATMEAL
page 42

SPICED BLUEBERRY-BRAN MUFFINS
page 45

FRUIT CUP

SERVES 2

375 calories

A KID'S FAVORITE BREAKFAST

~

Young and old alike will enjoy this delicious breakfast, centered around a variation of traditional French toast. Accompany it with two ounces of lean grilled ham and one small sliced orange per person for only 325 calories.

PINEAPPLE FRENCH TOAST
page 37

GRILLED HAM

FRESH ORANGE SLICES

SERVES 4

325 calories

HEARTY WINTER BREAKFAST

~

Cold winds and frosty mornings can make breakfast a comforting meal. This omelette serves two, but you can easily make more for a larger group. Breakfast Muffin Cake makes 16 slices — enough for a crowd, but it freezes well if you have leftovers (menu calories are based on one slice for a serving). Add half of a fresh grapefruit to round out this warming breakfast.

QUICK MOZZARELLA OMELETTE
page 39

BREAKFAST MUFFIN CAKE
page 44

GRAPEFRUIT HALF

SERVES 2

310 calories

SUNDAY BRUNCH FOR TWO

≈

This hearty brunch will start your day off right with only 365 calories. Extra egg whites are added to one egg yolk to make the omelette enough for two servings without increasing the cholesterol and fat content. Round off this meal with a toasted English muffin spread with one teaspoon of margarine, and one-half cup orange juice.

VEGETABLE OMELETTE
page 40

ENGLISH MUFFINS

ORANGE JUICE

SERVES 2
365 calories

SPEEDY SOUP AND SALAD I

≈

Whether you are short on time or just want to eat lightly, this lunch or supper menu is for you. The flavor of the soup actually improves if refrigerated and served the next day, making preparation for this meal even quicker. Add a crisp salad, a loaf of crusty French bread, and dessert (which can also be made the day ahead and reheated) to finish this meal. Menu calories are based on one serving of soup, salad, dessert, and a one-ounce slice of unbuttered French bread.

LENTIL SOUP: IT'S A ONE-BOWL MEAL
page 79

SUPER SALAD
page 64

FRENCH BREAD

WARM APPLE CRUNCH
page 258

SERVES 4
455 calories

SPEEDY SOUP AND SALAD II

∼

This speedy menu features Hearty Soup, a satisfying soup that is better the next day. Pretty Mixed Salad is simple to prepare, only requiring the ingredients to be tossed 15 minutes before serving time. Spiced Applesauce is a sweet-tasting applesauce made without sugar or sweeteners. Add one small dinner roll per person to complete the menu.

HEARTY SOUP
page 90

PRETTY MIXED SALAD
page 65

DINNER ROLLS

SPICED APPLESAUCE
page 280

SERVES 4

400 calories

SPEEDY SOUP AND SALAD III

∼

Try this interesting soup for lunch, made from celeriac, chicken stock, carrot juice, and seasonings. Accompany each serving with a slice of freshly baked rye bread (a dinner roll or one-ounce slice of French bread can be substituted), spinach salad, and one cup of mixed fresh fruit for dessert.

VELVETY-SMOOTH CELERY ROOT BISQUE
page 89

CRISP SPINACH SALAD
page 69

MAGNIFICENT RYE BREAD
page 232

MIXED FRESH FRUIT

SERVES 4

380 calories

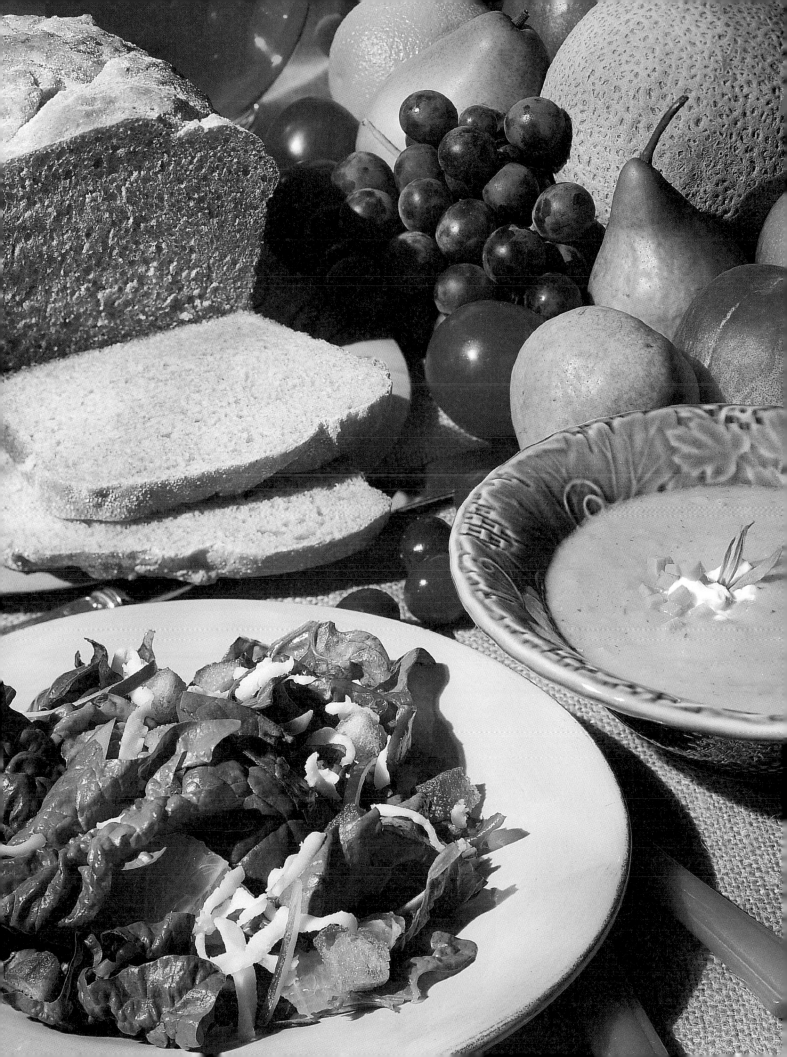

SUMMER PICNIC

~

Whether you picnic in the park, at the beach, or in your own backyard, this menu will be a welcome midday treat. Marinated Chicken Salad and Tofu Dip should be made the morning of your picnic and chilled a few hours before eating. Use hard rolls and wrap up slices of Apricot Spice Cake for a spicy and delicious dessert. Menu calories include one hard roll and one-half cup of raw vegetables with four teaspoons of dip per person.

MARINATED CHICKEN SALAD
page 70

RAW VEGETABLES WITH TOFU DIP
page 51

HARD ROLLS

APRICOT SPICE CAKE
page 272

SERVES 6
410 calories

SPRING LUNCHEON

~

Celebrate spring with this light and luscious menu featuring Tasty Tuna Salad, prepared with much less fat than traditional recipes for tuna salad. Accompany it with colorful Beet Relish and French rolls (one per person). For a refreshing beverage, mix four ounces of fruit juice with four ounces of chilled sparkling water and serve over ice in a tall glass for each guest.

TASTY TUNA SALAD
page 71

BEET RELISH
page 56

FRENCH ROLLS

FROZEN MIXED FRUIT MOUSSE
page 251

SPARKLING FRUIT JUICE SPRITZER

SERVES 4
355 calories

SAVORY MEAT LOAF DINNER

~

Cranberries add an exquisite taste to this family favorite dish. Mix the salad while the meat loaf and squash bake. For dessert, try Crunchy Cookies, which can be made a day ahead. Serve two cookies per person for a grand total of 535 calories for this delicious dinner.

CRANBERRY MEAT LOAF
page 159

STUFFED ACORN SQUASH
page 101

MIXED SALAD WITH SPROUTS
page 69

CRUNCHY COOKIES
page 254

SERVES 4
535 calories

ELEGANT COMPANY DINNER

~

Make any occasion special with this elegant menu. Toss your own blend of mixed greens with our dressing (two tablespoons per person) and use your own dinner rolls (one per person) to accompany the meal. Dessert can be made the day before to make lighter work of this meal.

ROMANTIC FILET MIGNON
page 154

RED-SKINNED POTATOES WITH SESAME SEED
page 111

RICH PUREE OF BROCCOLI
page 96

MIXED GREEN SALAD
WITH ALL-PURPOSE DRESSING
page 74

DINNER ROLLS

PRETTY POACHED PEARS IN CRANBERRY SAUCE
page 252

SERVES 4
790 calories

DELECTABLE THANKSGIVING DINNER

~

Guests will surely be surprised to see and taste a healthy holiday meal such as this one. Start with a well-seasoned turkey and wild rice stuffing. Continue with fresh baked onion rolls and green beans flavored with fresh basil. Make your own mixed green salad and use our dressing. Top it off with a twist on a traditional holiday dessert, Chocolate Pumpkin Pie. Menu calculations are based on one-half cup of dressing made without the veal, two tablespoons gravy, three ounces turkey, one roll, two tablespoons salad dressing, and one-twelfth of the pie per person. Enjoy the leftovers!

ROAST STUFFED TURKEY — THE MOST SUMPTUOUS EVER
page 150

FRENCHED GREEN BEANS WITH BASIL
page 97

TWENTY-FOUR ONION ROLLS AND ONE LOAF
page 228

MIXED GREEN SALAD WITH ALL-PURPOSE DRESSING
page 74

CHOCOLATE PUMPKIN PIE
page 255

SERVES 4

600 calories

SUNDAY CHICKEN DINNER

~

This is one of the easiest and quickest chicken recipes
you will ever make! The menu continues with My
Pet Potatoes, a lower-fat variation on French fries,
a salad, and a dinner roll for each person.
Sumptuous Chocolate Cake finishes the meal, sure
to be a favorite of all chocolate lovers.

BROCCOLI AND CHICKEN
page 132

MY PET POTATOES
page 113

FRESH MINT SALAD
page 62

DINNER ROLLS

SUMPTUOUS CHOCOLATE CAKE
WITH CREAMY CHOCOLATE FROSTING
pages 248 and 249

SERVES 4
785 calories

COME-HITHER FIRESIDE FARE

~

When it's cold and windy outside, who can resist the
allure of a glowing fire? When you feel drawn to
the fireplace, take this quick and delicious supper
with you. The entire menu can be made ahead —
even the day before! Start with a warming bowl of
Diced Chicken in a Pot. On the side try Miracle
Chicken Spread on a few crackers. Finish with
homemade Chocolate Pudding: The Way You Like
It. Menu calories are based on a serving of soup,
two tablespoons of spread, four to six snack crackers,
one serving of pudding, and four ounces of
hot apple cider.

DICED CHICKEN IN A POT
page 91

MIRACLE CHICKEN SPREAD ON CRACKERS
page 49

CHOCOLATE PUDDING: THE WAY YOU LIKE IT
page 250

HOT APPLE CIDER

SERVES 6
570 calories

SPECIAL-OCCASION DINNER

~

Make any birthday, anniversary, graduation, or other special occasion memorable with this delicious menu. Chicken and Ham Paillards with Madeira Glaze is an elegant dish usually served in restaurants, but now you can make it right in your own kitchen. Serve it with nutty-flavored Delicious Wild Rice I, Colorful Sautéed Zucchini, and dinner rolls. Hot Pink Sherbet is the cool ending to this meal with lots of spark!

CHICKEN AND HAM PAILLARDS WITH
MADEIRA GLAZE
page 124

DELICIOUS WILD RICE I
page 120

COLORFUL SAUTÉED ZUCCHINI
page 104

DINNER ROLLS

HOT PINK SHERBET
page 278

SERVES 4
585 calories

CHICKEN DINNER IN A SNAP

~

Here is the perfect menu for those times when you want to cook a wonderful meal with little effort. Aromatic Chicken simply simmers in its sauce for 45 minutes while you prepare Stunning Pasta Pearls as a side dish. Celeriac Salad can be made ahead of time, or even the day before serving. Try Speedy Spice Cake for dessert—all it requires is for the ingredients to be mixed and baked. Leftover slices can be frozen, or keep them handy for between-meal snacks!

AROMATIC CHICKEN
page 125

STUNNING PASTA PEARLS
page 108

CELERIAC SALAD
page 63

SPEEDY SPICE CAKE
page 273

SERVES 4
620 calories

OPEN HOUSE BUFFET, LIGHT-STYLE

~

An open house menu usually brings to mind fried finger foods, fatty dips, and rich pâtés. This menu, however, is for health-conscious people who like to eat light and still enjoy tasty food. The menu will serve eight if you double the recipes for Mix-and-Match Vegetable Salad and Stuffed Mushrooms. Add a platter of fresh assorted breads and rolls and tempt guests with Fabulous Cheesecake I. Menu calories have been calculated for one serving of salad, one kabob, three cocktail balls, three stuffed mushrooms, one roll or one slice of bread, and one serving of cheesecake.

MIX-AND-MATCH VEGETABLE SALAD
page 72

CORIANDER CHICKEN KABOBS
page 50

SAVORY VEAL COCKTAIL BALLS
page 54

LUSCIOUS STUFFED MUSHROOMS
page 52

ASSORTED BREADS AND ROLLS

FABULOUS CHEESECAKE I
page 238

SERVES 8
630 calories

FRIDAY NIGHT FAMILY FAVORITE

~

When you ask, "What do you want for supper?" a popular answer is a burger and a shake. This menu features lightened versions of these favorites. Serve the Curried Steakburger on a fresh two-ounce sandwich bun of your choice. Frosty Yogurt Milk Shake is our answer to the usual high-calorie and high-fat shakes. You will have to double the recipe or make two batches to serve four. This menu is a treat—any day of the week!

CURRIED STEAKBURGER WITH ONIONS AND MUSHROOMS ON A BUN
page 160

FENNEL COLESLAW
page 66

FROSTY YOGURT MILKSHAKE
page 280

SERVES 4
525 calories

SUPERB SNAPPER

~

The delicate yet full flavor of snapper makes it a favorite saltwater fish of many people. In this menu it is a dish to be remembered—baked in a sauce of herbs, stock, and sherry, and finished with a garnish of fresh grapes. Rice is always a good accompaniment to fish and here we have included Baked Rice in Red Wine—most of the alcohol is boiled off and all that remains is the savory flavor of the red wine. Add Brussels Sprouts with Mushrooms and one hard roll per person. Finish the meal with Enchanting Chocolate Chiffon Pie—a superb ending!

BAKED RED SNAPPER VERONIQUE
page 193

BAKED RICE IN RED WINE
page 117

BRUSSELS SPROUTS WITH MUSHROOMS
page 102

HARD ROLLS

ENCHANTING CHOCOLATE CHIFFON PIE
page 244

SERVES 4
635 calories

SCRUMPTIOUS SEAFOOD DINNER

~

This menu is simple enough to prepare for a family dinner, yet is special enough to serve company. Prepare the ingredients for Luscious Sautéed Shrimp and Vegetables ahead of time and stir-fry just before serving. Cook white rice and serve two-thirds cup per person. For an easy but elegant dessert, cut up fresh fruit and top with Yogurt Dessert Topping, allowing about one cup of fruit and three tablespoons of topping per person. Calories include one dinner roll per person. Prepare yourself for raves over this meal!

LUSCIOUS SAUTÉED SHRIMP AND VEGETABLES
page 196

WHITE RICE

WATERCRESS AND ENDIVE SALAD
page 66

DINNER ROLLS

FRESH FRUIT WITH YOGURT DESSERT TOPPING
page 213

SERVES 4
610 calories

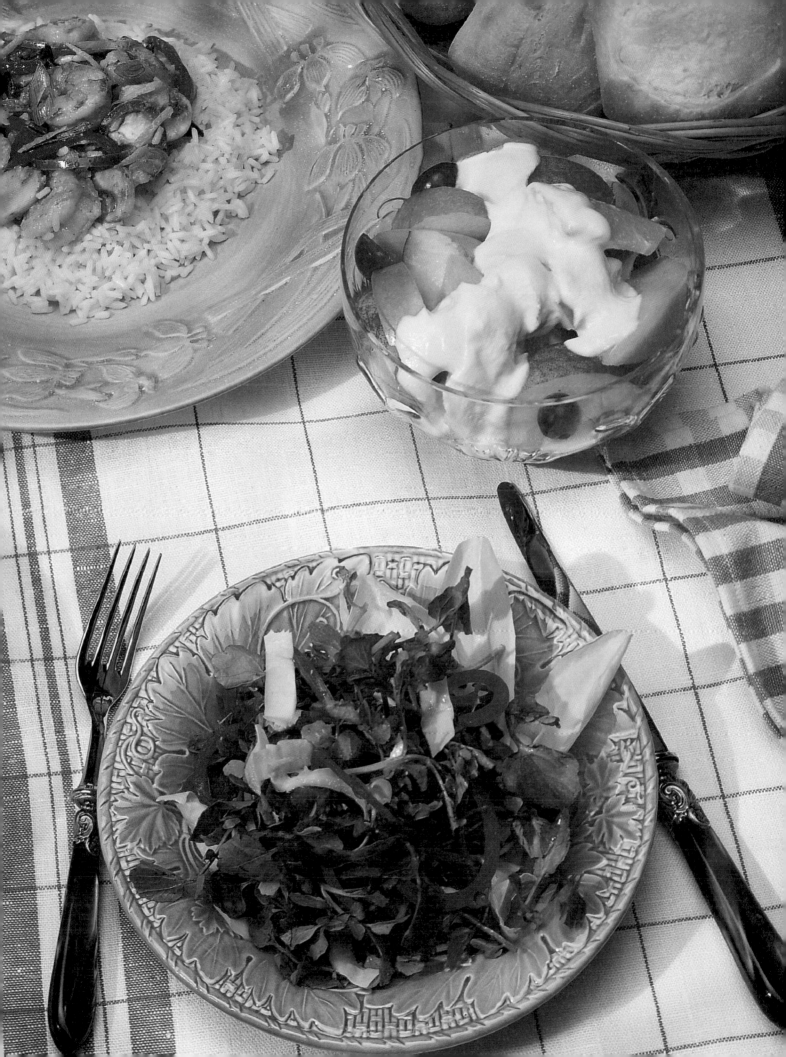

VEGETARIAN DELIGHT

~

You will love this meatless menu for either lunch or a light supper. Thick Vegetarian Chick-Pea Soup is delicately flavored, yet will satisfy the appetite of even the greatest meat lover. We have teamed it with one slice of Coriander Whole-Wheat Bread, a mixed green salad with two tablespoons of All-Purpose Salad Dressing, and Light Pineapple Tapioca for a refreshing dessert—all at only 415 calories!

THICK VEGETARIAN CHICK-PEA SOUP
page 84

CORIANDER WHOLE-WHEAT BREAD
page 224

MIXED GREEN SALAD WITH
ALL-PURPOSE SALAD DRESSING
page 74

LIGHT PINEAPPLE TAPIOCA
page 268

SERVES 6
415 calories

PAN FISH FRY

~

The old-fashioned fat-laden fish fry is a thing of the past in today's lighter eating style. But by using a nonstick skillet with a tiny amount of oil you'll be able to indulge in this family favorite—and without guilt! These fish steaks are coated in bread crumbs to give a crisp outside and a tender inside. The potatoes can be made ahead of time and finished just before serving. Menu calculations are for one serving of fish, potatoes and salad, one commercial dinner roll, and one serving of dessert.

SKILLET HALIBUT
page 178

SPINACH STUFFED POTATOES
page 110

ENDIVE AND MUSHROOM SALAD
WITH MINTY DRESSING
page 68

DINNER ROLLS

NEW CLASSIC APPLE TART
page 260

SERVES 4
650 calories

SPECIAL-TREAT SUPPER

~

If you like lamb, you are in for a treat with this menu. The presentation is subtle and sophisticated, but preparation is extremely easy—simply marinate the meat and roast! Accompany the delicious lamb entrée with Mashed Turnip with Yam, Sautéed Snow Peas and Mushrooms, and hard rolls (one per person). This colorful meal ends with Chocolate Chestnut Mousse with Strawberry Sauce, a special dessert that can be made the day ahead. Your guests will never forget this dining experience!

TANGY ROAST LEG OF LAMB
page 167

MASHED TURNIP WITH YAM
page 103

SAUTÉED SNOW PEAS AND MUSHROOMS
page 106

HARD ROLLS

CHOCOLATE CHESTNUT MOUSSE WITH
STRAWBERRY SAUCE
page 242

SERVES 4
660 calories

CLASSIC PORK CHOPS, UPTOWN STYLE

~

Here is an updated version of a classic family dish—pork chops. These pork chops are simmered with fruit juice and figs, creating a tasty, thick brown sauce during cooking. Browned Cabbage with Caraway and Pretty Pink Potatoes are perfect side dishes for this entrée, combining wonderfully with the flavors of the meat. Add one dinner roll per person and top off the meal with Frozen Chocolate Dessert. This is a meal you can serve to company as well as family.

PORK CHOPS WITH FRUIT
page 174

BROWNED CABBAGE WITH CARAWAY
page 99

PRETTY PINK POTATOES IN A CROCK
page 112

DINNER ROLLS

FROZEN CHOCOLATE DESSERT
page 279

SERVES 4
660 calories

Breakfast Foods

In our household, breakfast is the most important meal of the day, sending us soaring off into our full and active life. Lunch is light, a pleasant respite from the busy kitchen, the tapping typewriters, and the jangling phones. Psychologically, we simply can't afford to have dull repasts at either time. The following breakfast dishes—some of which double as luncheon dishes—are guaranteed to excite the taste buds and invigorate the psyche. Why not dream up more along these lines? The possibilities for wonderful breakfasts and lunches are virtually endless.

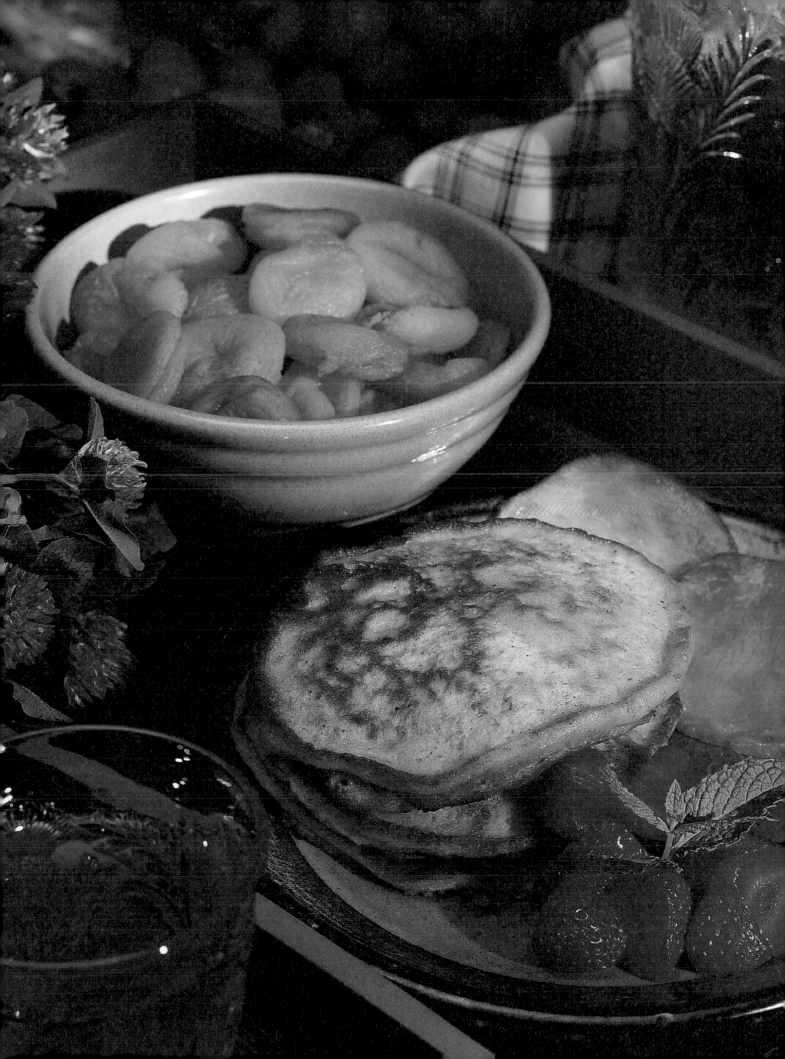

*S*piced Bran Griddle Cakes
~

YIELD: 16 PANCAKES (8 SERVINGS)

The griddle cake is an American institution, unchanged since its debut in the kitchens of the 13 colonies. Now savor the slight crunchiness of these breakfast beauties; you've never tasted that in a griddle cake before. In this innovative griddle cake, bran flakes are immersed in buttermilk and fruit juice concentrate for exactly 2 minutes before mixing with the rest of the ingredients, which include a bright new array of spices. Serve the cakes as soon as they're done, as is or topped with my Strawberry Sauce (see Serving Suggestions).

For 2 pancakes
Calories: 100
Carbohydrate: 14 g
Protein: 4 g
Fat: 3 g
Saturated fat: 1 g
Cholesterol: 22 mg
Dietary fiber: 1.1 g
Sodium: 171 mg
Exchanges: 1 starch/bread
½ fat

¾ cup unbleached flour

¼ teaspoon baking soda

1½ teaspoons baking powder

¼ teaspoon each cinnamon, ground cardamom (or nutmeg), and allspice

¾ tablespoon Italian olive oil or canola oil, plus 1½ teaspoons for pan

1 large egg

1½ cups low-fat buttermilk (preferably without salt)

2 tablespoons frozen pineapple juice concentrate

¾ cup bran flakes

¼ cup skim milk

1. Sift first 4 ingredients into a large bowl.

2. In a cup, blend 1 tablespoon oil with egg, beating with fork to blend.

3. In medium bowl, whisk together buttermilk and concentrate. Add bran flakes and stir to coat evenly. Let stand for 2 minutes.

4. Stir in sifted mixture. Then combine oil mix with batter, stirring until dry ingredients are moistened. Add skim milk and combine in a fold-over motion. Batter will be thick but pourable.

5. Prepare griddles in batches, using 1 or 2 large nonstick skillet(s). Place pan(s) over medium-high heat until a drop of cold water dances off. Using a ¼-cup measure, pour enough batter into pan(s) to make four 3-inch pancakes in each pan. Cook until bubbles form on top of pancakes. (A good turning test is to lift edges slightly with a spatula to see if they've browned.) Turn carefully and cook until lightly browned. Serve immediately—they won't wait.

SERVING SUGGESTIONS: Top with Strawberry Sauce (page 242), low-fat yogurt, and/or pureed canned pineapples (no sugar added).

VARIATION: Stir in ¼ cup crushed pineapples (no sugar added) at the end of step 4. Yield will be 18 pancakes.

$\mathcal{P}$ineapple French Toast

~

YIELD: SERVES 4

Per serving
Calories: 140
Carbohydrate: 14 g
Protein: 7 g
Fat: 7 g
Saturated fat: 1 g
Cholesterol: 69 mg
Dietary fiber: 0.3 g
Sodium: 65 mg
Exchanges: 1 starch/bread
  ½ lean meat
  1 fat

4 slices Light and Spongy Loaf
  (page 226) cut into ½-inch slices

3 eggs (use 1 egg yolk and 3 egg
  whites)

2 tablespoons crushed canned
  pineapple (no sugar added)

¼ cup evaporated skim milk

¼ teaspoon each ground coriander
  and cinnamon

2 dashes each ground cloves and red
  (cayenne) pepper

4 teaspoons Italian olive oil or
  canola oil

2 teaspoons date sugar
  (see page 297)

1. In large bowl, soak bread in lightly
  beaten mixture of eggs, pineapple,
  skim milk, and spices. Let stand
  until most of liquid is absorbed.

2. Heat 2 teaspoons oil in nonstick
  skillet until hot. Add bread,
  spooning with remaining liquid.
  Sauté over medium-high heat until
  browned on both sides, adding balance of oil (2 teaspoons) just before
  turning. Serve at once, sprinkled
  with date sugar, if desired.

NOTE: Good-quality commercial
  Italian or French bread may be
  substituted for Light and Spongy
  Loaf, bearing in mind that nutritional statistics will vary from
  mine.

Stewed Apricots
~

YIELD: SERVES 5

8 ounces dried apricots (unsulfured preferred) (see page 297)

1 cup apple juice (no sugar added)

½ cup water

1 teaspoon ground coriander

½ teaspoon each cinnamon and allspice

1. Place apricots in small heavy-bottom saucepan. Add balance of ingredients. Bring to boil. Remove from heat. Cover and let stand for 1 hour. Stir.

2. Re-cover. Bring to simmering point and cook over very low heat until apricots are tender (about 15 minutes). Remove from heat. Let stand, covered, until cooled.

3. Serve warm or chilled.

VARIATION: Just before serving, prepare Creamy Whipped Dessert Topping by pouring ¼ cup evaporated skim milk into large mixing bowl. Place bowl and whipping utensils in freezer. Chill until fine crystals begin to form around edges. Whip until stiff. Stir in ½ teaspoon finely grated orange zest and ⅛ teaspoon each ground cinnamon and coriander. Spoon over stewed apricots and serve immediately. Serves 7.

Per serving
Calories: 135
Carbohydrate: 31 g
Protein: 1 g
Fat: 0 g
Saturated fat: 0 g
Cholesterol: 0 mg
Dietary fiber: 4.5 g
Sodium: 6 mg
Exchanges: 2 fruit

Spiced Prunes
~

YIELD: ABOUT 24 PRUNES (8 SERVINGS)

1 8-ounce can prunes (no preservatives added)

¼ cup each apple juice (no sugar added) and water

1 teaspoon fresh lemon juice

½ teaspoon ground coriander

¼ teaspoon ground cardamom

1-inch slice orange zest

1. Place prunes in small, heavy-bottom saucepan. Add balance of ingredients. Bring to boil. Reduce heat, cover, and simmer for 10 minutes. Partially uncover and let prunes cool in pot. Discard orange zest.

2. Store in refrigerator in tightly closed glass jar. Serve chilled or at room temperature.

SERVING SUGGESTION:
Delicious served with cold cereal in the morning or with cottage cheese for lunch.

For 3 prunes
Calories: 60
Carbohydrate: 14 g
Protein: 1 g
Fat: trace
Saturated fat: 0 g
Cholesterol: 0 mg
Dietary fiber: 2.3 g
Sodium: 1 mg
Exchanges: 1 fruit

New Baked Apples

~

YIELD: SERVES 4

4 medium Cortland baking apples, washed and cored

2 tablespoons frozen apple juice concentrate

⅓ cup cranberry juice (no sugar added)

2 tablespoons water

½ teaspoon ground coriander

¼ teaspoon each freshly grated nutmeg, ground cardamom, and ground cinnamon

1 tablespoon raisins

1. Preheat oven to 350°F. Slit skins of apples to a depth of ⅓ of apple, starting from top center. Place in small shallow baking dish.

2. Combine balance of ingredients in heavy-bottom saucepan. Bring to simmering point and cook for 3 minutes. Spoon equal amounts over apples. Cover loosely with aluminum foil.

3. Bake for 30 to 40 minutes, basting every 10 minutes. Finished apples should be firm yet tender. (Do not overcook, or you'll have applesauce.)

4. Serve warm or chilled, with or without Creamy Vanilla Sauce (page 208).

Per serving
Calories: 78
Carbohydrate: 19 g
Protein: trace
Fat: trace
Saturated fat: trace
Cholesterol: 0 mg
Dietary fiber: 3.2 g
Sodium: 1 mg
Exchanges: 1 fruit

Quick Mozzarella Omelette

~

YIELD: SERVES 2

3 eggs (use 1 egg yolk and 3 egg whites)

2 teaspoons dried minced onion

½ teaspoon dried savory or tarragon leaves, crushed

3 dashes ground red (cayenne) pepper

¼ teaspoon smoked yeast (see page 297) (optional)

¼ teaspoon curry powder

1 tablespoon evaporated skim milk

2 tablespoons grated part-skim mozzarella cheese

¼ teaspoon Italian olive oil

1. In small bowl, combine and blend all ingredients except oil.

2. Using pastry brush, spread oil across and up sides of 8-inch nonstick skillet. Heat until hot (a drop of water should bounce off skillet). Pour egg mixture into pan. Let cook for 30 seconds. Then tilt pan in a complete circle so that residue will stick to sides of skillet. Cook until lightly browned on one side only (the center should remain moist).

3. Slide onto dish. Flip half over. Cut omelette in half and serve immediately.

Per serving
Calories: 99
Carbohydrate: 2 g
Protein: 11 g
Fat: 5 g
Saturated fat: 2 g
Cholesterol: 144 mg
Dietary fiber: 0.1 g
Sodium: 154 mg
Exchanges: 1½ lean meat

Vegetable Omelette

YIELD: SERVES 2

Per serving
Calories: 123
Carbohydrate: 7 g
Protein: 10 g
Fat: 6 g
Saturated fat: 1 g
Cholesterol: 137 mg
Dietary fiber: 1.8 g
Sodium: 107 mg
Exchanges: 1 medium-
        fat meat
        1 vegetable
        ½ fat

With 3 oz chicken or veal
Per serving
Calories: 193
Carbohydrate: 7 g
Protein: 24 g
Fat: 9 g
Saturated fat: 2 g
Cholesterol: 173 mg
Dietary fiber: 1.8 g
Sodium: 138 mg
Exchanges: 3 lean meat
        ½ fat

FOR THE FILLING:

1   teaspoon Italian olive oil

2   tablespoons each minced onion and sweet green or red pepper

1   clove garlic, minced

½   cup coarsely chopped fresh mushrooms (wash, dry, and trim them first)

½   cup coarsely chopped cored and seeded fresh tomatoes

1   teaspoon each minced fresh parsley and dill

½   teaspoon dried oregano, crushed

1   teaspoon tomato paste (no salt added) mixed with 1 tablespoon water

FOR THE OMELETTE:

3   eggs (use 1 egg yolk and 3 egg whites)

2   tablespoons evaporated skim milk

½   teaspoon crushed dried oregano

1   teaspoon each minced fresh parsley and dill

3   dashes ground red (cayenne) pepper

¼   teaspoon Italian olive oil

1. Prepare filling first. Using pastry brush, spread oil across an 8-inch nonstick skillet. Heat until hot. Sauté onion, pepper, garlic, and mushrooms over medium-high heat until lightly browned, stirring often. Add tomatoes, half of fresh herbs, dried oregano, and tomato paste mixture. Stir and cook for 3 minutes. Turn into small bowl. Cover to keep warm. Wipe out skillet.

2. To prepare omelette, combine all ingredients except oil in small bowl.

3. Follow instructions in step 2 for Quick Mozzarella Omelette (page 39) for preparation of omelette. Then slide onto warmed dish. Spoon filling on one-half of circle. Flip other half of circle over filling. Cut omelette in half and serve immediately.

NOTE: This delicious omelette could be your evening meal if you add a 3-ounce serving of cooked chicken or veal in step 1.

Appetizing Rice Omelette

YIELD: SERVES 2

Per serving
Calories: 131
Carbohydrate: 12 g
Protein: 8 g
Fat: 5 g
Saturated fat: 1 g
Cholesterol: 136 mg
Dietary fiber: 1.5 g
Sodium: 96 mg
Exchanges: 1 starch/bread
1 lean meat

FOR THE FILLING:

1 teaspoon Italian olive oil or canola oil

2 tablespoons minced onion

2 tablespoons minced celery

½ crisp sweet apple, peeled, cored, and coarsely chopped

¼ cup cooked brown rice, chilled

¼ teaspoon each ground cinnamon and freshly grated nutmeg

3 dashes ground red (cayenne) pepper

FOR THE OMELETTE:

3 eggs (use 1 egg yolk and 3 egg whites)

1 tablespoon each evaporated skim milk and water

¼ teaspoon each cinnamon and nutmeg

1 dash ground red (cayenne) pepper

¼ teaspoon Italian olive oil or canola oil

1. Prepare filling first. Using pastry brush, spread oil across an 8-inch nonstick skillet. Heat until hot. Sauté onion, celery, and apple until lightly browned (about 3 minutes).

2. Stir in rice, breaking up congealed pieces with spoon. Sprinkle with spices and cook until rice is heated through, and apple is tender. Transfer to plate. Cover to keep warm. Wipe out skillet.

3. To prepare omelette, combine all ingredients except oil in small bowl.

4. Follow instructions in step 2 for Quick Mozzarella Omelette (page 39) for preparation of omelette. Then slide onto warmed dish. Spoon filling on one-half of circle. Flip other half of circle over filling. Cut omelette in half and serve immediately.

Smooth and Satisfying Cream of Wheat

~

YIELD: SERVES 3

1   cup each water and skim milk

¼   cup apple juice (no sugar added)

¼   teaspoon each ground cinnamon and cardamom

3   dashes ground cloves

⅓   cup regular enriched Cream of Wheat cereal

2   tablespoons unprocessed bran, or oat bran

¼   teaspoon pure vanilla extract

1.   Combine water, milk, juice, and spices in heavy-bottom saucepan. Bring to slow boil. Sprinkle with Cream of Wheat, stirring constantly. Reduce heat to simmering and cook uncovered for 4 minutes.

2.   Sprinkle bran into mixture, stirring to blend. Continue cooking for 2 minutes more. Remove from heat. Stir in vanilla and serve.

Per serving
Calories: 157
Carbohydrate: 31 g
Protein: 7 g
Fat: trace
Saturated fat: 0 g
Cholesterol: 1 mg
Dietary fiber: 3.5 g
Sodium: 55 mg
Exchanges: 1½ starch/bread
            ½ milk

Sweet and Chunky Oatmeal

~

YIELD: SERVES 2

¼   cup apple juice (no sugar added)

1¼   cups water

¼   teaspoon each freshly grated nutmeg and allspice

½   teaspoon ground coriander

⅔   cup old-fashioned rolled oats

2   teaspoons date sugar (see page 297) (optional)

1.   Combine all ingredients except oats in heavy-bottom saucepan. Bring to boil. Stir in oats. Turn heat down and simmer gently for 8 to 10 minutes, stirring often.

2.   Cover and let stand for 2 minutes before serving. Sprinkle with date sugar, if desired.

Per serving
Calories: 200
Carbohydrate: 37 g
Protein: 7 g
Fat: 3 g
Saturated fat: trace
Cholesterol: 0
Dietary fiber: 2.5 g
Sodium: 426 mg
Exchanges: 1 starch/bread
            ½ fruit

This recipe contains a moderate amount of sugar and should be used only occasionally. It should be carefully worked into your individual meal plan.

Bulgur Breakfast Pudding

~

YIELD: SERVES 6 AS BREAKFAST PUDDING;

SERVES 10 AS DESSERT TREAT

For 6 servings

Per serving

Calories: 89

Carbohydrate: 20 g

Protein: 2 g

Fat: trace

Saturated fat: 0 g

Cholesterol: 0 mg

Dietary fiber: 1.9 g

Sodium: 11 mg

Exchanges: ½ starch/bread

½ fruit

For 10 servings

Per serving

Calories: 53

Carbohydrate: 11 g

Protein: 1 g

Fat: trace

Saturated fat: 0 g

Cholesterol: 0 mg

Dietary fiber: 1.1 g

Sodium: 7 mg

Exchanges: ½ starch/bread

1¾ cups water

1 cup diet orange soda or water

2 tablespoons each frozen orange and apple juice concentrates

½ teaspoon ground cinnamon

1 teaspoon ground coriander

¼ teaspoon freshly grated nutmeg

½ cup bulgur

2 tablespoons each buckwheat and brown rice flours (see page 297)

¼ cup raisins (optional)

1. Combine first 6 ingredients in top of double boiler. Bring to boil over direct heat. Add bulgur and flours. Stir to blend. Bring to simmering point. Cover and cook for 5 minutes. Add raisins. Re-cover.

2. Half-fill bottom section of double boiler with water. Bring to simmering point. Combine pots, and cook over simmering water for 20 minutes. Remove from heat. Partially uncover and let stand for 10 minutes.

3. Spoon into small bowls. Serve hot or warm.

NOTE: Refrigerate any leftover pudding and reheat to perfection in your double boiler.

SERVING SUGGESTION: Serve smaller portions as a delicious sweet-tasting dessert topped with Creamy Whipped Dessert Topping (see Variation, page 38).

VARIATION: Add 2 tablespoons rinsed and picked-over fresh cranberries in step 1, and simmer, covered, for 3 minutes before bulgur is added. Pudding will be less sweet and cranberry flavored. No extra exchanges for the cranberries—they're free for you to enjoy.

Breakfast Muffin Cake
~

YIELD: 16 SLICES (1 LOAF)

Per slice
Calories: 150
Carbohydrate: 23 g
Protein: 3 g
Fat: 5 g
Saturated fat: 1 g
Cholesterol: 17 mg
Dietary fiber: 2.5 g
Sodium: 110 mg
Exchanges: 1 starch/bread
½ fruit
1 fat

This recipe contains a moderate amount of sugar and should be used only occasionally. It should be carefully worked into your individual meal plan.

½ cup fully ripe mashed bananas

⅓ cup chopped prunes (about 6 pitted prunes)

1 cup unprocessed bran

½ cup date sugar (see page 297)

⅔ cup buttermilk (preferably without salt)

⅓ cup sweet soft corn oil margarine, plus ½ teaspoon for pan

3 tablespoons granulated fructose (see page 297)

2 eggs (use 1 egg yolk and 2 egg whites)

½ teaspoon pure vanilla extract

1½ cups unbleached flour

2½ teaspoons baking powder

¼ cup coarsely chopped walnuts

1. Combine first 4 ingredients in bowl. Pour buttermilk into mixture, stirring to blend. Let stand for 5 minutes.

2. Add ⅓ cup margarine and fructose. Beat until well blended. Add eggs and beat until smooth.

3. Add banana mixture and vanilla and blend briefly.

4. Sift flour with baking powder. Spoon ½ cup at a time into batter, blending after each addition. Stir in nuts.

5. Spread mixture into 9-inch lightly greased loaf pan. Bake in preheated 350°F oven for 50 minutes. Place pan on rack and let cool for 15 minutes.

6. Carefully remove from pan. Serve warm or at room temperature.

NOTE: This cake freezes very well. Slice entire loaf; wrap each slice in waxed paper, then in aluminum foil, and freeze.

Spiced Blueberry-Bran Muffins
~

YIELD: 12 MUFFINS

Per muffin
Calories: 117
Carbohydrate: 16 g
Protein: 3 g
Fat: 4 g
Saturated fat: 1 g
Cholesterol: 23 mg
Dietary fiber: 1.4 g
Sodium: 109 mg
Exchanges: 1 starch/bread
1 fat

½   cup whole-wheat flour

¾   cup unbleached flour

1   teaspoon ground coriander

½   teaspoon ground cinnamon

2½ teaspoons baking powder

¼   cup each date sugar and oat bran (see page 297)

2   eggs (use 1 egg yolk and 2 egg whites)

3   tablespoons Italian olive oil

1   tablespoon grated orange zest (preferably from navel orange)

1   cup low-sodium buttermilk (preferably without salt)

½   teaspoon pure vanilla extract

1   cup fresh blueberries (picked over, washed, and patted dry with paper toweling)

½   teaspoon sweet soft corn oil margarine

1. Preheat oven to 400°F. Sift flours, spices, and baking powder into bowl. Stir in date sugar and oat bran (pulverized in food blender before measuring for light-textured muffin). Set aside.

2. In large mixing bowl, beat eggs, oil, and orange zest with whisk until blended.

3. Add flour mixture alternately with buttermilk, stirring (not beating) with wooden spoon until all flour is absorbed. Then stir in vanilla and fold in blueberries.

4. Half-fill margarine-greased 3-inch muffin pans with batter. Bake for 20 to 22 minutes, until browned.

5. Remove pan from oven. Place on rack for 5 minutes. With blunt knife, loosen muffins from sides of pan and remove. Let cool for 5 minutes before serving.

NOTE: These muffins freeze to perfection. To reheat, wrap in aluminum foil and bake in preheated 400°F oven for 15 to 20 minutes. Uncover and let cool a few minutes before serving.

Hors d'oeuvres and Condiments

HORS D'OEUVRES

CONDIMENTS

What do you want hors d'oeuvres and condiments to do for you? Stimulate your appetite? Or graciously add to the enjoyment of your food without compelling you to take just one more bite... and one more... and one more? My hors d'oeuvres and condiments are in the latter category. Without sugar or salt (the two most powerful appetite stimulants), they gratify your taste without expanding your waist.

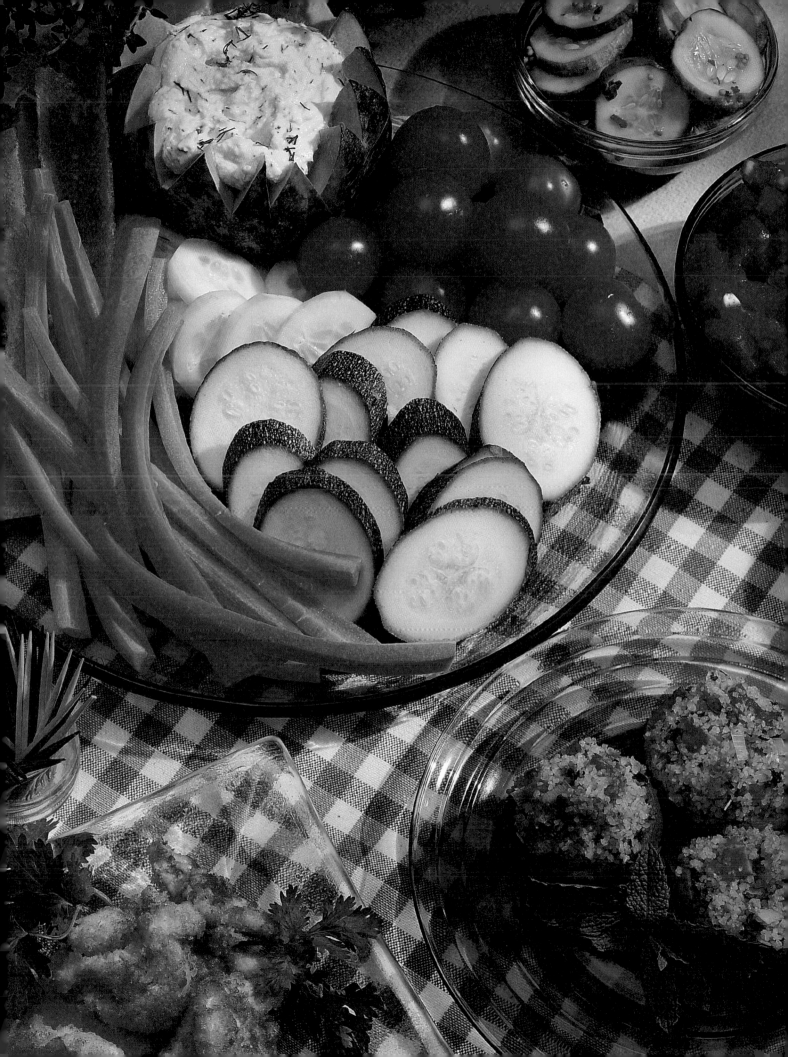

Hors d'oeuvres

Sliced Stuffed Cucumbers

~

YIELD: ABOUT 32 SLICES

2 straight firm cucumbers, about 6 inches long, well scrubbed

½ cup dry curd cottage cheese (no salt added) or drained low-fat cottage cheese (no salt added)

1 tablespoon each grated onion and carrot

2 tablespoons each minced fresh dill and parsley

½ teaspoon Worcestershire sauce

¼ teaspoon chili con carne seasoning

2 tablespoons Ketchup Taste-Alike (page 58)

Ground red (cayenne) pepper to taste (2–3 dashes)

1. Cut ⅜ inch off one end of cucumbers. Using small melon scooper, carefully scoop out centers.

2. Mash together balance of ingredients in small bowl. Stuff cucumbers. Chill well.

3. Cut into ⅜-inch slices. Serve immediately.

Per slice
Calories: 5
Carbohydrate: 1 g
Protein: 1 g
Fat: 0 g
Saturated fat: 0 g
Cholesterol: trace
Dietary fiber: 0.3 g
Sodium: 1 mg
Exchanges: free
   (4 slices = 1 vegetable)

Miracle Chicken Spread
~

YIELD: 1¼ CUPS

For 2 tablespoons
Calories: 58
Carbohydrate: 6 g
Protein: 5 g
Fat: 1 g
Saturated fat: trace
Cholesterol: 7 mg
Dietary fiber: 0.9 g
Sodium: 8 mg
Exchanges: ½ starch/bread
　　　　　 ½ lean meat

½　cup dried chick-peas

2　cups water

¾　cup diced cooked chicken

1　tablespoon fresh lemon juice

3　large shallots, minced

2　tablespoons minced fresh parsley or dill

¼　teaspoon ground cumin seed

½　teaspoon chili con carne seasoning

4　dashes ground red (cayenne) pepper

2　tablespoons tomato juice (no salt added)

2　tablespoons Mayonnaise-Type Salad Dressing (page 75) or Real Tomato Mayonnaise (page 73)

1.　Soak chick-peas overnight in cold water to cover. Drain. Place in small heavy-bottom saucepan. Add 2 cups water. Bring to boil. Reduce heat to simmering and cook, partially covered, until tender (about 2 hours), stirring from time to time. Mash in bowl while warm.

2.　Add chicken to bowl. Sprinkle with lemon juice, mashing mixture to blend. Add shallots, parsley, and spices. Stir in tomato juice until well incorporated into mixture. Then blend in mayonnaise.

3.　Serve at room temperature or chilled as a sandwich spread, appetizer (served in lettuce cups), or as a canapé spread on thinly sliced triangles of any of my breads (pages 218–235) or on commercial low-sodium bread.

NOTES:
1.　Spread may be quickly prepared in food processor fitted with steel blade. Here's how: Place cooked chick-peas, diced chicken, lemon juice, and peeled and halved shallots in work bowl. Process on/off 3 times, scraping down sides of bowl after, if necessary. Add parsley and spices. Process on/off once. Add tomato juice and mayonnaise. Process once.

2.　The nutrition analysis for this recipe is calculated at a serving size of 2 tablespoons only because exchange values could not be calculated using a smaller serving size. Using a smaller serving size will satisfy your taste buds just as much as 2 tablespoons, and will save you unwanted calories as well.

Coriander Chicken Kabobs
~

YIELD: SERVES 8

Per serving
Calories: 95
Carbohydrate: 2 g
Protein: 14 g
Fat: 3 g
Saturated fat: 1 g
Cholesterol: 36 mg
Dietary fiber: 0
Sodium: 41 mg
Exchanges: 2 lean meat

1   pound chicken breasts, boned and skinned, flattened to ¼-inch thickness

1   tablespoon each dry vermouth, wine vinegar, and fresh lime juice

¼   cup pineapple juice (no sugar added)

½   teaspoon ground coriander

¼   teaspoon ground cardamom

2   teaspoons minced dried onion

⅓   cup toasted Magnificent Rye Bread crumbs (page 232)

3   teaspoons Italian olive oil

1. Wash chicken and dry thoroughly with paper toweling. Cut into 1- to 1½-inch pieces. (There should be 24 pieces.)

2. Combine vermouth, vinegar, lime juice, and next 4 ingredients in bowl, beating with fork to blend. Add chicken, turning to coat. Let stand, covered, at room temperature for 1 hour, or refrigerated for several hours. Drain.

3. Spread half of crumbs across large plate. Lay chicken pieces on crumbs. Sprinkle with balance of crumbs. Coat evenly.

4. Heat 1½ teaspoons oil over medium-high heat in large non-stick skillet until hot. Sauté chicken on first side until golden brown (about 2 minutes). Add balance of oil (1½ teaspoons), turn, and sauté until browned. Do not overcook.

5. Arrange on serving platter. Pierce kabobs with colorful cocktail picks, and serve hot out of the skillet.

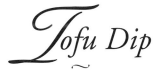

Tofu Dip

YIELD: ¾ CUP

Per teaspoon
Calories: 6
Carbohydrate: trace
Protein: 1 g
Fat: trace
Saturated fat: 0 g
Cholesterol: 0 mg
Dietary fiber: 0 g
Sodium: 2 mg
Exchanges: free

1   **cake tofu (½ pound bean curd)**

1   **teaspoon each fresh lemon juice and wine vinegar**

2   **tablespoons apple juice (no sugar added)**

1   **tablespoon low-fat cottage cheese (no salt added)**

1   **teaspoon prepared Dijon mustard**

½   **teaspoon paprika**

1   **clove garlic, minced**

2   **shallots, minced**

1   **tablespoon minced fresh parsley or dill**

1. Drain tofu on paper toweling. Cut into small cubes. Place in blender or food processor. Add lemon juice, vinegar, and apple juice. Blend until smooth.

2. Add balance of ingredients. Blend only until well combined. Pour into jar. Cover and chill for 3 hours or more before using.

NOTES:

1. Two tablespoons finely minced scallion (including green part) or fresh chives may be substituted for shallots and garlic.

2. Low-sodium Norwegian flatbreads are delicious with this dip.

3. Up to 3 teaspoons, this is a free food. At 4 teaspoons, it's worth ½ lean meat exchange.

VARIATION: Add 2 tablespoons tomato juice (no salt added) in step 2.

Luscious Stuffed Mushrooms

~

YIELD: 12 STUFFED MUSHROOMS

For 3 stuffed mushrooms
Calories: 88
Carbohydrate: 12 g
Protein: 2 g
Fat: 3 g
Saturated fat: trace
Cholesterol: 0 mg
Dietary fiber: 2.3 g
Sodium: 9 mg
Exchanges: ½ starch/bread
1 vegetable
½ fat

¼ cup bulgur

¾ cup water

12 large fresh mushrooms (about ½ pound), washed, dried, and trimmed

1 tablespoon Italian olive oil

1 leek, white part only, well washed, trimmed, and minced

2 cloves garlic, minced

½ teaspoon each dried sage leaves, crushed, and chili con carne seasoning

3 dashes ground red (cayenne) pepper

2 teaspoons dry sherry

1 tablespoon minced fresh mint leaves, plus 2 teaspoons

3 teaspoons minced fresh parsley

1 tablespoon minced drained pimento (no salt added)

1. Soak bulgur in water for 30 minutes. Then bring to boil and slow-boil for 8 minutes. Drain. Preheat oven to 400°F.

2. Gently separate stems from mushroom caps. Mince stems. Set caps aside.

3. Heat 1½ teaspoons oil in nonstick skillet until hot. Sauté minced stems, leek, and garlic over medium-high heat until lightly browned. Add bulgur, stirring to combine.

4. Sprinkle mixture with sage, chili con carne seasoning, ground red pepper, and sherry, stirring to blend. Cook for 1 minute. Remove from heat.

5. Stir in 1 tablespoon mint, parsley, and pimento, blending well. Transfer to bowl. Wipe out skillet.

6. Heat balance of oil (1½ teaspoons) in skillet until hot. Sauté mushroom caps on both sides for 1½ minutes. Transfer to small baking dish. Fill with bulgur mixture. Sprinkle with balance of mint (2 teaspoons).

7. Bake for 10 to 15 minutes until mushroom caps are heated through. Serve hot.

NOTE: Minced fresh dill may be substituted for fresh mint.

Delicious Turkey Bundles

~

YIELD: ABOUT 12 BUNDLES

Per serving
Calories: 41
Carbohydrate: trace
Protein: 8 g
Fat: 1 g
Saturated fat: trace
Cholesterol: 20 mg
Dietary fiber: 0.1 g
Sodium: 19 mg
Exchanges: 1 lean meat

½ teaspoon smoked yeast (see page 297)

⅛ teaspoon ground cumin seed

3 dashes ground red (cayenne) pepper

½ pound thinly sliced roast turkey breast, chilled

1 bunch crisp arugula, each leaf well washed and dried (see Note 1)

8 fresh asparagus tips, cooked and chilled

1. Combine smoked yeast, cumin, and ground red pepper in small cup, blending well. Set aside.

2. Cut turkey slices into about 12 easy-to-roll pieces. Sprinkle and rub each piece with spice mixture. Lay one arugula leaf on top of each hors d'oeuvre.

3. Cut each asparagus tip in half. Lay equal amounts in each hors d'oeuvre. Roll up and secure with colorful cocktail picks. Serve chilled.

NOTES:
1. Arugula is an Italian green. It is meaty in texture and pleasantly bitter. If you can't locate it, substitute crisp Belgian endive leaves or watercress leaves.

2. If you're buying turkey breast, be certain it's turkey—*not* turkey roll, which is turkey mixed with salt and other objectionable ingredients.

Savory Veal Cocktail Balls

YIELD: 28 COCKTAIL BALLS

Per cocktail ball
Calories: 48
Carbohydrate: 1 g
Protein: 4 g
Fat: 3 g
Saturated fat: 1 g
Cholesterol: 17 mg
Dietary fiber: 0.2 g
Sodium: 21 mg
Exchanges: ½ lean meat
½ fat

1 pound lean ground veal

¼ cup finely chopped walnuts

2 tablespoons minced fresh parsley

1 whole egg

½ cup dry red wine, divided

2 teaspoons tomato paste (no salt added)

1 teaspoon prepared Dijon mustard

½ teaspoon ground ginger

1 tablespoon minced dried onion

2 slices No-Fuss Cracked-Wheat Bread (page 234), crusts removed, lightly toasted and torn into small pieces

1 tablespoon Italian olive oil

½ cup Easy Chicken Stock (page 216)

1. Place meat in large bowl. Blend in nuts and 1 tablespoon parsley. Set aside.

2. In small bowl, combine egg and ¼ cup wine. Beat with fork or whisk until blended. Add 1 teaspoon tomato paste, mustard, ginger, and onion. Whisk again.

3. Add bread, coating well. Let stand for 5 minutes. Pour into meat mixture, mixing well. Shape into 28 compact balls. Cover and refrigerate for 15 minutes or longer. (Mixture may be prepared up to this point well in advance of cooking time.)

4. Heat oil over medium heat in well-seasoned nonstick skillet until hot. Sauté meatballs, turning gingerly with spatula, until browned on all sides (about 4 minutes). Do not overcook. Pour off any remaining oil and exuded fat from skillet.

5. Add balance of wine (¼ cup), stock, balance of tomato paste (1 teaspoon), and balance of parsley (1 tablespoon) to skillet. Heat to simmering point. Reduce heat. Cover and simmer for 10 minutes, spooning with sauce several times.

6. Uncover, raise heat under skillet, and cook until most of sauce is reduced, turning often. Serve hot, pierced with colorful cocktail picks, or in small individual plate servings.

NOTE: I've used my No-Fuss Cracked-Wheat Bread in this recipe to give the meat a crunchy yet light texture. But you may use the commercial variety, bearing in mind that the sodium content in each meatball will increase by about 5 mg.

ALTERNATIVE SERVING SUGGESTION: Serve as a main course. During step 5, cook for 15 minutes. With slotted spoon, transfer meatballs to warmed, covered bowl. Raise heat and reduce sauce by half. Pour over meat and serve immediately. Lovely over cooked pasta or grains. Serves 4.

Spicy Orange Shrimp on Toast

YIELD: SERVES 4

Per serving
Calories: 175
Carbohydrate: 18 g
Protein: 19 g
Fat: 3 g
Saturated fat: 1 g
Cholesterol: 140 mg
Dietary fiber: 0.5 g
Sodium: 296 mg
Exchanges: 1 starch/bread
2 lean meat

1　pound fresh shrimp, shelled and deveined

1　teaspoon fresh lime juice

¼　teaspoon each dried tarragon leaves, crushed, and ground cumin seed

2　teaspoons Italian olive oil

2　large shallots, minced

1　tablespoon dry vermouth

1　tablespoon frozen orange juice concentrate

½　teaspoon each ground cumin seed and mild curry powder

⅛　teaspoon cinnamon

3　tablespoons evaporated skim milk

4　slices Light and Spongy Loaf (page 226), lightly toasted, or good-quality thin-sliced commercial bread

1　tablespoon minced fresh parsley

1.　Dry shrimp well with paper toweling. Transfer to bowl. Sprinkle with lime juice, turning to coat. Let stand for 10 minutes. Then pat dry with paper toweling. Sprinkle and rub with tarragon and cumin. Coarsely chop.

2.　Heat oil over medium heat in non-stick skillet until hot. Spread shallots across skillet. Sauté for 1 minute. Sprinkle chopped shrimp on shallots. Sauté until delicately pink on all sides, turning often. (Cooking time will be about 2½ to 3 minutes.)

3.　Combine vermouth, orange juice concentrate, and spices in small bowl. Beat with fork to blend. Pour over shrimp. Bring to simmering point and simmer for 1 minute. Stir in milk. Bring to simmering point. (Do not boil.)

4.　Pour over just-toasted slices of bread. Sprinkle with parsley and serve.

Beet Relish

~

YIELD: SERVES 4

1   bunch beets (about 1¼ pounds)

1   tablespoon apple cider vinegar
    plus ½ cup apple cider or wine vinegar

2   tablespoons fresh lemon juice

¼   cup apple juice (no sugar added)

½   teaspoon ground coriander

1   tablespoon pickling spices

¼   cup chopped onion

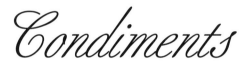

Condiments

1. Wash beets and cut off leaves 1 inch from beets. Place in saucepan with 1 tablespoon apple cider vinegar and water to cover. Cook until tender (10 to 20 minutes, depending upon size of beets). Drain, reserving ¼ cup cooking juices. Peel and dice. Place in bowl with reserved cooking juices.

2. Combine balance of ingredients, except onion, in heavy-bottom saucepan. Bring to simmering point. Partially cover and simmer for 15 minutes.

Strain into bowl with beets. Add onion, stirring to blend. Let cool.

3. Transfer to jar. Cover and refrigerate overnight. Drain and serve chilled.

Per serving
Calories: 45
Carbohydrate: 10 g
Protein: 1 g
Fat: 0 g
Saturated fat: 0 g
Cholesterol: 0 mg
Dietary fiber: 3 g
Sodium: 57 mg
Exchanges: 2 vegetable

Mildly Pickled Mushrooms and Artichokes

~

YIELD: SERVES 6

Per serving
Calories: 28
Carbohydrate: 5 g
Protein: 1 g
Fat: 0 g
Saturated fat: 0 g
Cholesterol: 0 mg
Dietary fiber: 1.6 g
Sodium: 22 mg
Exchanges: 1 vegetable

1   9-ounce box frozen artichoke hearts

¼   cup each wine vinegar, apple cider vinegar, dry vermouth, and water

1   tablespoon fresh lemon juice

2   cloves garlic, minced

½   teaspoon each ground cumin seed and curry powder

1   tablespoon minced fresh parsley

1   tablespoon minced dried onion

½   pound fresh small snow-white mushrooms, washed, dried, ends trimmed

½   teaspoon granulated fructose (see page 297)

½   teaspoon grated orange zest (preferably from navel orange)

1. Bring saucepan of water to rolling boil. Add frozen artichokes. Bring to boil and continue to boil for 2 minutes. Drain.

2. Combine vinegars, vermouth, water, lemon juice, garlic, spices, parsley, and dried onion in 1½-quart saucepan. Bring to boil and cook for 1 minute. Add artichokes and mushrooms. Bring mixture to boil and cook for 3 minutes, gently pushing artichokes down into liquid.

3. Transfer to bowl. Stir in fructose, if desired. Then stir in orange zest. Let cool.

4. Transfer to tightly covered jar and refrigerate overnight. Drain and serve.

Ketchup Taste-Alike

YIELD: ⅔ CUP

Per tablespoon
Calories: 7
Carbohydrate: 1 g
Protein: trace
Fat: 0 g
Saturated fat: 0 g
Cholesterol: 0 mg
Dietary fiber: 0.3 g
Sodium: 6 mg
Exchanges: free

½ cup tomato puree, preferably without salt

1 tablespoon tomato paste (no salt added)

4 dashes ground red (cayenne) pepper, or more to taste

⅛ teaspoon freshly grated nutmeg

¼ teaspoon ground ginger

1 tablespoon minced fresh parsley

½ teaspoon granulated fructose (see page 297) dissolved in 1 teaspoon warm water

1. In small bowl, combine and whisk all but last ingredient until well blended.

2. Stir in dissolved fructose. Let mixture stand for 5 minutes. Taste. Add more ground red pepper if desired.

3. Store in glass jar in refrigerator. It will keep for up to 4 days.

Super No-Salt Pickles

~

YIELD: SERVES 4

Per serving
Calories: 16
Carbohydrate: 4 g
Protein: 1 g
Fat: 0 g
Saturated fat: 0 g
Cholesterol: 0 mg
Dietary fiber: 1.5 g
Sodium: 2 mg
Exchanges: free

1 pound Kirby cucumbers, well scrubbed, cut into ¼-inch slices

1 teaspoon fresh lemon juice

1¼ cups apple cider vinegar

¼ cup wine vinegar

4 teaspoons pickling spices

½ teaspoon dry mustard

2 teaspoons ground coriander

½ teaspoon dried chervil leaves, crumbled

¼ teaspoon freshly grated nutmeg

1 large sprig parsley

1. Place sliced cucumbers in medium-size bowl.

2. Combine balance of ingredients in heavy-bottom saucepan. Bring to simmering point. Partially cover and simmer for 10 minutes. Strain into cucumbers. Stir. Let cool. Transfer to jar and refrigerate overnight. Drain and serve chilled.

NOTE: I prefer my pickles without sweetener. But if you prefer a sweeter taste, add 1 teaspoon granulated fructose after cooking liquid has cooled (step 2).

Salads and Salad Dressings

Would you like to know the simplest weight-control trick in the world? Just eat your salad slowly before your main dish. As you eat, that empty feeling diminishes, and you can't eat as much of the higher-calorie entrée. But the trick only works if the salad dressings are as low as you can get in calories without sacrificing taste. Mine are.

What I'm discussing, of course, are green salads, which need not necessarily be green. As a matter of fact, one of my favorite green salads, Mix-and-Match Vegetable Salad, is a palette of colors emanating from carrots, corn, squash, onions, peppers—any vegetables of your choice. But there's another kind of salad that can be a weight and health watcher's nightmare—and that's the salad served as an entrée.

That kind of salad is built around meat, fowl, fish, and shellfish—all of which add calories and/or salt. Even some fruit salads, when they're made with coconut, contain quantities of fat and saturated fat that a prudent food lover should avoid. Add to all these no-no ingredients high-calorie dressings, and eating that kind of salad for lunch or dinner could be a first-class nutritional mistake. You won't make that mistake when you enjoy my two entrée salads in this book, Marinated Chicken Salad and Tasty Tuna Salad (pages 70 and 71).

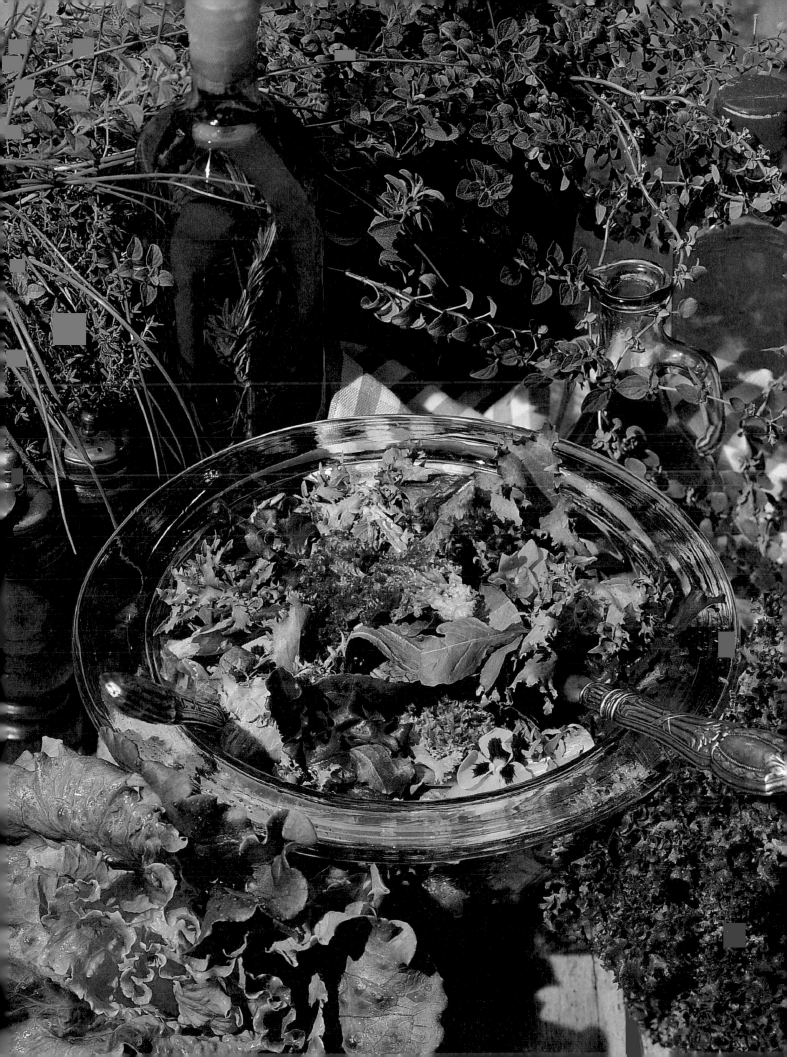

Salads

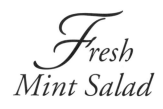

Fresh Mint Salad

~

YIELD: SERVES 4

4   egg tomatoes, cored, seeded, and cut into
    ½-inch cubes

3   medium Kirby cucumbers, peeled, and
    cut into ½-inch cubes

1   medium onion, thinly sliced, separated
    into rings

2   tablespoons peeled and coarsely grated carrot

1   tablespoon each apple cider vinegar,
    wine vinegar, and fresh lemon juice

4½ teaspoons Italian olive oil

3   tablespoons tomato juice (no salt added)

¼   teaspoon each ground cumin seed and mild
    curry powder

3   dashes ground red (cayenne) pepper (optional)

½   teaspoon dried tarragon leaves, crushed

2   tablespoons minced fresh mint

1. Place first 4 ingredi-
    ents in salad bowl.
    Toss.

2. Combine balance of
    ingredients in jar,
    shaking to blend.
    Pour over vegetables;
    toss. Let stand for
    30 minutes. Stir
    twice before serving.

Per serving
Calories: 108
Carbohydrate: 10 g
Protein: 1 g
Fat: 7 g
Saturated fat: 1 g
Cholesterol: 0 mg
Dietary fiber: 4.2 g
Sodium: 10 mg
Exchanges: 2 vegetable
1 fat

Celeriac Salad

YIELD: SERVES 8

There was a king of France in the days of yore who, tired of the same old gourmet meals of veal, beef, or chicken day after day, ordered his master chef to invent a new animal to cook. Like that king, you're probably fed up with the same old dishes, particularly salads.

So can you come up with something new? Yes, you can. It's celeriac, also known as knob celery. It's one of the ugliest vegetables on this planet: Wartlike knobs of all sizes emerge from a fibrous peel. But beneath its uncouth exterior (it doesn't even _resemble_ celery), celeriac conceals a unique crunchiness and a flavor that you'll find new and exciting.

Per serving
Calories: 52
Carbohydrate: 6 g
Protein: 1 g
Fat: 3 g
Saturated fat: trace
Cholesterol: 1 mg
Dietary fiber: 1.4 g
Sodium: 58 mg
Exchanges: 1 vegetable
½ fat

½	lemon
1	pound celeriac (celery root)
1	small carrot, peeled, ends trimmed, shredded
½	cup thin-sliced scallions, including tender green section
3	tablespoons chopped fresh coriander or 2 tablespoons minced parsley
½	cup tomato juice, preferably without salt
1	teaspoon dried oregano
¼	teaspoon dry mustard
2	tablespoons fresh orange juice
1	teaspoon onion powder
2	dashes cayenne pepper
½	teaspoon granulated fructose (see page 297)
4	tablespoons unseasoned rice wine vinegar
1½	tablespoons Italian olive oil
1	tablespoon freshly grated Parmesan cheese (optional)

1. Squeeze lemon juice into a 2-quart saucepan. Half-fill pan with water. Peel celeriac. Rinse, then dip into lemon water. Set on a cutting board and cut into ¼-inch slices; then cut slices into ¼-inch strips, dropping them into the lemon water as they're cut (this prevents them from turning brown). Set pot over high heat and bring liquid to a rolling boil. Cook, uncovered, for 1 minute. Pour into colander. Cool briefly under cold running water. When well drained, transfer strips to a large salad bowl.

2. Toss with carrot, scallion, and coriander (or parsley).

3. In a small bowl, whisk together tomato juice, oregano, mustard, orange juice, onion powder, cayenne, fructose, and 3 tablespoons vinegar. Let mixture stand for 2 minutes. Then pour over salad, and gently toss. Let stand for 10 minutes.

4. Drizzle with oil and toss. Add remaining vinegar to taste, and top with Parmesan cheese if desired. Serve right away.

NOTE: Refrigerate leftovers and bring to room temperature before serving next day. A few turns of your pepper mill and a few drops of vinegar will brighten its taste.

Super Salad

YIELD: SERVES 4

Per serving
Calories: 66
Carbohydrate: 4 g
Protein: 1 g
Fat: 4 g
Saturated fat: 1 g
Cholesterol: 0 mg
Dietary fiber: 2.0 g
Sodium: 9 mg
Exchanges: 1 vegetable
    1 fat

Variation
Per serving
Calories: 107
Carbohydrate: 6 g
Protein: 8 g
Fat: 5 g
Saturated fat: 1 g
Cholesterol: 3 mg
Dietary fiber: 2.0 g
Sodium: 238 mg
Exchanges: 1 lean meat
    1 vegetable
    1 fat

2   heads Bibb or Boston lettuce, leaves separated, well washed and dried

10   sprigs arugula or watercress, tough stalks removed, well washed and dried

1   medium sweet red onion, peeled and thinly sliced, separated into rings

1   small sweet red pepper, seeded and cut into ¼-inch slivers

4   fresh mushrooms, washed, dried, trimmed, and thinly sliced

1   ounce alfalfa sprouts (about ½ cup)

  All-Purpose Salad Dressing (page 74)

4   large radishes, well washed, trimmed, cut into rosettes for garnish

1. Cut away any tough centers of lettuce leaves. Break (do not cut) into bite-size pieces. Place in large salad bowl. Add next 5 ingredients and toss gently.

2. Add only enough salad dressing to moisten salad, allowing up to 1½ tablespoons per serving. Toss to coat.

3. Arrange in individual salad plates, garnished with one radish rosette in center.

VARIATION: Serve as a tempting luncheon salad course. Add ¼ cup low-fat cottage cheese (no salt added) or part-skim ricotta cheese to each salad plate before garnishing with radishes.

*P*retty Mixed Salad

~

YIELD: SERVES 4

Per serving
Calories: 134
Carbohydrate: 11 g
Protein: 3 g
Fat: 8 g
Saturated fat: 2 g
Cholesterol: 3 mg
Dietary fiber: 2.8 g
Sodium: 93 mg
Exchanges: 2 vegetable
1½ fat

6   small scallions, trimmed, cut diagonally into ½-inch slices

4   egg tomatoes, cut into ½-inch chunks

1   rib celery, diced

1   small sweet red pepper, seeded, cut into ¼-inch slivers

3   tablespoons peeled, coarsely grated carrot

½   crisp sweet apple, peeled, cored, and diced

2   large fresh mushrooms, washed, dried, trimmed, and thinly sliced

5   tablespoons All-Purpose Salad Dressing (page 74)

1   tablespoon fresh lemon juice

3   tablespoons coarsely grated part-skim mozzarella cheese

2   tablespoons minced fresh basil

1. Combine first 7 ingredients in bowl, stirring to blend.

2. Add salad dressing and lemon juice, tossing to blend. Let stand for 15 minutes at room temperature, stirring once.

3. Sprinkle with mozzarella cheese and fresh basil. Toss lightly. Serve immediately.

NOTE: Fresh herbs taste best in this salad. If fresh basil isn't available, substitute minced fresh tarragon, dill, or mint.

Fennel Coleslaw

~

YIELD: SERVES 10

1 small head green cabbage (1 pound), shredded or thinly sliced

1 medium carrot, peeled and grated

1 medium onion, grated

1 large sweet red or green pepper (¼ pound), seeded and minced

2 tablespoons minced fresh parsley

1 tablespoon each fresh lemon juice and apple cider vinegar

2 teaspoons prepared Dijon mustard

½ teaspoon each ground coriander and cinnamon

3 tablespoons apple juice (no sugar added)

½ teaspoon fennel seed, well crushed

⅛ teaspoon ground red (cayenne) pepper

⅔ cup buttermilk (preferably without added salt)

1. In large bowl, combine first 5 ingredients. Toss to blend. Add lemon juice, vinegar, and mustard. Stir.

2. In a cup, combine spices with apple juice. Beat with fork to blend. Stir into cabbage mixture.

3. Add fennel, ground red pepper, and buttermilk. Blend. Place in covered container and refrigerate for several hours before serving, stirring from time to time.

Per serving
Calories: 27
Carbohydrate: 5 g
Protein: 1 g
Fat: trace
Saturated fat: trace
Cholesterol: 1 mg
Dietary fiber: 1.3 g
Sodium: 19 mg
Exchanges: 1 vegetable

Watercress and Endive Salad

~

YIELD: SERVES 4

1 bunch crisp fresh watercress, tough ends removed, well washed and dried

2 medium Belgian endives, washed, dried, and thinly sliced

1 small sweet red pepper, seeded and cut into ¼-inch slivers

All-Purpose Salad Dressing (page 74)

1 tablespoon each minced fresh dill or rosemary, and minced chives

1. Place first 3 ingredients in salad bowl, tossing to combine.

2. Add salad dressing, allowing up to 1½ tablespoons per serving. Sprinkle with dill and chives; serve.

Per serving
Calories: 101
Carbohydrate: 3 g
Protein: 1 g
Fat: 10 g
Saturated fat: 1 g
Cholesterol: trace
Dietary fiber: 1.5 g
Sodium: 13 mg
Exchanges: 1 vegetable
2 fat

Eggplant and Bean Salad

~

YIELD: SERVES 6

Per serving
Calories: 111
Carbohydrate: 14 g
Protein: 3 g
Fat: 4 g
Saturated fat: 1 g
Cholesterol: 0 mg
Dietary fiber: 3.6 g
Sodium: 5 mg
Exchanges: ½ starch/bread
1 vegetable
1 fat

½ cup washed dried red beans

2 cups water

1 pound eggplant

¼ cup minced onion or green onions

⅓ cup sweet red pepper (¼-inch slivers)

1 large tomato, cored, seeded, and coarsely chopped

2 tablespoons each wine vinegar and apple cider vinegar

2 tablespoons Italian olive oil

½ teaspoon each curry powder and ground cumin seed

⅛ teaspoon ground red (cayenne) pepper

½ teaspoon dried mint leaves, crumbled

¼ cup minced fresh basil leaves

1 tablespoon minced fresh parsley

1. Combine beans and water in waterless cooker or stainless steel pot. Cover and bring to boil. Cook for 10 minutes. Remove from heat and let stand, covered, for 2 hours. Then bring to boil again. Slow-boil until tender (40 to 45 minutes). Drain.

2. Prick eggplant all around with sharp-pronged fork. Place on baking sheet and bake in preheated 400°F oven for 45 minutes. Let cool. Peel off skin (it will come off easily), and cut eggplant into ½-inch cubes.

3. In a large bowl, combine beans, eggplant, onion, sweet red pepper, and tomato. Toss gently.

4. Combine vinegars, oil, curry powder, cumin, and dried mint leaves in jar, shaking to blend. Pour over salad and stir briefly until mixture is coated.

5. Fold in basil and parsley. Serve warm or at room temperature.

Endive and Mushroom Salad with Minty Dressing

YIELD: SERVES 4

Per serving
Calories: 124
Carbohydrate: 7 g
Protein: 1 g
Fat: 10 g
Saturated fat: 1 g
Cholesterol: 0 mg
Dietary fiber: 2.1 g
Sodium: 14 mg
Exchanges: 1 vegetable
2 fat

FOR THE DRESSING:

1   tablespoon minced fresh mint

2   tablespoons minced fresh dill

2   shallots, minced

2   tablespoons wine vinegar

2   tablespoons Italian olive oil

1   tablespoon each fresh lemon juice and apple juice (no sugar added)

¼   teaspoon dry mustard

FOR THE SALAD:

2   large crisp Belgian endives (½ pound), washed, dried, and thinly sliced

¼   pound large fresh snow-white mushrooms, washed, dried, trimmed, and thinly sliced

1   medium carrot, peeled, then pared into pieces with swivel-bladed paring utensil

1. Prepare salad dressing first. Combine all ingredients in jar and shake well to blend. Let stand for 30 minutes at room temperature before using.

2. Combine endives, mushrooms, and carrot in bowl. Pour salad dressing over them a little at a time while stirring to blend. Serve immediately for the freshest taste and crunchiest texture.

Mixed Salad with Sprouts

~

YIELD: SERVES 4

2   bunches scallions (about 12), trimmed, cut diagonally into ½-inch slices

¼   pound firm fresh snow-white mushrooms, washed, dried, trimmed, and thinly sliced

2   ounces alfalfa sprouts (about 1 cup)

⅓   cup All-Purpose Salad Dressing (page 74)

½   teaspoon chili con carne seasoning

6   dashes ground red (cayenne) pepper

½   teaspoon each dried tarragon and chervil leaves, crumbled

2   tablespoons minced parsley

1. Prepare salad just before serving. Place scallions and mushrooms in a salad bowl. Pull alfalfa sprouts apart (they tend to absorb too much oil when tightly packed), and add to bowl.

2. In a jar, combine salad dressing with chili con carne seasoning, ground red pepper, and dried herbs. Shake well to blend. Let stand for a minute, then shake again. Pour half of mixture over salad while tossing with fork. Pour balance of mixture over salad slowly, adding only enough to coat lightly. Serve immediately.

Per serving
Calories: 128
Carbohydrate: 11 g
Protein: 2 g
Fat: 8 g
Saturated fat: 1 g
Cholesterol: trace
Dietary fiber: 2.2 g
Sodium: 10 mg
Exchanges: 2 vegetable
                1½ fat

Crisp Spinach Salad

~

YIELD: SERVES 5

1¼ pounds fresh spinach, tough ends removed, well washed

1   large sweet red onion, peeled, cut into ¼-inch slices

1   large navel orange, peeled, cut into ½-inch cubes

⅓   cup All-Purpose Salad Dressing (page 74)

½   teaspoon chili con carne seasoning

⅓   cup toasted bread croutons made from any of my breads (pages 218–235)

¼   cup coarsely grated part-skim mozzarella cheese

1. Dry spinach flat on paper toweling. Do not wring. Tear into bite-size pieces. Place in salad bowl with onion and orange. Gently toss.

2. In a jar, combine salad dressing with chili con carne seasoning, shaking to blend. Pour ⅓ cup over salad while tossing with fork, using only enough to lightly coat mixture.

3. Stir croutons into salad. Add balance of dressing, if necessary, to coat.

4. Serve in individual salad bowls, sprinkled with mozzarella cheese.

NOTE: Good-quality commercial bread may be used, bearing in mind that the nutritional statistics are likely to be less desirable.

Per serving
Calories: 149
Carbohydrate: 9 g
Protein: 5 g
Fat: 9 g
Saturated fat: 2 g
Cholesterol: 5 mg
Dietary fiber: 4.8 g
Sodium: 132 mg
Exchanges: ½ starch/bread
                1 vegetable
                2 fat

Marinated Chicken Salad

YIELD: SERVES 6

Per serving
Calories: 179
Carbohydrate: 5 g
Protein: 20 g
Fat: 8 g
Saturated fat: 1 g
Cholesterol: 48 mg
Dietary fiber: 2.3 g
Sodium: 47 mg
Exchanges: 2½ lean meat
1 vegetable

FOR THE MARINADE:

⅓ cup wine vinegar

2 tablespoons Italian olive oil

¼ cup tomato juice (no salt added)

½ teaspoon each ground cumin seed, mild curry powder, dry mustard and smoked yeast (see page 297)

6 dashes ground red (cayenne) pepper

½ teaspoon Worcestershire sauce

1 teaspoon minced dried onion

FOR THE SALAD:

3 cups chilled cooked skinned chicken, cut into ½-inch cubes

¼ pound fresh snow peas, washed, stems and strings removed

1 small sweet red pepper, seeded and cut into ¼-inch slivers

1 medium zucchini, well scrubbed, cut into ½-inch cubes

¼ pound fresh snow-white mushrooms, washed, dried, trimmed, and cut into ¼-inch slices

2 large shallots, minced

2 tablespoons minced fresh parsley or fresh coriander

2 tablespoons blanched slivered almonds

8 cherry tomatoes

1. Prepare marinade first. Combine all ingredients in a jar, shaking well to blend. Let stand for 15 minutes, shaking from time to time.

2. Combine all salad ingredients except almonds and tomatoes in salad bowl. Toss gently to combine. Pour marinade over salad, stirring to coat. Cover and refrigerate for at least 2 hours, stirring from time to time.

3. Remove from refrigerator. Toss gently. Sprinkle almonds across mixture. Garnish with cherry tomatoes and serve.

VARIATION: Stir in 2 tablespoons low-fat plain yogurt to mixture at beginning of step 3.

Tasty Tuna Salad

~

YIELD: SERVES 4

Per serving
Calories: 97
Carbohydrate: 4 g
Protein: 11 g
Fat: 4 g
Saturated fat: 1 g
Cholesterol: 13 mg
Dietary fiber: 1.3 g
Sodium: 104 mg
Exchanges: 1½ lean meat
           1 vegetable

1   6½-ounce can tuna packed in water (no salt added)

1   tablespoon fresh lemon juice

1   hard-cooked egg white, chopped

1   rib celery, minced

2   tablespoons minced sweet red pepper

1   medium onion, minced

1   tablespoon coarsely grated carrot

1   teaspoon minced fresh mint or ½ teaspoon dried mint, crumbled

1   tablespoon finely minced fresh dill

¼   teaspoon ground cumin seed

5   dashes ground red (cayenne) pepper, or to taste

2   tablespoons Mayonnaise-Type Salad Dressing (page 75)

⅓   cup cooked fresh peas

1. Drain tuna. Place in bowl. Sprinkle with lemon juice. Mash.

2. Stir in next 7 ingredients.

3. Blend cumin and ground red pepper with mayonnaise dressing. Stir into mixture. Carefully fold in peas. Serve chilled.

SERVING SUGGESTION: Delicious spooned into crisp lettuce cups and garnished with radishes and sliced cucumbers.

VARIATION: Blanched snow peas, cut crosswise into ⅜-inch strips, may be substituted for fresh peas.

Mix-and-Match Vegetable Salad

~

YIELD: SERVES 4

Per serving
Calories: 88
Carbohydrate: 14 g
Protein: 2 g
Fat: 3 g
Saturated fat: 1 g
Cholesterol: 1 mg
Dietary fiber: 1.3 g
Sodium: 20 mg
Exchanges: ½ starch/bread
1 vegetable
½ fat

½ cup cooked sliced carrots

¾ cup cooked brown rice

¾ cup cooked broccoli florets

2 scallions, trimmed, cut diagonally into 1-inch slices

2 tablespoons any minced fresh green herb (such as tarragon, rosemary, dill, or basil), or to taste

½ teaspoon ground coriander

4 dashes ground red (cayenne) pepper, or to taste

1 teaspoon wine vinegar

2 teaspoons Italian olive oil

¼ cup low-fat plain yogurt

1. Have vegetables at room temperature or chilled. Place first 7 ingredients in large bowl. Toss gently to combine.

2. Combine vinegar and oil in a cup and whisk to blend. Dribble over mixture, then blend gently.

3. Fold in yogurt. Serve immediately or refrigerate until ready to serve.

Salad Dressings

Real Tomato Mayonnaise
~

YIELD: 1¼ CUPS

1	egg yolk (see Note)
1	teaspoon prepared Dijon mustard
1	scant cup Italian olive oil
1	tablespoon fresh lemon juice
1	teaspoon apple cider vinegar
3	dashes ground red (cayenne) pepper
½	teaspoon dried tarragon or basil, crumbled
¼	cup tomato juice (no salt added)

1. Combine egg with mustard and 1 tablespoon oil in food blender. Blend on high speed until smooth. Add lemon juice, vinegar, and ground red pepper. Blend for 30 seconds.

2. With machine running, add balance of oil by dribbling it in ever so slowly until it's all absorbed and mayonnaise is thick.

3. With machine still running, sprinkle with tarragon or basil, and very slowly add tomato juice.

4. Pour into jar and refrigerate. Mayonnaise will thicken to spreadable consistency when well chilled.

NOTE: I recommend using organic eggs in making mayonnaise.

Per teaspoon
Calories: 30
Carbohydrate: trace
Protein: trace
Fat: 3 g
Saturated fat: 1 g
Cholesterol: 5 mg
Dietary fiber: 0 g
Sodium: trace
Exchanges: ½ fat

All-Purpose Salad Dressing

YIELD: ABOUT ⅔ CUP

Per tablespoon
Calories: 58
Carbohydrate: 0 g
Protein: 0 g
Fat: 6 g
Saturated fat: 1 g
Cholesterol: trace
Dietary fiber: 0 g
Sodium: 1 mg
Exchanges: 1 fat

⅓ cup Italian olive oil

2 tablespoons wine vinegar

1 tablespoon apple cider vinegar

2 tablespoons Easy Chicken Stock (page 216)

6 dashes ground red (cayenne) pepper

¼ teaspoon dry mustard

1 teaspoon minced dried onion

1 teaspoon dried fine herbs (see Note 2 below)

1. Place all ingredients in jar, shaking well to blend. Let stand for at least 1 hour before serving. Shake again before using.

NOTES:

1. This dressing will stay fresh for 2 or 3 days in tightly closed jar, well refrigerated.

2. Fine herbs are a prepared mixture of thyme, oregano, rosemary, marjoram, and basil. It's available in spice racks of supermarkets.

VARIATION: Add ½ teaspoon chile con carne seasoning to mixture, increase dry mustard measurement to ½ teaspoon, and substitute ½ teaspoon ground marjoram for fine herbs.

Mayonnaise-Type Salad Dressing

YIELD: 1½ CUPS

Per tablespoon
Calories: 44
Carbohydrate: trace
Protein: trace
Fat: 5 g
Saturated fat: 1 g
Cholesterol: 11 mg
Dietary fiber: 0 g
Sodium: 2 mg
Exchanges: 1 fat

¼ cup each Thirty-Minute Chicken Broth (page 215) or Easy Chicken Stock (page 216) and tomato juice (no salt added)

1 tablespoon arrowroot flour

1 egg yolk (see Note, page 73)

1 teaspoon prepared Dijon mustard (no salt added)

½ cup Italian olive oil or canola oil

1 tablespoon fresh lemon juice

1 teaspoon apple cider vinegar

4 dashes ground red (cayenne) pepper

½ teaspoon dried tarragon or basil leaves, crumbled

1. Combine stock and tomato juice in saucepan. Heat until warm. Whisk in arrowroot flour until well blended and dissolved. Let cool.

2. Combine egg with mustard and 1 tablespoon oil in food blender. Blend on high speed until smooth. Add lemon juice, vinegar, and ground red pepper. Blend for 30 seconds.

3. With machine running, dribble in balance of oil very slowly until well absorbed (mayonnaise will thicken). Then sprinkle with tarragon or basil. Slowly pour in cooled broth mixture.

4. Pour into jar and refrigerate for 4 to 5 hours. Mayonnaise will thicken to consistency of thick sour cream after well chilled.

Soups

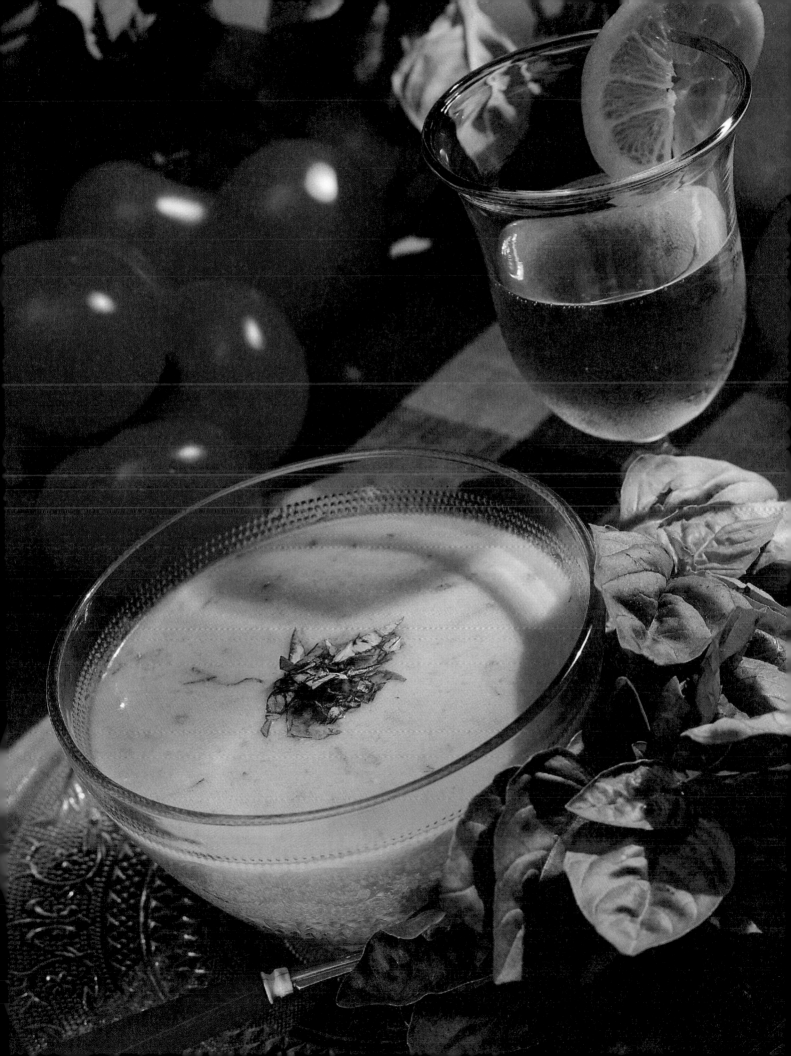

Cucumber-Tomato Soup
~

YIELD: SERVES 4

One of my favorite food games is "What's that taste?" It's easy to play; you simply ask your guests to identify the ingredients of a dish. Play the game with this dish, and you'll baffle even the most discerning gourmets. And that proves once again that in great cooking the whole is tastier than its parts.

Per serving (about 1 cup)
Calories: 90
Carbohydrate: 11 g
Protein: 3 g
Fat: 4 g
Saturated fat: 1 g
Cholesterol: 5 mg
Dietary fiber: 2.5 g
Sodium: 88 mg
Exchanges: 2 vegetable
             1 fat

2   large shallots, minced
2   large cloves garlic, minced
1   large onion, minced
2   large scallions, minced
2   teaspoons Italian olive oil
1   tablespoon wine vinegar
2   medium cucumbers, peeled, seeded, and coarsely chopped (3 cups)
2   medium tomatoes, peeled, cored, seeded, and coarsely chopped
⅓   cup loosely packed, coarsely chopped fresh basil leaves, or 2 teaspoons oregano, crushed

½   teaspoon dried savory leaves, crushed
6   dashes ground red (cayenne) pepper
3   sprigs fresh parsley
2½ cups Easy Chicken Stock (page 216)
⅓   cup apple juice (no sugar added)
1   tablespoon regular Cream of Wheat

1. Combine first 4 ingredients in measuring cup. These should equal 1 cup minced ingredients. If not, add more shallots or onions to fill out the cup.

2. Heat oil in waterless cooker or stainless steel pot until moderately hot. Add minced ingredients and cook until onion is translucent (about 3 minutes).

3. Add vinegar. Cook for 30 seconds. Add cucumbers and balance of ingredients except Cream of Wheat. Bring to simmering point.

Sprinkle with Cream of Wheat. Stir to blend. Cover partially and simmer for 25 minutes, stirring from time to time.

4. Pour into food mill and puree. Most of solids will strain through. Discard balance of solids that don't puree. Reheat and serve.

VARIATION: Chill soup. Whisk in 3 tablespoons low-fat plain yogurt just before serving. Serves 5.

*L*entil Soup: It's a One-Bowl Meal

YIELD: SERVES 8

*L*entils are one of the tastiest and most nutritious of all legumes. In this elegant and delectable thick soup, I've combined tender morsels of chicken and beef with a mélange of vegetables and herbs. It's original, exciting, and irresistible.

Per serving (about 1 cup)
Calories: 165
Carbohydrate: 18 g
Protein: 14 g
Fat: 3 g
Saturated fat: 1 g
Cholesterol: 26 mg
Dietary fiber: 3.4 g
Sodium: 36 mg
Exchanges: 1 starch/bread
              1 lean meat
              1 vegetable

1   cup lentils

2   teaspoons Italian olive oil

¼   pound lean beef such as top round, well trimmed, cut into ¼-inch cubes

1   small chicken leg and thigh (about ½ pound), skinned and disjointed

1   whole leek, well washed, minced

4   large cloves garlic, minced

¼   pound fresh mushrooms, well washed, dried, trimmed, and coarsely chopped

1   tablespoon wine vinegar

1   small carrot, diced

½   cup loosely packed minced fresh basil leaves, or 2 teaspoons crumbled dried basil leaves

1   cup canned Italian plum tomatoes (no salt added), chopped

½   teaspoon ground ginger

1   teaspoon ground marjoram

⅛   teaspoon crushed red (cayenne) pepper

¼   cup dry vermouth

5   cups water

1. Rinse, then soak lentils in water to cover for 1 hour. Repeat procedure. Then soak in water to cover overnight.

2. Heat oil in large stainless steel pot or waterless cooker. Add meat and chicken and sauté for 3 minutes, stirring and turning so that ingredients don't stick. Add leek, garlic, and mushrooms. Sauté and stir over medium-high heat until wilted but not brown.

3. Add vinegar. Stir and cook for 1 minute. Add balance of ingredients, including drained and rinsed lentils. Stir well to blend. Bring to simmering point. Cover and simmer for 1½ hours, removing scum that rises to top during first 10 minutes. Stir ingredients from time to time to prevent sticking. Remove from heat and let stand for 15 minutes.

4. Remove chicken from bones. Cut into bite-size pieces. Reheat if necessary, and serve.

NOTES:
1. Flavor of soup is improved if refrigerated and served the next day.

2. Soup freezes very well if packaged in airtight containers or heat-sealed plastic bags.

Shrimp Gumbo

YIELD: SERVES 4

Okra has become one of my favorite foods since I learned how to rid it of its mucilagelike texture. My secret: For fresh okra, sprinkle with vinegar and let stand for 30 minutes; for frozen okra, cook briefly in vinegar and water before using. These techniques are put to use with striking effectiveness in the following three recipes. The first is an original gumbo enhanced by pearl-size pieces of succulent shrimp; the second is a light version of traditional Chicken Gumbo that you'll find as appealing as it is economical; and the third is an elegantly delectable Tomato-Okra Soup.

Per serving (about 1 cup)
Calories: 210
Carbohydrate: 23 g
Protein: 16 g
Fat: 6 g
Saturated fat: 1 g
Cholesterol: 91 mg
Dietary fiber: 3.9 g
Sodium: 157 mg
Exchanges: 1 starch/bread
      1 lean meat
      2 vegetable
      ½ fat

½   **pound fresh okra, ends trimmed (see Note)**

2   **tablespoons white vinegar**

3   **teaspoons Italian olive oil**

1   **medium sweet green pepper, minced**

1   **medium leek, well washed, tough pieces discarded, and minced**

3   **cloves garlic, minced**

¼   **cup raw brown rice**

1   **cup canned Italian plum tomatoes (no salt added)**

2   **cups Easy Chicken Stock (page 216)**

4   **dashes ground red (cayenne) pepper**

½   **teaspoon curry powder**

½   **teaspoon each thyme and rosemary leaves, crushed**

   Bouquet garni (1 sprig parsley, 1 bay leaf, tied together with white thread)

2   **large shallots, minced**

½   **pound fresh unshelled shrimp (shell, devein, and coarsely chop)**

1. Wash okra under cold running water. Place in bowl. Sprinkle with vinegar, turning to coat. Let stand for 30 minutes. Rinse under cold running water. Drain and slice. Place in waterless cooker or stainless steel pot. Set aside.

2. Heat 2 teaspoons oil in nonstick skillet until hot. Sauté green pepper, leek, and garlic until just wilted (don't brown). Add rice, stirring to coat. Cook for 1 minute.

3. Pour mixture into waterless cooker with okra. Add tomatoes, stock, ground red pepper, curry, herbs, and bouquet garni. Bring to simmering point. Cover and simmer gumbo for 20 minutes.

4. Five minutes before gumbo is finished cooking, wipe out skillet. Heat balance of oil (1 teaspoon) until hot. Spread minced shallots across skillet. Sauté for 1 minute. Sprinkle chopped shrimp on top of shallots. Sauté, turning often, until just delicately pink. Remove from heat.

5. Add shrimp to gumbo. Bring to simmering point. Simmer uncovered for 1 minute. Remove bouquet garni, pressing out juices. Serve immediately.

NOTE: If fresh okra isn't available, you may substitute a 10-ounce box of frozen okra. Replace step 1 with the following step: Place okra, 1 cup water, and ¼ cup white vinegar in small saucepan. Bring to boil. Reduce heat to slow boil. Cook uncovered for 3 minutes. Drain and slice.

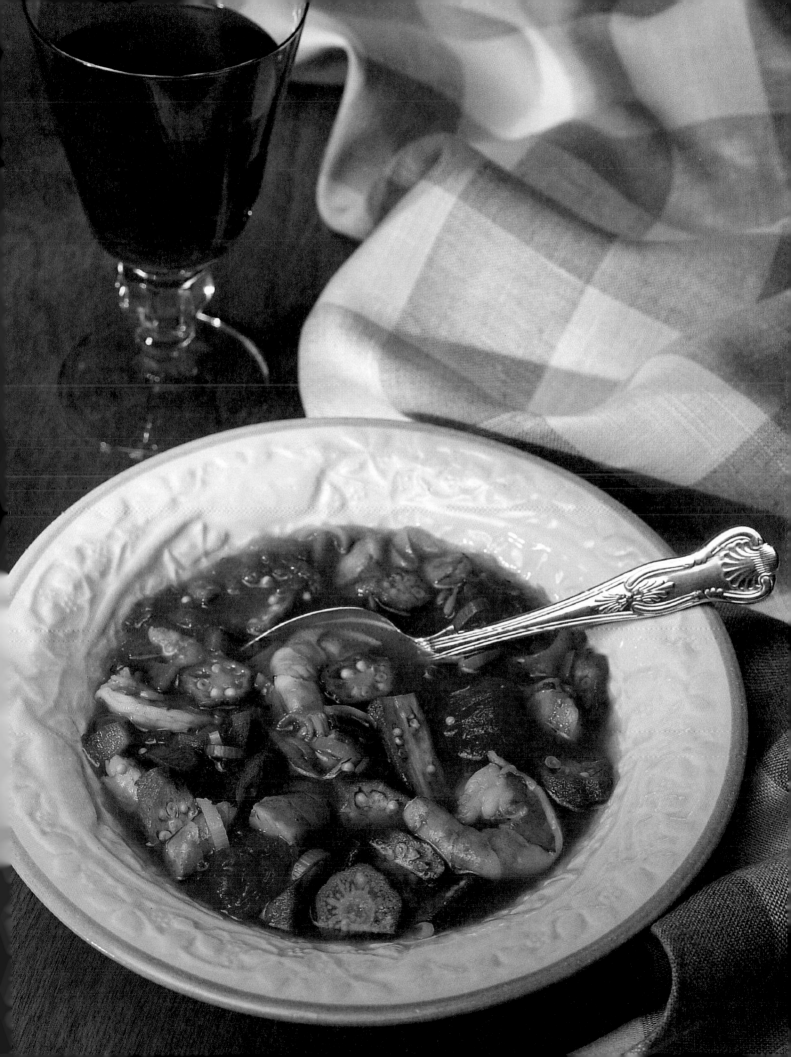

Chicken Gumbo
~

YIELD: SERVES 6

Per serving (about 1 cup)
Calories: 183
Carbohydrate: 13 g
Protein: 19 g
Fat: 6 g
Saturated fat: 1 g
Cholesterol: 51 mg
Dietary fiber: 3.1 g
Sodium: 59 mg
Exchanges: ½ starch/bread
1 lean meat
½ vegetable

½ pound fresh okra, ends trimmed

2 tablespoons white vinegar

1 small broiling chicken (2½ pounds), skinned, cut into eighths

2 cups water

1 medium onion, minced

1 small carrot, peeled and diced

½ teaspoon dried thyme leaves, crushed

Bouquet garni (1 sprig parsley, 1 bay leaf, tied together with white thread)

2 teaspoons Italian olive oil

1 medium sweet green pepper, seeded and coarsely chopped

2 large cloves garlic, minced

1 leek, white part only, well washed and sliced

¼ cup raw brown rice

2 cups canned Italian plum tomatoes (no salt added)

1 cup tomato juice (no salt added)

6 dashes ground red (cayenne) pepper

½ teaspoon chili con carne seasoning

1. Follow directions for preparing okra in step 1 of Shrimp Gumbo (preceding recipe). Set aside.

2. Place chicken and water in kettle or waterless cooker. Bring to boil. Reduce to simmering. Cool, uncovered, 2 minutes, removing scum that rises to top. Add onion, carrot, thyme, and bouquet garni. Cover and simmer for 40 minutes, shifting chicken pieces from time to time so that they cook evenly. Remove chicken from pot. Cut into bite-size pieces. Return to pot.

3. Heat oil in nonstick skillet until hot. Sauté green pepper, garlic, and leek until wilted but not brown, stirring often. Add rice and sauté for 1 minute. Pour into waterless cooker with chicken.

4. Add tomatoes, tomato juice, okra, and seasonings. Bring to simmering point. Cover and simmer for 20 minutes. Turn off heat. Let stand for 10 minutes. Remove bouquet garni, pressing out juices, and serve.

Tomato-Okra Soup

YIELD: SERVES 4

Per serving (about 1 cup)
Calories: 110
Carbohydrate: 16 g
Protein: 3 g
Fat: 3 g
Saturated fat: 1 g
Cholesterol: 4 mg
Dietary fiber: 3.9 g
Sodium: 67 mg
Exchanges: ½ starch/bread
2 vegetable
½ fat

1	10-ounce box frozen whole okra
1	tablespoon white vinegar
2	teaspoons Italian olive oil
3	large cloves garlic, minced
2	teaspoons peeled and shredded fresh ginger
1	medium onion, minced
2	tablespoons minced sweet green pepper
1	tablespoon wine vinegar
2	cups Easy Chicken Stock (page 216)
½	cup apple juice (no sugar added)
1	cup canned Italian plum tomatoes (no salt added), chopped
1	tablespoon tomato paste (no salt added)
½	teaspoon each dried rosemary and thyme leaves and fennel seed, crushed
⅛	teaspoon ground red (cayenne) pepper
2	tablespoons barley
	Bouquet garni (1 sprig parsley, 1 bay leaf, tied together with white thread)

1. Bring saucepan of water to rolling boil. Add okra and white vinegar. Boil for 2 minutes. Drain. Cut into ½-inch slices. Set aside.

2. Heat oil in waterless cooker or stainless steel pot. Sauté garlic, ginger, onion, and green pepper over medium-high heat until lightly browned.

3. Add wine vinegar and cook for 30 seconds. Add balance of ingredients. Bring to simmering point. Partially cover and simmer for 1 hour, stirring from time to time. Turn heat off. Let stand, covered, for 15 minutes. Remove bouquet garni, pressing out juices. Reheat, if necessary, and serve.

Thick Vegetarian Chick-Pea Soup

~

YIELD: SERVES 8

Vegetarians: You'll marvel at the delicate flavor and chewy texture of this glorious soup. But meat lovers, don't pass it over. You'll never believe there's no meat here.

Per serving (about 1 cup)
Calories: 127
Carbohydrate: 20 g
Protein: 5 g
Fat: 3 g
Saturated fat: trace
Cholesterol: 0 mg
Dietary fiber: 4.3 g
Sodium: 19 mg
Exchanges: 1 starch/bread
          1 vegetable
          ½ fat

½ cup each dried chick-peas and lentils

1 quart water

1 tablespoon Italian olive oil

2 medium onions, minced

4 large cloves garlic, minced

1 rib celery, diced

4 large fresh mushrooms, washed, dried, trimmed, and coarsely chopped

1 cup peeled and diced eggplant (½-inch cubes)

1 teaspoon each ground cumin seed and dried thyme leaves, crushed

1 tablespoon mild curry powder

4 dashes ground red (cayenne) pepper

1 cup canned Italian plum tomatoes (no salt added), chopped

1 tablespoon wine vinegar

1 tablespoon tomato paste (no salt added)

2½ cups water

1½ cups tomato juice (no salt added)

¼ cup just-snipped fresh dill

1. Rinse chick-peas and lentils. Place in saucepan with 1 quart water. Bring to boil. Slow-boil, partially covered, for 15 minutes. Remove from heat and let stand for 2 hours. Drain. Rinse under cold running water. Transfer to stainless steel pot or waterless cooker.

2. Heat oil in well-seasoned iron skillet until hot. Sauté onions, garlic, celery, and mushrooms over medium-high heat for 3 minutes, stirring often. Add eggplant. Sprinkle with cumin, thyme, curry, and ground red pepper. Stir and continue sautéing until ingredients are lightly browned.

3. Add tomatoes and vinegar. Bring to a simmering point. Cook for 1 minute. Combine with chick-peas and lentils.

4. Add water, tomato juice, and dill. Bring to boil. Reduce heat to sim-

mering. Cover and cook for 1¼ hours, stirring often. Remove from heat. Let stand, covered, for 30 minutes. Reheat, if necessary, and serve.

SUBSTITUTION: One pound fresh ripe Italian plum tomatoes, skinned, cored, seeded, and coarsely chopped, may be substituted for canned tomatoes.

NOTES:
1. Chick-peas and lentils may be soaked in water to cover overnight. Drain next day, and they're ready to use.

2. Entire cooking process may be done in an enameled cast-iron skillet.

SERVING SUGGESTION: Sprinkle each portion with 1 teaspoon freshly grated Parmesan cheese. (This will add about 30 mg of sodium per serving.)

Bean and Vegetable Soup

YIELD: SERVES 6

Leg of lamb is so delicious, but it does contain an inedible bone for which you have to pay. Why not get your money's worth by putting the bone to work? In this recipe, that's just what you do. Add the cooked lamb bone to this slightly sweet amalgam of herbed-and-spiced beans and vegetables, and a rich meatiness permeates the mix—without the cost of extra meat.

½   cup each lentils and Great Northern or baby white beans

2   ribs celery including leaves

1   bay leaf

⅓   cup peeled and diced yellow turnip (rutabaga)

1   small carrot, diced

1   large onion, coarsely chopped

3   large cloves garlic, minced

1   crisp Greening or Washington State apple, peeled, cored, and coarsely chopped

2   teaspoons each apple cider vinegar and wine vinegar

1   cup each Easy Chicken Stock (page 216) and apple juice (no sugar added)

1   cup canned Italian plum tomatoes (no salt added), chopped

1   cup water

1   cooked leg of lamb bone

½   teaspoon each dried sage and savory leaves, crushed

⅛   teaspoon crushed red (cayenne) pepper

Per serving (about 1 cup)
Calories: 146
Carbohydrate: 28 g
Protein: 7 g
Fat: 1 g
Saturated fat: trace
Cholesterol: 1 mg
Dietary fiber: 5.6 g
Sodium: 62 mg
Exchanges: 1½ starch/bread
            1 vegetable

1. Rinse, then soak lentils and beans in water to cover for 1 hour. Repeat procedure. Then soak in water to cover overnight. Rinse and drain. Transfer to kettle or waterless cooker.

2. Make a bouquet garni by breaking off celery leaves and wrapping around bay leaf. Tie with white thread into neat bundle. Add to pot. Coarsely chop celery.

3. Add balance of ingredients. Bring to boil. Reduce to simmering. Cover and cook for 1½ hours, stirring from time to time. Remove from heat and let stand, covered, for 10 minutes.

4. Discard bouquet garni, pressing out juices. Cut any meat from bone into bite-size pieces and add

to soup. Reheat, if necessary, and serve.

SUGGESTION FOR QUICK PREPARATION: Minced ingredients can be jiffy-prepared if you use a food processor. Cut turnip and carrots into large chunks. Process on/off twice. Add quartered onion, whole garlic cloves, and quartered apple. Process on/off twice. They are now ready for step 3.

VARIATION: If you prefer to prepare this satisfying soup without a lamb bone, increase stock measurement to 2 cups and eliminate water.

*B*utternut-Brown Bean Soup

~

YIELD: SERVES 6

*T*his lovely-to-look-at, lusty, sharply spiced soup comes to your table with a promise of lasting satisfaction—and fills that promise.

Per serving (about 1 cup)
Calories: 171
Carbohydrate: 30 g
Protein: 8 g
Fat: 2 g
Saturated fat: trace
Cholesterol: 2 mg
Dietary fiber: 4.7 g
Sodium: 47 mg
Exchanges: 2 starch/bread

½   cup each dried lentils and Great Northern or baby white beans

2   teaspoons Italian olive oil

½   medium sweet green pepper, seeded and minced

1   medium onion, minced

2   scallions, minced

1   teaspoon peeled and shredded fresh ginger

3   large cloves garlic, minced

1   small carrot, minced

½   teaspoon dried rosemary leaves, crushed

1   teaspoon dried basil leaves, crushed

1   teaspoon chili con carne seasoning

⅛   teaspoon crushed red (cayenne) pepper

1   tablespoon apple cider vinegar

1   cup apple juice (no sugar added)

1½   cups each Easy Chicken Stock (page 216) or Thirty-Minute Chicken Broth (page 215), and tomato juice (no salt added)

2   cups water

Bouquet garni (1 sprig each parsley and dill, 1 bay leaf, tied together with white thread)

¼   cup bulgur

1. Rinse, then soak lentils and beans in water to cover for 1 hour. Repeat procedure. Then soak in water to cover overnight.

2. Heat oil in heavy-bottom stainless steel pot or waterless cooker until hot. Sauté green pepper, onion, scallions, ginger, garlic, and carrot over medium-high heat until very lightly browned (about 4 minutes). Sprinkle with herbs and seasonings, stirring to blend. Add vinegar. Cook and stir for 30 seconds.

3. Add drained and rinsed lentils and beans, and balance of ingredients, except bulgur. Bring to boiling point. Reduce heat to simmering. Cover and simmer for 1 hour.

4. Stir in bulgur. Reduce to simmering point. Cover and simmer for 20 minutes. Remove from heat and let stand, covered, for 10 minutes.

5. Remove bouquet garni, pressing out juices, and serve.

Three-Way Beet Soup

YIELD: SERVES 6

Enjoy this adventurous dish three ways—as a hot soup; as a hot side dish; and chilled, as a relish— and you'll wonder why beets seem to be banned from gourmet restaurant menus.

Per serving (about 1 cup)
Calories: 138
Carbohydrate: 17 g
Protein: 9 g
Fat: 4 g
Saturated fat: 2 g
Cholesterol: 24 mg
Dietary fiber: 3.5 g
Sodium: 104 mg
Exchanges: ½ starch/bread
　　　　　　1 lean meat
　　　　　　2 vegetable

¼ cup baby white beans

3¾ cups water

½ pound lean stewing veal, cut into ½-inch cubes

2½ cups Easy Chicken Stock (page 216)

1 cup apple juice (no sugar added)

1 tablespoon each apple cider vinegar and fresh lemon juice

4 teaspoons tomato paste (no salt added)

4 beets with tops, beets peeled and cubed, greens washed and chopped

1 medium carrot, peeled and diced

4 cloves garlic, minced

1 small leek, well washed, minced

5 whole cloves, crushed

1 teaspoon ground coriander

¼ teaspoon crushed red (cayenne) pepper

Bouquet garni (1 sprig parsley, 1 bay leaf, tied together with white thread)

Low-fat plain yogurt for garnish

1. Wash beans. Place in small saucepan with 2¼ cups water. Bring to rolling boil. Turn off heat and let stand for 1 hour. Bring to boil again. Cover and simmer for 1 hour, taking care not to scorch beans during last 10 minutes cooking time. Drain any remaining cooking liquid. Set aside.

2. Place veal and balance of water (1½ cups) in kettle or waterless cooker. Bring to boil. Reduce heat. Partially cover and simmer for 20 minutes, removing scum as it rises to top.

3. Add balance of ingredients, except cooked beans and yogurt. Bring to simmering point. Cover and simmer until meat and vegetables are tender (about 45 minutes).

4. Stir in cooked beans. Re-cover and simmer for 5 minutes. Remove bouquet garni, pressing out juices. Serve with yogurt on the side.

NOTES:

1. If beet greens aren't attached to your beets when you buy them, substitute 1 cup coarsely shredded cabbage.

2. This soup is vegetable-thick. Additional stock may be added to thin down to desired consistency. Refer to nutritional statistics for Easy Chicken Stock (page 216) to calculate increase in sodium.

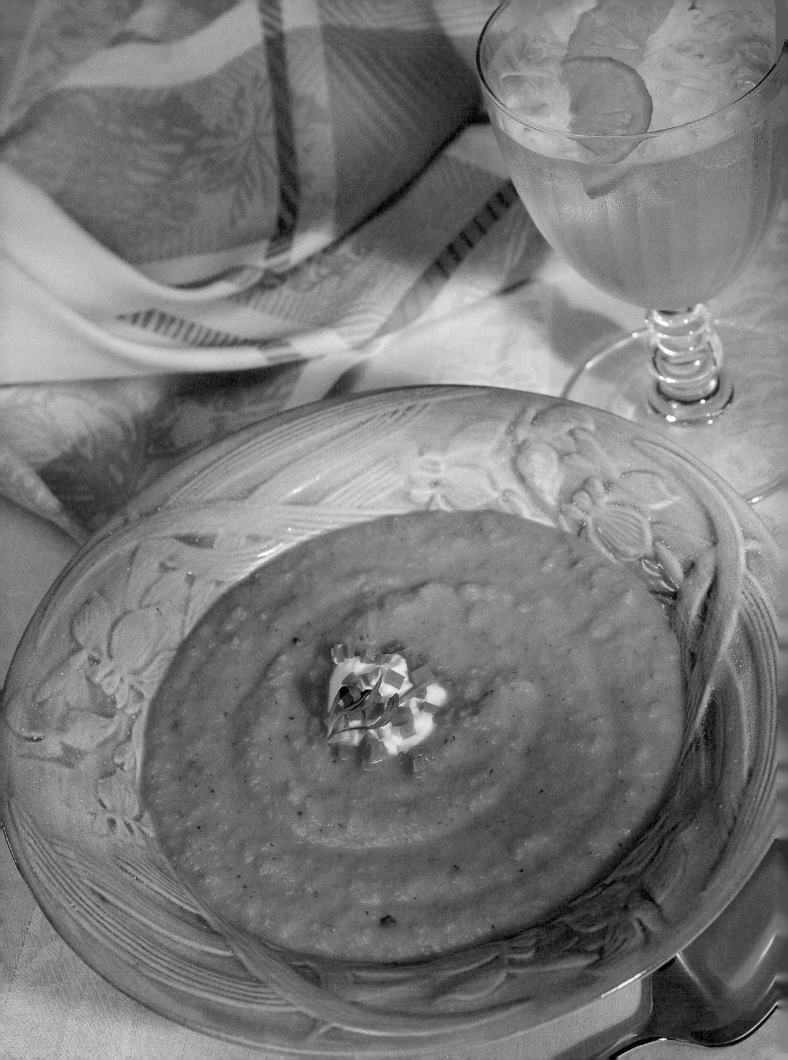

Velvety-Smooth Celery Root Bisque

~

YIELD: SERVES 7

"Never judge a book by its cover," my mother used to say, as she cut up a knobby celery root. Probably the least attractive of all root vegetables, it's often passed over by the shopper who doesn't know that its remarkable taste belies its disagreeable appearance. Combine it with shallots, garlic, sweet carrot juice, stock, and innovative seasonings, and you have a four-star starter for dinner, or a full-bodied, one-bowl course for lunch.

Per serving (about ⅔ cup)
Calories: 104
Carbohydrate: 14 g
Protein: 2 g
Fat: 4 g
Saturated fat: 2 g
Cholesterol: 3 mg
Dietary fiber: 2.3 g
Sodium: 137 mg
Exchanges: ½ starch/bread
   1 vegetable
   1 fat

2 tablespoons fresh lemon juice

1½ pound celeriac (celery knob), ends trimmed, peeled, cut into ½-inch cubes

1 tablespoon Italian olive oil

½ cup coarsely chopped shallots

1 teaspoon minced garlic

2 teaspoons peeled and minced fresh ginger

½ cup coarsely chopped red bell pepper

¼ cup short-grain Italian rice (Arborio), well rinsed and drained

3 cups Easy Chicken Stock (page 216)

1 cup fresh or canned carrot juice

2 teaspoons dried tarragon leaves, crumbled

1½ teaspoons mild curry powder

Florets from 4 large sprigs parsley

¼ cup reduced-fat sour cream

Freshly ground white or black pepper to taste

Minced parsley or shredded carrot for garnish

1. Pour lemon juice into a large bowl. Put celery root pieces into the bowl as they're cut, turning to coat. (This prevents it from blackening.)

2. Heat oil in a heavy-bottom saucepan until hot. Over medium heat, sauté shallots, garlic, ginger, and red pepper until softened without browning. Stir in rice and cook for 1 minute, stirring continually. Then add celery root with any residual lemon juice. Continue stirring and cook for 1 minute.

3. Pour in 2 cups stock, half the carrot juice, tarragon, and curry. Bring to a boil. Reduce heat to simmering. Cover and simmer for 40 minutes, stirring from time to time. Mixture will be thick. Remove from heat. Uncover and let stand for 10 minutes.

4. Transfer to workbowl of food processor that has been fitted with steel blade (or puree in batches in a blender). Add parsley and puree until smooth. Pour back into the saucepan.

5. Whisk in remaining cup of stock, balance of carrot juice (½ cup), sour cream, and pepper. Reheat over lowest temperature, whisking often. Serve at once.

NOTE: Chilled leftovers will be thick. To reheat without scorching, spoon into the top of a double boiler, and cook uncovered over simmering water, stirring often.

Hearty Soup

YIELD: SERVES 6

Replete with peas, lentils, and barley, and heady with flavor, this satisfying soup, enriched with stock and, of all things, apple juice, could be your perfect answer to that wintertime craving for a hot, hearty dish. Bonus: It's better the second day.

Per serving (about 1 cup)
Calories: 120
Carbohydrate: 16 g
Protein: 6 g
Fat: 4 g
Saturated fat: 1 g
Cholesterol: 6 mg
Dietary fiber: 3.0 g
Sodium: 17 mg
Exchanges: 1 starch/bread
          1 fat

With Easy Chicken Stock
Per serving (about 1 cup)
Calories: 135
Carbohydrate: 16 g
Protein: 6 g
Fat: 5 g
Saturated fat: 1 g
Cholesterol: 10 mg
Dietary fiber: 3.0 g
Sodium: 72 mg
Exchanges: 1 starch/bread
          1 fat

¼ cup each dried split peas and lentils

2 tablespoons barley

¾ cup water

1 fresh ham bone (or leg of lamb or veal bone)

Bouquet garni (1 sprig parsley, 1 bay leaf, tied together with white thread)

3 teaspoons Italian olive oil

¼ pound fresh mushrooms, washed, dried, and coarsely chopped

3 large cloves garlic, minced

1 medium onion, minced

½ carrot, peeled and coarsely chopped

⅓ cup peeled and diced yellow turnip (rutabaga)

½ teaspoon each dried rosemary, thyme, and mint leaves, crushed

⅛ teaspoon crushed red (cayenne) pepper

1 tablespoon apple cider vinegar

4½ cups water, or 3 cups water and 1½ cups Easy Chicken Stock (page 216)

½ cup apple juice (no sugar added)

2 tablespoons tomato paste (no salt added)

1. Wash and drain split peas, lentils, and barley. Place in kettle or waterless cooker with water. Let soak for 30 minutes. Most of liquid will be absorbed. Pour into strainer and drain. Rinse under cold running water. Return to kettle. Add bone and bouquet garni.

2. Heat 1½ teaspoons oil in nonstick skillet until hot. Sauté mushrooms for 1½ minutes, stirring often and taking care that they don't brown. Push to side of skillet.

3. Heat balance of oil. Sauté garlic and onion for 1 minute. Add carrot and turnip, stirring and sautéing for 1 minute. Sprinkle with herbs and crushed red pepper.

4. Add balance of ingredients. Bring to simmering point. Pour into kettle with beans and bone. Bring to simmering point again. Cover partially and simmer gently for 1 hour, stirring from time to time.

5. Turn off heat. Let soup stand tightly covered for 10 minutes. Remove bone, cutting off any tidbits of meat and returning to soup. Remove bouquet garni, pressing out juices. Reheat if necessary, and serve.

Diced Chicken in a Pot

~

YIELD: SERVES 6

*P*repare *this chicken-bean soup the night before, then sit down in luxurious leisure to a one-dish meal that makes the word "homespun" synony-mous with "Hurray!"*

Per serving (about 1 cup)
Calories: 167
Carbohydrate: 23 g
Protein: 15 g
Fat: 2 g
Saturated fat: trace
Cholesterol: 22 mg
Dietary fiber: 3.7 g
Sodium: 54 mg
Exchanges: 1 starch/bread
           1 lean meat
           1 vegetable

¾ cup dried lentils

¼ cup split peas

1 small chicken breast (about ½ pound), boned and skinned

3 large cloves garlic, minced

3 shallots, minced, or 1 small sharp onion, minced

½ cup ½-inch diced yellow turnip (rutabaga)

1 tablespoon apple cider vinegar

3 cups water

1½ cups Easy Chicken Stock (page 216)

½ cup apple juice (no sugar added)

1 tablespoon tomato paste (no salt added)

1 teaspoon chili con carne seasoning

1 teaspoon each dried rosemary leaves and cumin seed, crushed

½ teaspoon ground marjoram

Bouquet garni (1 sprig parsley, 1 bay leaf, tied together with white thread)

1. Early in the day, soak lentils in water to cover for 1 hour. Repeat procedure. Then soak in water to cover for at least 5 hours. Drain and rinse. Wash peas. Place lentils and peas in waterless cooker or stainless steel pot.

2. Add balance of ingredients. Bring to boil. Reduce heat to simmering. Cover and simmer for 1½ hours. Remove from heat and let stand for 15 minutes.

3. Cut chicken into bite-size pieces. Return to soup. Stir to distribute evenly. Remove bouquet garni, pressing out juices. Reheat, if necessary, and serve.

*Vegetables,
Grains,
and Pasta*

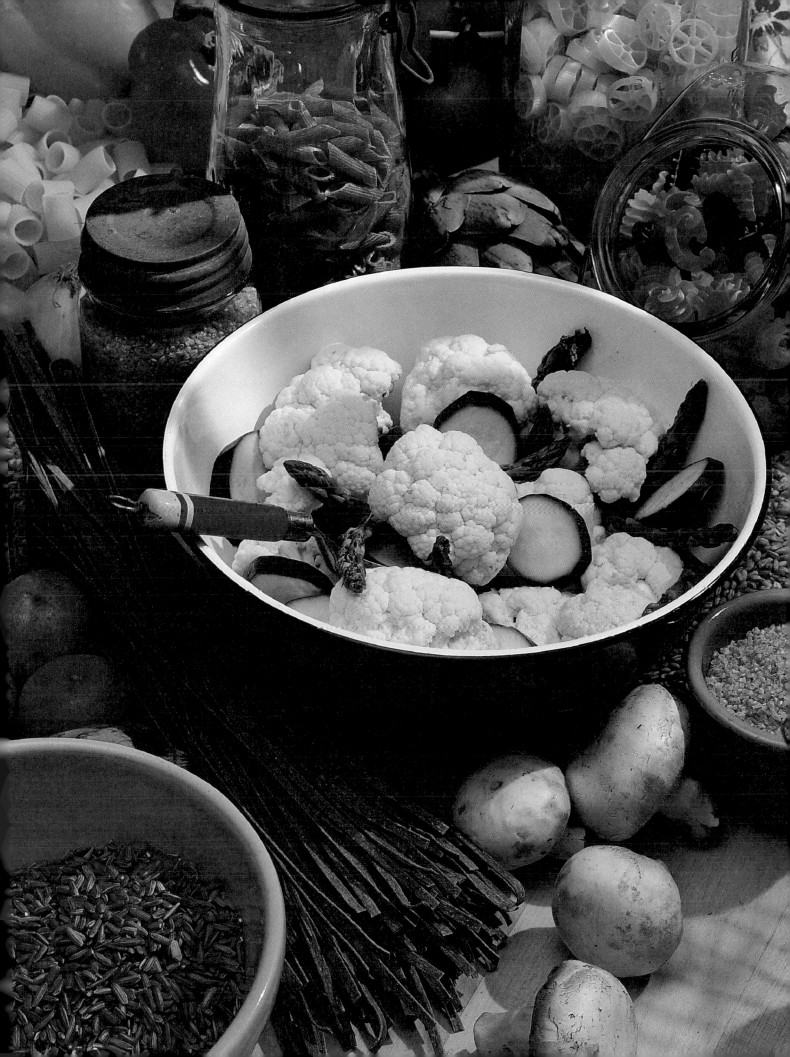

Poached Asparagus with Orange Sauce

~

YIELD: SERVES 4

*I*sn't it nice when other people think the same way as you do? Of course it is. So when I ask, "What's your favorite vegetable?" I'm thrilled when most people answer, "Asparagus." Here it's cooked to crunchy goodness in stock and orange juice concentrate, then topped with toasted pine nuts. As excitingly tasteful as it's innovative.

1½ pounds fresh asparagus, well washed, tough ends removed

¾ cup Thirty-Minute Chicken Broth (page 215)

1 tablespoon orange juice concentrate

3 large shallots, minced

½ teaspoon crushed dried tarragon

1 sprig fresh parsley

2 tablespoons evaporated skim milk

2 tablespoons toasted pine nuts or skinned sliced almonds, chopped (see Note)

1 tablespoon minced fresh coriander or parsley

Per serving
Calories: 86
Carbohydrate: 10 g
Protein: 4 g
Fat: 3 g
Saturated fat: 1 g
Cholesterol: 1 mg
Dietary fiber: 3.3 g
Sodium: 27 mg
Exchanges: 2 vegetable
        ½ fat

1. Place asparagus in wide, heavy-bottom saucepan. Combine and blend broth, orange juice concentrate, shallots, and tarragon. Pour over asparagus. Add parsley sprig. Bring to simmering point. Cover and poach for 7 to 8 minutes, spooning twice with poaching liquid. Cooked asparagus should remain firm. With slotted spatula, transfer to warmed serving plate. Cover to keep warm.

2. Strain poaching liquid, pressing out juices. Pour back into pot. Bring to boil and reduce to ¼ cup. Remove from heat. Stir in milk. Heat briefly to just under simmering point.

3. Pour sauce over asparagus. Sprinkle with nuts and serve immediately.

NOTE: To toast nuts, heat nonstick skillet until hot. Add nuts and toast over medium heat until lightly browned (about 4 minutes), shaking skillet from time to time. Then coarsely chop.

Poached Artichokes

YIELD: SERVES 4

Artichokes have been food lovers' delights ever since the fifteenth century, and in the ensuing years have been prepared in numerous titillating ways. But the way to eat an artichoke has remained unchanged. You pull off the leaves one by one, dip them into the sauce, draw the leaves between your teeth, then remove the fuzzy "choke," and finally uncover the tender heart. It's a ceremony that should be observed without the distractions of accompanying dishes. That's why I serve this magnificent vegetable in solitary splendor as an appetizer. Try it hot, or prepare it a day in advance and serve it cold. Either way, it's an unforgettable adventure in fine eating.

Per serving
Calories: 115
Carbohydrate: 18 g
Protein: 4 g
Fat: 3 g
Saturated fat: 1 g
Cholesterol: 1 mg
Dietary fiber: 5.7 g
Sodium: 93 mg
Exchanges: 2 vegetable
　　　　　 ½ fat

4　small fresh artichokes, trimmed, stems removed

4　teaspoons each minced fresh parsley and mint

2　large cloves garlic, minced

4　large shallots, minced

2　teaspoons Italian olive oil

½　teaspoon dried thyme leaves, crushed

¼　cup each dry vermouth, Easy Chicken Stock (page 216) or Thirty-Minute Chicken Broth (page 215), apple juice (no sugar added), and water

1. Wash and drain artichokes. In a small bowl, combine parsley, mint, garlic, and shallots. Using 1 teaspoon for each artichoke, push mixture down between leaves.

2. Heat oil in small kettle or waterless cooker until hot. Sauté artichokes on all sides for 5 minutes, taking care not to scorch.

3. Sprinkle with thyme. Add liquids. Bring to simmering point. Cover and simmer until tender (about 30 minutes), spooning liquid into artichokes from time to time. Transfer to bowl, pouring any liquid over artichokes (most of liquid will have been absorbed). Serve hot or chilled.

NOTE: Check pot from time to time. If liquid evaporates before artichokes have finished cooking, add small amount of water.

Rich Puree of Broccoli
~

YIELD: SERVES 6

*H*ere's how to get the most taste from a bunch of fresh broccoli: Cut off florets with 1 inch of stalk. Peel skin off 1-inch portion. Then cut thick skin away from remaining stalks. Cut each peeled stalk into ½-inch cubes. Drop cubes into rapidly boiling water and cook for 3 to 4 minutes. Add florets to pot, and cook until they just begin to lose their bright green color (3 to 4 minutes). Quickly drain and rinse under cold running water to stop cooking action. Broccoli can now be set aside and final preparation resumed when you're ready.

Per serving

Calories: 109
Carbohydrate: 10 g
Protein: 8 g
Fat: 4 g
Saturated fat: 2 g
Cholesterol: 62 mg
Dietary fiber: 3.3 g
Sodium: 73 mg
Exchanges: 1 lean meat
        2 vegetable

1   large bunch broccoli (1½ pounds), cooked

3   shallots, peeled, trimmed, and halved

¼   cup each tomato juice (no salt added) and evaporated skim milk

½   teaspoon mild curry powder

⅛   teaspoon ground red (cayenne) pepper

¼   teaspoon freshly grated nutmeg

1   teaspoon fresh lemon juice

2   eggs

½   cup part-skim ricotta cheese

2   tablespoons low-fat plain yogurt

½   teaspoon sweet soft corn oil margarine

1. Instructions are for food processor, but broccoli and shallots may be easily knife-chopped, and balance of ingredients combined by hand. In work bowl of food processor, combine cooked broccoli, shallots, tomato juice, skim milk, spices, and lemon juice. Process on/off twice (do not overprocess).

2. Add eggs, cheese, and yogurt. Process on/off twice.

3. Pour into 1-quart margarine-greased casserole. Place casserole, covered, in larger bowl or pan. Add ½ inch boiling water, and bake in preheated 350°F oven for 45 minutes. Serve immediately.

ALTERNATIVE COOKING METHOD: Pour prepared mixture into margarine-greased 1-quart ring mold. Bake according to instructions in step 3. Chill overnight. Just before serving, gently unmold on a bed of crisp romaine lettuce leaves. Garnish with cherry tomatoes and carrot curls. Serve cold.

NOTE: Mixture will hold its shape in unmolding, but does not slice. Use large serving spoon to serve.

*F*renched Green Beans with Basil

~

YIELD: SERVES 4

*B*asil is that sweet, spicy, clove-tasting herb with an enticing aroma, and when it's blended with fresh or frozen green beans, you'll get a scented sensation that will delight all vegetable lovers. But that will only happen when you use one recipe for the fresh and another for the frozen. Both recipes follow.

Per serving
Calories: 53
Carbohydrate: 9 g
Protein: 1 g
Fat: 1 g
Saturated fat: trace
Cholesterol: 1 mg
Dietary fiber: 3.1 g
Sodium: 13 mg
Exchanges: 2 vegetable

USING FRESH GREEN BEANS:

1   pound fresh green beans, washed, trimmed, French cut (sliced lengthwise)

½   teaspoon wine vinegar

1   teaspoon tomato paste (no salt added)

¼   cup Easy Chicken Stock (page 216)

1   teaspoon sweet soft corn oil margarine

1   clove garlic, minced

2   shallots, minced

4   dashes ground red (cayenne) pepper

½   teaspoon dried fine herbs, crushed (see Note 2, page 297)

¼   cup minced fresh basil or dill

USING FROZEN BEANS:

1½   10-ounce boxes French-style green beans partially thawed

½   cup plus 2 tablespoons Easy Chicken Stock (page 216)

1   large shallot, minced

1   clove garlic, minced

½   teaspoon wine vinegar

½   teaspoon dried fine herbs, crushed

4   dashes ground red (cayenne) pepper

1   teaspoon tomato paste (no salt added)

¼   cup minced fresh basil or dill

1. Steam green beans until just tender. Drain; to completely dry, roll up beans on paper toweling.

2. In small heavy-bottom saucepan, combine and blend vinegar, tomato paste, and stock. Slow-boil until mixture is reduced by half. Set aside.

3. Heat margarine in nonstick skillet. Sauté garlic and shallots for 2 minutes over medium heat (do not brown). Add green beans. Sprinkle with ground red pepper and fine herbs. Stir and sauté for 30 seconds. Spoon stock mixture over green beans. Stir and cook for 30 seconds over medium-high heat.

4. Turn into serving dish. Sprinkle with basil or dill and serve immediately.

1. In nonstick skillet, combine partially thawed beans, ½ cup stock, shallot, garlic, and vinegar. Bring to simmering point. Partially cover and simmer until beans are cooked (about 8 minutes).

2. Sprinkle with fine herbs and ground red pepper. Stir.

3. Combine balance of stock (2 tablespoons) with tomato paste. Spoon mixture over green beans. Stir and sauté for 30 seconds over medium-high heat.

4. Turn into serving dish. Sprinkle with basil or dill and serve immediately.

Pan-Fried Escarole

YIELD: SERVES 4

This somewhat bitter green plays a dual role in my kitchen. Its fresh, crisp, tender leaves add sophistication to many a salad bowl, and on their own cook into a vegetable that satisfies our craving for something beyond the commonplace. Most panned escaroles derive their flavor from bacon fat, butter, salt, and pepper. My version is based on a careful selection of herbs and spices and just the right amount of corn oil margarine and Italian olive oil. It should come as no surprise that my healthful version is the better tasting.

Per serving
Calories: 35
Carbohydrate: 3 g
Protein: 1 g
Fat: 2 g
Saturated fat: trace
Cholesterol: 0 mg
Dietary fiber: 1.6 g
Sodium: 13 mg
Exchanges: 1 vegetable

2 teaspoons each sweet soft corn oil margarine and Italian olive oil

3 cloves garlic, minced

1 medium onion, minced

1 head escarole, leaves washed, well dried, and finely chopped (4 cups)

1 teaspoon dried tarragon leaves, crushed

¼ teaspoon paprika

⅛ teaspoon ground red (cayenne) pepper

1 teaspoon wine vinegar or balsamic vinegar

2 tablespoons minced fresh parsley

1. Heat oil and margarine in well-seasoned iron skillet until hot. Add garlic and onion. Sauté for 30 seconds.

2. Add chopped escarole, spreading across skillet. Raise heat under skillet and sauté for 5 minutes, stirring often.

3. Sprinkle with balance of ingredients, and continue to sauté, stirring constantly for 5 minutes more. Volume of escarole will be reduced. Serve immediately.

NOTE: If you own a food processor, chopping can be done in a jiffy with this magic machine. Fit with steel blade. Place halved garlic cloves, quartered onion, parsley florets, and torn escarole leaves in work bowl, taking care not to overload. Process on/off 3 times, or until finely chopped.

VARIATION: Add 2 teaspoons tomato paste (no salt added) in step 3.

Browned Cabbage with Caraway

YIELD: SERVES 6

Cabbage too tough for you? Not when it's sautéed to melting tenderness. So overpowering that you can't taste anything else? Not when its flavor is subdued by sweet herbs and spices. Too cabbagey? Not when it's married to caraway, the seed that helps make Jewish and Norwegian rye breads so delicious. Even if you've been a cabbage hater all your life, you'll love this cabbage. And if you're a cabbage lover—well!

Per serving
Calories: 70
Carbohydrate: 9 g
Protein: 1 g
Fat: 3 g
Saturated fat: trace
Cholesterol: 0 mg
Dietary fiber: 3.6 g
Sodium: 29 mg
Exchanges: 2 vegetable
          ½ fat

1   head (1½ pounds) green cabbage

2   teaspoons each Italian olive oil and sweet soft corn oil margarine

2   large cloves garlic, minced

1   medium onion, minced

1   small sweet red pepper, seeded, cut into ¼-inch slivers

¼   teaspoon freshly grated nutmeg

⅛   teaspoon ground red (cayenne) pepper

½   teaspoon ground marjoram

1   teaspoon grated orange zest (preferably from navel orange)

1½   teaspoons caraway seed, partially crushed

2   teaspoons apple cider vinegar

2   tablespoons apple juice (no sugar added)

1. Cut cabbage into quarters. Cut away tough center section. Shred or thinly slice cabbage with food processor or with sharp knife.

2. Heat oil and margarine in well-seasoned iron skillet until hot (do not brown). Add cabbage, garlic, onion, and sweet red pepper. Combine and stir with fork. Sprinkle with spices and marjoram. Stir and sauté over medium-high heat, uncovered, until reduced and browned (about 30 to 35 minutes).

3. Sprinkle with orange zest and caraway seed. Stir to blend. Then add vinegar and apple juice; blend. Cook for 2 minutes, or until well heated through. Serve very hot.

Three-Vegetable Medley

YIELD: SERVES 4

Do you like carrots? Snow peas? Mushrooms? If your answers are yes, yes, yes, you'll love this medley. And if your answers are no, no, no, you'll love it, too— because in my gourmet cuisine of health, the whole is always tastier than its parts. This dish is delicious made in a saucepan and fabulous in a wok. Here are instructions for cooking with either utensil.

Per serving
Calories: 65
Carbohydrate: 9 g
Protein: 2 g
Fat: 2 g
Saturated fat: trace
Cholesterol: trace
Dietary fiber: 2.7 g
Sodium: 27 mg
Exchanges: 2 vegetable

3 medium carrots (6 ounces), trimmed and peeled, cut into ½-inch matchstick-shaped pieces

2 ounces fresh snow peas, washed, stems and strings removed

2 teaspoons Italian olive oil

2 large shallots, minced

2 cloves garlic, minced

½ teaspoon minced fresh ginger

¼ pound fresh mushrooms, washed, dried, trimmed, and thinly sliced

4 dashes ground red (cayenne) pepper

½ teaspoon each ground mild curry powder and dried tarragon leaves, crushed

3 tablespoons Thirty-Minute Chicken Broth (page 215) or Easy Chicken Stock (page 216)

1 teaspoon finely grated orange zest (preferably from navel orange)

1 tablespoon minced fresh parsley

1. In saucepan, boil carrots in water to cover until tender but firm (8 to 10 minutes). Pour into colander and drain, reserving cooking liquid. Return cooking liquid to saucepan. Bring to boil.

2. Drop snow peas into boiling liquid and cook for 1 minute. Pour into colander with carrots and drain. (Reserve cooking liquid for soups and sauces—it's delicious and vitamin rich.) Run cold water over vegetables to stop cooking action. Let drain in colander.

3. Heat oil over medium heat in non-stick skillet until hot. Sauté shallots, garlic, ginger, and mushrooms for 3 minutes, stirring constantly, adjusting heat so that mixture doesn't brown.

4. Add carrots and snow peas, stirring gently. Sprinkle with spices and tarragon. Sauté over medium-high heat until vegetables are heated through (about 1 minute). Stir in stock. Cook for 30 seconds.

5. Remove from stove. Sprinkle with orange zest and parsley, and serve piping hot.

NOTES:

1. This dish is particularly delicious if prepared in a wok. Here's how. In step 3, heat wok over high heat for 1½ minutes. Pour oil around rim of wok. When oil drips down add shallots, garlic, ginger, and mushrooms. Stir-fry for 1½ minutes. Continue with recipe, taking care not to overcook vegetables.

2. If fresh snow peas are not available, substitute ¼ pound fresh green beans. (I shun frozen snow peas because salt is ordinarily added and their natural crunchy texture is destroyed by the freezing process.) French-cut fresh green beans and cook with carrots in steps 1 and 2.

Stuffed Acorn Squash
~

YIELD: SERVES 4

Stuff this stick-to-the-ribs edible with other vegetables and herbs and spices, and you create an exquisite dish like no other squash dish you've ever tasted. Added bonus: Acorn squash is one of the two last truly inexpensive vegetables left. The other, as you may have guessed, is the turnip. During the winter months when you yearn for vegetables with potatolike texture, keep your food bin well-stocked with both.

Per serving
Calories: 72
Carbohydrate: 10 g
Protein: 2 g
Fat: 3 g
Saturated fat: trace
Cholesterol: trace
Dietary fiber: 2.5 g
Sodium: 18 mg
Exchanges: 2 vegetable
       ½ fat

2   acorn squash (¾ pound each)

2   shallots, coarsely chopped

1   tablespoon coarsely chopped celery

2   tablespoons coarsely grated carrot

1   tablespoon minced fresh parsley, dill, or basil

½   teaspoon caraway seed, partially crushed

2   tablespoons dark seedless raisins

1   tablespoon each Coriander Whole-Wheat or Magnificent Rye Bread crumbs (pages 224 and 232, and Note, page 235), and toasted regular wheat germ

½   teaspoon each ground coriander and cinnamon

4   dashes ground red (cayenne) pepper

2   tablespoons apple juice (no sugar added)

1½   teaspoons Italian olive oil or melted sweet soft corn oil margarine

1. Pick squash with uniform dark green color. (They've begun to age when there are visible orange spots on skin.) Cut in half. Remove seeds and pulp. Trim stem and blossom ends so that halves stand upright. Stand in shallow baking dish or pan. Preheat oven to 400°F.

2. Combine next 6 ingredients in a bowl.

3. Combine crumbs, wheat germ, and spices. Sprinkle, then stir into mixture. Add apple juice, a spoonful at a time, and stir until ingredients are all moistened. Fill squash cavities, spreading some of the filling over cut edges of each half.

4. Add ½ inch boiling water to baking dish. Cover loosely with aluminum foil and bake for 10 minutes. Drizzle with oil or margarine. Re-cover and bake for 35 minutes. Serve hot.

Brussels Sprouts with Mushrooms

~

YIELD: SERVES 4

A sk my husband Harold what his least favorite vegetable is and he'll say "Brussels sprouts." I prepared them one evening in this simple but unique manner, and sat by amused while he polished off two portions. The point? There's no such thing as a "least-favored vegetable" when it's prepared the way it should be.

Per serving
Calories: 78
Carbohydrate: 10 g
Protein: 3 g
Fat: 2 g
Saturated fat: trace
Cholesterol: 0 mg
Dietary fiber: 3.9 g
Sodium: 24 mg
Exchanges: 2 vegetable
         ½ fat

¾ pound fresh Brussels sprouts, well trimmed, or a 10-ounce box frozen Brussels sprouts

1 tablespoon wine vinegar

1 teaspoon dried basil leaves, crushed

½ teaspoon ground marjoram

2 teaspoons Italian olive oil

¼ pound fresh mushrooms, washed, dried, trimmed and sliced

1 clove garlic, minced

2 shallots, minced

1 small sweet red pepper, seeded, and cut into ¼-inch slivers

1. Cook Brussels sprouts until tender but not oversoft. Drain. Place in a bowl. Sprinkle with vinegar, turning to coat. Then sprinkle with basil and marjoram. Stir. Let stand for 10 minutes.

2. Heat oil in nonstick skillet until hot. Sauté mushrooms, garlic, shallots, and sweet red pepper until tender but still crunchy.

3. Add Brussels sprouts to skillet. Combine all ingredients, and cook, uncovered, over medium heat until well heated. Serve immediately.

NOTE: Step 1 may be completed well in advance of cooking time and ingredients refrigerated until ready to complete cooking. Cover skillet in step 3, and cook until well heated.

Mashed Turnip with Yam

YIELD: SERVES 4

Recently when I was a guest on a national radio call-in show, a woman telephoned and said, "I just had to tell you why your cooking is so wonderful. You make familiar foods taste so different." I was glad to hear her comment, because that was what I had set out to do. Here's a perfect example of how two of the most familiar of all American foods can taste as haute cuisine as any exotic dish.

1	1-pound yellow turnip (rutabaga), peeled, cut into ½-inch cubes, cooked
2	teaspoons Italian olive oil
2	shallots, minced
2	cloves garlic, minced
1	medium yam (½ pound), baked
½	teaspoon each dried thyme and rosemary leaves, crushed, and ground coriander
¼	teaspoon freshly grated nutmeg
⅛	teaspoon ground red (cayenne) pepper
2	tablespoons minced fresh parsley
2	tablespoons low-fat plain yogurt
2	tablespoons chopped fresh chives

Per serving
Calories: 120
Carbohydrate: 23 g
Protein: 2 g
Fat: 2 g
Saturated fat: trace
Cholesterol: 1 mg
Dietary fiber: 4.1 g
Sodium: 69 mg
Exchanges: 1 starch/bread
1 vegetable

1. Place turnip in large kettle. Partially cover with water, and boil briskly until tender (45 to 50 minutes). Drain in colander. Let stand uncovered in colander for 10 minutes. Mash or put through food mill. Place in bowl.

2. Heat oil over medium heat in nonstick skillet until hot. Sauté shallots and garlic until wilted but not brown. Add to bowl.

3. Scoop out yam from skin and blend with turnip, using a fork. Stir in dried herbs, spices, and parsley.

4. Fold in yogurt and chives. Return mixture to nonstick skillet and reheat. Serve immediately.

ALTERNATIVE COOKING METHOD: Mixture may be prepared well in advance, piled into 4 lightly oiled ovenproof crocks, and baked in a preheated 400°F oven until heated through. (Use no more than ½ teaspoon Italian olive oil for crocks.)

Colorful Sautéed Zucchini

~

YIELD: SERVES 4

True or false: Zucchini is an exotic Italian vegetable. False. It's a native American squash. But it does taste and look like a haute cuisine import in this delectable dish, which appeals to the eye as much as to the palate. We like it so much that we set some of it aside at dinner and enjoy the zucchini cold next day at lunch.

1 tablespoon Italian olive oil

2 large cloves garlic, minced

1 large onion, thinly sliced, separated into rings

1 small sweet red pepper, seeded, cut into ⅜-inch slivers

2 zucchini (¾ pound), ends trimmed, scrubbed, cut into ½-inch cubes

1 large crisp apple (such as Washington State), cored, peeled, quartered, and sliced

¼ teaspoon each ground marjoram and coriander

6 dashes ground red (cayenne) pepper

2 teaspoons apple cider vinegar

2 tablespoons Easy Chicken Stock (page 216) (optional)

2 tablespoons cognac or medium-dry sherry

2 tablespoons minced fresh basil leaves

Per serving
Calories: 63
Carbohydrate: 7 g
Protein: 1 g
Fat: 3 g
Saturated fat: trace
Cholesterol: 0 mg
Dietary fiber: 1.9 g
Sodium: 4 mg
Exchanges: 1 vegetable
  ½ fat

1. Heat oil in large, well-seasoned iron skillet or wok. (I prefer to use the wok because the pure texture and taste of the vegetables are retained.) Add garlic, onion, and sweet red pepper. Sauté for 2 minutes, stirring often.

2. Add zucchini and apple, stirring well to coat. Sprinkle with marjoram and spices. Stir and sauté for 3 minutes.

3. Add vinegar. Stir quickly to blend. Add optional stock and cognac or sherry. Cook over high heat for 1 minute.

4. Turn onto serving plate. Sprinkle with basil and serve at once.

NOTE: Fresh herbs taste best here. If fresh basil isn't available, substitute fresh dill, tarragon, or rosemary.

Fabulous Zucchini Boats

~

YIELD: SERVES 4

*B*ulgur, mixed with tender cubed chicken breasts and a palette of herbs and spices, is the rich cargo of these boat-shaped delights. This is a delicate dish, yet one that will satisfy your appetite for hours and hours—perhaps because bulgur is parboiled whole wheat. Good for lunch or for dinner.

Per serving
Calories: 150
Carbohydrate: 13 g
Protein: 14 g
Fat: 4 g
Saturated fat: 1 g
Cholesterol: 26 mg
Dietary fiber: 3.3 g
Sodium: 35 mg
Exchanges: ½ starch/bread
1 lean meat
1 vegetable
½ fat

¼ cup bulgur

2 firm zucchini (about 1½ pounds)

6 ounces skinned and boned chicken breasts, cut into ½-inch cubes

½ teaspoon each ground sage and marjoram

6 dashes ground red (cayenne) pepper

3 teaspoons Italian olive oil

2 tablespoons minced sweet red pepper

2 scallions, trimmed and minced

1 teaspoon peeled and minced fresh ginger

¼ pound fresh mushrooms, washed, dried, trimmed, and coarsely chopped

2 tablespoons dry vermouth

1 tablespoon tomato paste (no salt added)

⅓ cup coarsely chopped, loosely packed fresh basil leaves

1. Place bulgur in bowl. Add cold water to cover. Stir. Let stand for 30 minutes. Drain in strainer, pressing out water. Turn into large bowl and set aside. Preheat oven to 425°F.

2. Scrub zucchini. Cut each zucchini in half lengthwise. Insert serrated knife through pulp to a depth of ¼ inch from skin. Cut around entire half vegetable. Remove pulp with melon scraper, taking care not to puncture skin. Coarsely chop pulp. Lay shells in baking dish.

3. Sprinkle and rub chicken on all sides with dried herbs and ground red pepper. Heat 1½ teaspoons oil over medium-high heat in nonstick skillet until hot. Sauté chicken on all sides until just lightly browned (about 3 minutes). Do not overcook. Transfer to plate.

4. Heat balance of oil (1½ teaspoons) in skillet until hot. Sauté sweet red pepper, scallions, ginger, and mushrooms for 2 minutes, turning constantly. Add zucchini pulp. Sauté for 2 minutes, turning constantly.

5. Combine vermouth with tomato paste. Add to skillet. Cook for 30 seconds. Add basil and browned chicken. Combine and sauté all ingredients for 30 seconds. Pour into bowl with bulgur. Blend.

6. Pile into zucchini shells, smoothing tops with moist knife. Bake, uncovered, for 15 minutes. Remove from oven and cover loosely with aluminum foil to prevent browning. Return to oven and bake for 10 minutes. Zucchini shells should be firm but fork-tender. Serve immediately.

SERVING SUGGESTIONS: Serve with Fresh Basil Tomato Sauce (page 209) or sprinkle with 1 tablespoon freshly grated Parmesan cheese.

Sautéed Snow Peas and Mushrooms

~

YIELD: SERVES 4

As everyone knows, there are no peas in snow peas (they're so tiny as to be negligible). But there is a pod—a bright green, flavorful, crunchy pod that has delighted Oriental epicures for centuries, and now is commonplace in our supermarkets. Snow peas are marvelous textural counterpoints to fish, fowl, meat, rice, grains, tofu— and, in this recipe, mushrooms. Here snow peas are treated with all the tender loving care they deserve— and that's a treat for you.

Per serving
Calories: 69
Carbohydrate: 7 g
Protein: 2 g
Fat: 3 g
Saturated fat: trace
Cholesterol: 0 mg
Dietary fiber: 2.9 g
Sodium: 8 mg
Exchanges: 2 vegetable
            ½ fat

1   tablespoon Italian olive oil

½   teaspoon peeled and minced fresh ginger

2   large cloves garlic, minced

1   leek, white part plus 1 inch green part, well washed, dried, and minced

½   pound fresh mushrooms, washed, dried, trimmed, and thinly sliced

¼   pound fresh snow peas, washed, dried, stems and strings removed

1   teaspoon dried tarragon leaves, crumbled

4   dashes ground red (cayenne) pepper

½   teaspoon chili con carne seasoning

1   tablespoon minced fresh parsley

2   teaspoons fresh lemon juice

1. For the most delicious results, have all ingredients measured and ready to add to skillet before starting recipe. Heat oil in well-seasoned iron skillet until hot. Sauté ginger, garlic, and leek over high heat for 1 minute.

2. Add mushrooms. Stir and sauté for 2 minutes. Mushrooms will give up their juices and mixture will be moist.

3. Add snow peas, tarragon, seasonings, and parsley. Continue to sauté over high heat, stirring constantly for 2 minutes. Total cooking time is 5 minutes.

4. Sprinkle with lemon juice. Stir to blend. Serve immediately.

VARIATION: Prepare in wok and serve as luncheon dish. For the most delicious results have all ingredients measured and ready to add to wok before starting recipe. Heat wok for 1½ minutes over high heat. Pour oil around rim of wok. Add ingredients as listed, following instructions. (Because of the size, shape, and intense heat of wok, cooking time will be slightly reduced and vegetables will give up less juices and be more crunchy than with the iron skillet.) Add ¼ cup Easy Chicken Stock (page 216) at end of step 3. Then sprinkle with lemon juice. Combine 2 teaspoons cornstarch with 1 tablespoon water. Dribble into hot mixture. Stir in 2 teaspoons medium-dry sherry. Serve immediately.

Nuovo Risotto

YIELD: SERVES 4

Unless Marco Polo did it when he visited the lands of the Great Khan, I may be the first cook to prepare an Italian dish in a wok. And it works! Nuovo Risotto translates to "New Style Italian Rice"—and "new style" means I don't use rice, I use bulgur and still get that special Italian flavor. With a wok, the bulgur retains its al dente texture; the mushrooms cook to simultaneous perfection; and the spices, herbs, juices, and other vegetables blend into utter harmony. If you're not wok-wise yet, use a large nonstick skillet, and allow more time for each sequence.

Per serving
Calories: 162
Carbohydrate: 26 g
Protein: 6 g
Fat: 3 g
Saturated fat: 1 g
Cholesterol: trace
Dietary fiber: 6.2 g
Sodium: 14 mg
Exchanges: 1 starch/bread
        2 vegetable
        ½ fat

¾   cup bulgur

1   tablespoon Italian olive oil

2   large cloves garlic, minced

2   scallions, trimmed, cut into ½-inch diagonal slices

½   pound fresh mushrooms, washed, dried, trimmed, and thinly sliced

¼   pound fresh snow peas, washed, dried, stems and strings removed

½   teaspoon each ground ginger and caraway seed, lightly crushed

⅛   teaspoon ground red (cayenne) pepper

½   teaspoon dried tarragon leaves, crumbled

1   teaspoon fresh lemon juice

3   tablespoons Easy Chicken Stock (page 216) or apple juice (no sugar added)

2   tablespoons minced fresh parsley

1. In small heavy-bottom saucepan, soak bulgur in water to cover for 30 minutes. Bring to boil. Slow boil for 8 minutes. Drain. Set aside.

2. Heat wok over high heat for 1½ minutes. Pour oil around rim of wok. When oil drips down, add garlic and stir-fry for 1 minute.

3. Add scallions, mushrooms, and snow peas. Stir-fry for 2 minutes.

4. Add bulgur, stirring quickly to combine. Sprinkle with ginger, caraway seed, ground red pepper, and tarragon. Stir-fry for 1 minute.

5. Sprinkle with lemon juice. Stir in stock and parsley. Stir-fry for 30 seconds. Serve at once.

Stunning Pasta Pearls

~

YIELD: SERVES 6

How can you make flour and water taste hundreds of different ways without adding a single other ingredient? By changing the shape, as every pasta lover knows. I enhance the varied tastes of each form of pasta with a compatible sauce. Here's a subtle herb sauce for pasta pearls, and in the following recipe there's a delicate mushroom sauce for the fine strands of linguine. Bonus: These pastas, like so many others, contain no added sugar, salt, eggs, fat, or artificial coloring.

Per serving
Calories: 166
Carbohydrate: 28 g
Protein: 5 g
Fat: 3 g
Saturated fat: 1 g
Cholesterol: 1 mg
Dietary fiber: 2.4 g
Sodium: 38 mg
Exchanges: 1½ starch/bread
           1 vegetable
           ½ fat

4	teaspoons Italian olive oil
2	small sweet green peppers, cored, seeded, and minced
2	medium onions, minced
2	teaspoons peeled and minced fresh ginger
4	large cloves garlic, minced
1	small rib celery, minced
½	pound cherry tomatoes, cored and coarsely chopped
2	teaspoons wine vinegar

1	cup Easy Chicken Stock (page 216)
3	tablespoons tomato paste (no salt added)
2	teaspoons each chili con carne seasoning and smoked yeast (see page 297)
⅛	teaspoon ground red (cayenne) pepper
¼	cup finely minced fresh parsley
8	ounces pasta pearls (see Note)

1. Heat oil over medium heat in well-seasoned iron skillet until hot. Sauté sweet green peppers, onions, ginger, garlic, and celery over medium-high heat, stirring constantly until lightly browned.

2. Add tomatoes, stirring to combine. Then stir in vinegar. Cook for 1 minute.

3. Add balance of ingredients except pasta. Bring to simmering point. Cover and simmer gently for 45 minutes, stirring from time to time.

4. Ten minutes before sauce is done, bring a pot of water to rolling boil. Add pasta pearls. Continue to boil, stirring occasionally, for 10 to 12 minutes. Drain. Pour pasta back into pot. Pour sauce over pasta; stir briefly to combine.

5. Turn into well-heated serving bowl and serve.

NOTE: Pasta pearls is my name for a commercial pasta product called Acini Pepe 44, an enriched durum wheat product with no salt added. It's available in supermarkets. Orzo-47, a rice-size pasta, may be substituted.

VARIATION: Sprinkle with 1 tablespoon freshly grated Parmesan or finely grated part-skim mozzarella cheese before serving.

Piquant Mushroom Sauce over Whole-Wheat Pasta
~

YIELD: SERVES 6

Per serving
Calories: 221
Carbohydrate: 40 g
Protein: 6 g
Fat: 4 g
Saturated fat: 1 g
Cholesterol: 0 mg
Dietary fiber: 3.3 g
Sodium: 16 mg
Exchanges: 2 starch/bread
　　　　　　1 vegetable
　　　　　　1 fat

½ ounce dark dried imported mushrooms, well washed, broken up

¼ cup freshly snipped dill

2 cups canned Italian plum tomatoes (no salt added)

4 teaspoons tomato paste (no salt added)

4 teaspoons Italian olive oil

1 large sweet green pepper, minced

1 tablespoon peeled and minced fresh ginger

3 large cloves garlic, minced

2 medium leeks, white part and 1 inch of green part, well washed and minced

2 tablespoons peeled and grated carrot

½ teaspoon each dried savory, thyme, and marjoram leaves, crushed

5 dashes ground red (cayenne) pepper

¼ cup dry vermouth

2 teaspoons fresh lemon juice

⅓ cup apple juice (no sugar added)

12 ounces whole-wheat linguine (no salt added) (see Note)

1. Soak mushrooms in ¼ cup water for 30 minutes. Set aside.

2. Combine dill, tomatoes, and tomato paste in food blender. Puree until smooth. Set aside.

3. Heat oil in large, well-seasoned iron skillet until hot. Add green pepper, ginger, garlic, leeks, and carrot; sauté over medium heat until softened (about 7 minutes), stirring often. Sprinkle with dried herbs and ground red pepper. Sauté for 1 minute.

4. Add vermouth. Simmer for 2 minutes. Add mushrooms with soaking liquid, pureed tomato mixture, and lemon and apple juices. Stir to blend. Bring to simmering point. Cover and simmer gently for 1 hour, stirring every 15 minutes. Uncover, and cook over medium-high heat (just below boiling point) for 5 minutes to reduce liquid.

5. Ten minutes before sauce is finished cooking, bring large pot of water to rolling boil. Ease linguine into pot and cook for 8 to 10 minutes (*al dente*—firm to the bite). Do not overcook. Drain. Transfer to large serving bowl. Pour hot sauce over pasta. With 2 large spoons, combine sauce with pasta, and serve.

NOTE: To serve four, prepare 8 ounces linguine, use two-thirds of the sauce, and freeze balance of sauce for another meal for two.

VARIATION: In step 5, sprinkle sauce with 1 tablespoon freshly grated Parmesan cheese before combining with pasta.

Spinach-Stuffed Potatoes

YIELD: SERVES 4

As a member of the Popeye generation, I was a spinach victim. "Eat it," my mother would order. "It will make you big and strong." If that's the way to get big and strong, I told my mother, I'd rather stay small and weak. But I couldn't resist my mother, and I grew up hating spinach. Yet it is a wonderfully nutritious vegetable, so what to do? First, I had to get rid of its disagreeable aftertaste, and I did that by mixing it with potatoes. Then, I had to elevate it to an irresistible delight, and I did that by adding carrot, herbs, spices, yogurt, and cheese. The result is likely to convert any spinach hater into a spinach lover at first taste.

Per serving
Calories: 147
Carbohydrate: 29 g
Protein: 4 g
Fat: 2 g
Saturated fat: trace
Cholesterol: 1 mg
Dietary fiber: 4.9 g
Sodium: 87 mg
Exchanges: 1 starch/bread
2 vegetable

1 medium carrot, peeled and diced

1 10-ounce box frozen leaf spinach, or 1 pound fresh spinach, tough sections removed

2 large shallots, minced

2 Idaho potatoes (1 pound), well scrubbed, baked

½ teaspoon each ground cinnamon and mild curry powder

4 dashes ground red (cayenne) pepper, or to taste

2 tablespoons minced fresh parsley

3 tablespoons low-fat plain yogurt

1 teaspoon Italian olive oil (optional)

3 teaspoons freshly grated Parmesan cheese

1. Place carrot in heavy-bottom saucepan or enameled pot. Add water to barely cover and boil until tender (about 10 minutes). Drain and mash. Set aside in bowl. Preheat oven to 425°F.

2. Place frozen spinach in saucepan with shallots. Add ¼ cup water and cook, partially covered, until done (about 8 minutes). If using fresh spinach, wash thoroughly. Add no water to pot. Cover and cook until tender, stirring often. Drain in colander, pressing out juices. Chop. Add to carrot mixture and combine.

3. Carefully cut each potato in half lengthwise. Scoop out centers into small bowl. Add spices, parsley, yogurt, and oil, if desired. Mash until smooth. Combine with spinach mixture and blend.

4. Stuff each potato half with mixture, smoothing tops with knife, then running fork tip over mixture to create a striated pattern. Brush with oil. Then sprinkle with cheese. Place on nonstick baking surface and bake, uncovered, until heated through and lightly browned. Serve immediately.

NOTE: Potatoes may be stuffed ahead of time and refrigerated until ready to complete last step. Bake for 10 minutes in preheated 400°F oven. Then brush with oil and sprinkle with cheese. Raise heat to 450°F and bake for 5 minutes or until tops are lightly browned.

Red-Skinned Potatoes with Sesame Seed

~

YIELD: SERVES 4

This recipe and the two that follow were created for people who are bored to tears with the same old plain boiled or baked potato time after time. In this recipe, the natural sweetness of red-skinned potatoes is enhanced with sweet spices and marjoram, then sautéed to a crunchy goodness with sesame seed. In the next recipe, white potatoes are combined with yams and just a hint of Indian spices to make exquisite Pretty Pink Potatoes in a Crock. And in the third recipe — well, why not flip a few pages and find out about a new kind of potato that could very well make you forget French fries. No wonder they're My Pet Potatoes.

Per serving
Calories: 155
Carbohydrate: 29 g
Protein: 2 g
Fat: 3 g
Saturated fat: trace
Cholesterol: 0 mg
Dietary fiber: 3.2 g
Sodium: 10 mg
Exchanges: 1½ starch/bread
　　　　　½ fat

8	small red-skinned potatoes (about 1¼ pounds)
2	teaspoons Italian olive oil
3	large shallots, minced
½	teaspoon each ground coriander and ginger
4	dashes ground red (cayenne) pepper
¼	teaspoon ground marjoram
1	tablespoon unshelled sesame seed (see page 297)

1. Cook potatoes in water to cover until almost tender. Drain. Let cool completely before peeling.

2. Heat oil in nonstick skillet until hot. Add shallots and sauté for 1 minute.

3. Add potatoes. Sprinkle with spices and marjoram, turning potatoes to coat evenly. Sauté over medium-high heat for 1 minute.

4. Sprinkle with sesame seed. Roll potatoes back and forth in skillet so that most of seeds will adhere. Sauté until seeds and potatoes are lightly and evenly browned, rolling potatoes every minute. Skillet will become dry; do not add more oil. Serve immediately.

Pretty Pink Potatoes in a Crock

YIELD: SERVES 4

Per serving
Calories: 173
Carbohydrate: 34 g
Protein: 3 g
Fat: 3 g
Saturated fat: trace
Cholesterol: 1 mg
Dietary fiber: 3.8 g
Sodium: 26 mg
Exchanges: 2 starch/bread
½ fat

1 pound Idaho potatoes, peeled

1 small yam (½ pound), peeled

1 teaspoon each Italian olive oil and sweet soft corn oil margarine, plus ½ teaspoon for crocks

2 large shallots, minced

1 large clove garlic, minced

½ teaspoon ground cardamom

¼ teaspoon each ground cumin seed and mild curry powder

3 dashes ground red (cayenne) pepper

2 tablespoons low-fat plain yogurt

½ teaspoon caraway seed, partially crushed

2 tablespoons minced fresh basil

1. Cut Idaho potatoes and yam into ½-inch cubes. Boil together, uncovered, in heavy-bottom saucepan in water to cover until tender (about 12 minutes). Drain well. Transfer to bowl. Mash until smooth.

2. Heat 1 teaspoon each oil and margarine in saucepan until hot. Sauté shallots and garlic until just wilted (do not brown). Add to potatoes, stirring to blend.

3. Add spices, yogurt, and caraway seed, stirring to blend. Fold in fresh basil.

4. Pile into 4 margarine-greased ovenproof crocks (or 1½ quart casserole), striating top(s) with a fork. Bake in preheated 400°F oven for 20 minutes. Mixture will puff up. Serve immediately.

VARIATION: Substitute equal amount of fresh tarragon or dill for fresh basil.

My Pet Potatoes

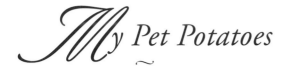

YIELD: SERVES 4

2 large Idaho potatoes (1 pound), peeled, cut into 1-inch-thick French-fry strips

1 tablespoon Italian olive oil

2 large cloves garlic, minced

3 large shallots, minced

¼ teaspoon each dried tarragon, marjoram, and thyme leaves, crushed

¼ teaspoon ground ginger

6 dashes ground red (cayenne) pepper

½ teaspoon wine vinegar

1 tablespoon minced fresh parsley

Of all my potato recipes this is, as the title proclaims, my very favorite. It starts with French-fry strips, then takes a quantum leap into a gastronomic paradise. Subtly seasoned and meticulously sautéed for crispness and succulence, these American sautées could replace French fries on your menu. They have on ours.

Per serving
Calories: 112
Carbohydrate: 18 g
Protein: 2 g
Fat: 3 g
Saturated fat: trace
Cholesterol: 0 mg
Dietary fiber: 2.4 g
Sodium: 15 mg
Exchanges: 1 starch/bread
    ½ fat

1. Lay potato strips on doubled paper toweling. Dry well.

2. Heat oil in well-seasoned iron skillet. Add garlic and shallots. Sauté about 30 seconds. Add potatoes. Sauté over medium-high heat for 2 minutes, turning twice.

3. Sprinkle with herbs and spices. Partially cover. Reduce heat to medium and cook for 10 minutes, turning often.

4. Sprinkle with vinegar and parsley. Stir and sauté, uncovered, until nicely browned and tender (about 5 minutes). Serve immediately.

Corn and Beans

YIELD: SERVES 4

1 teaspoon Italian olive oil

1 large clove garlic, minced

2 large shallots, minced

1 small sweet red pepper, seeded, cut into ¼-inch slivers

1 cup cooked fresh corn

1 cup cooked dried baby white beans

1 teaspoon mild curry powder

4 dashes ground red (cayenne) pepper

½ teaspoon dried tarragon leaves, crushed

1 teaspoon apple cider vinegar

1 tablespoon minced fresh parsley

Except when it's piping hot off the cob, corn needs a companionable vegetable, doesn't it? In this recipe, I've introduced corn to baby white beans; and in the next recipe, to carrots. When you're ravenous, try this one; when you're in the mood for a lighter accompaniment, try the next one. Both innovative dishes are subtly flavored.

Per serving
Calories: 113
Carbohydrate: 20 g
Protein: 4 g
Fat: 2 g
Saturated fat: trace
Cholesterol: 0 mg
Dietary fiber: 5.1 g
Sodium: 22 mg
Exchanges: 1 starch/bread
    1 vegetable

1. Spread oil across nonstick skillet and heat until hot over medium heat. Sprinkle garlic, shallots, and sweet red pepper across skillet. Sauté until wilted but not brown (about 3 minutes).

2. Add corn and beans. Sprinkle with spices and tarragon. Stir until well blended. Sauté until mixture is well heated.

3. Add vinegar and cook for 1 minute. Turn into warmed serving bowl. Sprinkle with parsley and serve.

Corn and Carrots

YIELD: SERVES 4

Per serving
Calories: 83
Carbohydrate: 14 g
Protein: 1 g
Fat: 3 g
Saturated fat: trace
Cholesterol: 0 mg
Dietary fiber: 3.3 g
Sodium: 20 mg
Exchanges: ½ starch/bread
1 vegetable
½ fat

2   large carrots, trimmed, well scrubbed (peeled if desired)

2   fresh ears of small-kerneled corn, cleaned

2   teaspoons Italian olive oil

2   large shallots, minced

½   teaspoon dried tarragon leaves, crushed

2   dashes ground red (cayenne) pepper

½   teaspoon mild curry powder

½   teaspoon tarragon vinegar or wine vinegar

1   tablespoon minced fresh mint or fresh basil

1. Slit carrots in half lengthwise. Place in pot with corn and enough water to cover. Bring to a boil. Partially cover and cook until just tender. Drain. (Vegetables may also be steamed until tender.) Stand cobs upright on cutting board. Cut kernels from cob with serrated knife. Thinly slice or dice carrots.

2. Heat oil over medium heat in non-stick skillet until hot. Add shallots. Sauté for 2 minutes, taking care not to brown. Add corn and carrots. Combine and stir.

3. Sprinkle with tarragon and spices. Stir and sauté for 30 seconds. Sprinkle with vinegar. Stir.

4. Turn onto warmed serving plate. Top with fresh mint, and serve.

VARIATION: At the end of step 3, add 2 tablespoons low-fat plain yogurt to skillet. Stir and cook briefly until heated through. Turn onto warmed serving plate. Sprinkle with mint and serve.

Lentil and Bulgur Medley

~

YIELD: SERVES 6

Not too long ago, it was considered gauche to serve two starchy vegetables together. Not anymore, particularly when the vegetables contain a satisfying quota of fiber, as they do here. Bulgur is parboiled whole wheat, and lentils are those wondrous tasty legumes for which Esau of the Bible sold his birthright (no, it wasn't "pottage"). Together, in a rich mixture of herbs, spices, fruit juices, and other vegetables, they make a dish as memorable as it is original. And you'll find an equally delectable bulgur-based medley in the recipe that follows.

Per serving
Calories: 185
Carbohydrate: 33 g
Protein: 9 g
Fat: 2 g
Saturated fat: trace
Cholesterol: 1 mg
Dietary fiber: 4.5 g
Sodium: 28 mg
Exchanges: 2 starch/bread
    1 vegetable

¾ cup lentils

5 cups water

1 cup apple juice (no sugar added)

1 sprig fresh parsley

¾ cup bulgur

2 teaspoons Italian olive oil

3 cloves garlic, minced

1 leek, white part only, well washed, minced

1 rib celery, minced

1 teaspoon peeled and minced fresh ginger

¼ pound fresh snow-white mushrooms, washed, dried, trimmed, and sliced

⅛ teaspoon ground red (cayenne) pepper

2 teaspoons chili con carne seasoning

½ teaspoon dried thyme leaves, crushed

½ cup Easy Chicken Stock (page 216)

¼ cup grated carrot

2 tablespoons minced fresh parsley

1. In a pot, soak lentils in 2 cups water for 2½ hours. Pour into strainer. Rinse under cold running water for 1 minute. Return lentils to pot. Add balance of water, apple juice, and parsley sprig. Bring to boil. Reduce heat to simmering. Partially cover and simmer for 20 minutes.

2. Add bulgur and simmer for 15 minutes. Pour into strainer and drain. Let cool. Set aside.

3. Heat oil in nonstick skillet until hot. Add garlic, leek, celery, and ginger. Sauté for 2 minutes, stirring often. Add mushrooms and sauté over medium-high heat until lightly browned.

4. Sprinkle with spices and thyme. Stir. Add lentils and bulgur mixture, stirring to combine. Then add stock and carrot. Cover and cook briefly until heated through.

5. Turn into heated serving bowl. Sprinkle with parsley and serve at once.

ALTERNATIVE COOKING METHOD: Complete step 1. Pour lentils into a 2-quart casserole. Add bulgur, stirring to blend. Cover and bake in preheated 350°F oven for 20 minutes. Follow step 3. Then turn ingredients in skillet into casserole together with spices, thyme, stock, and carrot. Stir. Re-cover and bake for 10 minutes. Sprinkle with parsley and serve immediately.

Okra-Bulgur Casserole

YIELD: SERVES 6

Per serving
Calories: 89
Carbohydrate: 16 g
Protein: 3 g
Fat: 2 g
Saturated fat: trace
Cholesterol: trace
Dietary fiber: 3.0 g
Sodium: 17 mg
Exchanges: ½ starch/bread
              1 vegetable

1   10-ounce box whole frozen okra

2   cups water

¼   cup white vinegar

2   teaspoons Italian olive oil

2   large cloves garlic, minced

2   shallots, minced

2   tablespoons coarsely chopped sweet green or red pepper

½   teaspoon each dried savory and rosemary leaves, and caraway seed, crushed

6   dashes ground red (cayenne) pepper

½   cup bulgur

½   cup apple juice (no sugar added)

1   cup canned Italian plum tomatoes (no salt added), chopped

1   sprig fresh dill

2   teaspoons freshly grated Parmesan cheese

1. Preheat oven to 350°F. Place okra, 1 cup water, and vinegar in small saucepan. Bring to boil. Reduce heat to slow boil. Cook uncovered for 3 minutes. Drain. Set aside.

2. Heat oil over medium heat in non-stick skillet until hot. Sauté garlic, shallots, and sweet pepper until wilted (do not brown), stirring often. Sprinkle with herbs, seed, and ground red pepper.

3. Add bulgur, stirring to coat. Cook for 1 minute.

4. Add balance of water (1 cup), apple juice, tomatoes, and dill sprig. Bring to simmering point. Pour into 1¾-quart ovenproof casserole. Bake for 15 minutes. Sprinkle with cheese. Return to oven until cheese melts (about 5 minutes).

5. Discard dill sprig, stir, and serve.

Baked Rice in Red Wine

~

YIELD: SERVES 6

Wine, admittedly, does wonders for food, but too often no-salt cooking relies solely on it—with disappointing results. The secret is to use wine as only one theme in a rhapsody of flavors. But here it's the dominant theme, and that gives distinction to this dish. (When wine is cooked all the alcohol is boiled off, and all that remains is the flavor.)

1 tablespoon Italian olive oil

¼ pound fresh mushrooms, washed, dried, trimmed, and thinly sliced

1 teaspoon peeled and minced fresh ginger

3 large cloves garlic, minced

½ cup enriched rice

½ teaspoon each dried sage and oregano leaves, crushed

⅛ teaspoon ground red (cayenne) pepper

½ cup dry red wine

¼ cup apple juice (no sugar added)

¾ cup water or vegetable juice (see Note)

1 cup canned Italian plum tomatoes (no salt added), chopped

Bouquet garni (1 sprig parsley, 1 bay leaf, tied together with white thread)

Per serving
Calories: 99
Carbohydrate: 17 g
Protein: 2 g
Fat: 2 g
Saturated fat: trace
Cholesterol: 0 mg
Dietary fiber: 1.8 g
Sodium: 7 mg
Exchanges: 1 starch/bread
　　　　　　 1 vegetable

1. Preheat oven to 400°F. Heat oil in well-seasoned iron skillet until hot. Sauté mushrooms, ginger, and garlic over medium-high heat, turning constantly, until mixture is lightly browned.

2. Add rice. Stir and sauté for 2 minutes.

3. Sprinkle with sage, oregano, and ground red pepper. Sauté for 30 seconds.

4. Stir in balance of ingredients except bouquet garni. Bring to simmering point. Transfer to 1½-quart ovenproof casserole. Add bouquet garni, pushing down into liquid. Bake for 35 minutes, fluffing with fork midway.

5. Remove from oven. Let stand for 5 minutes. Discard bouquet garni and serve.

NOTE: If you've saved vegetable cooking juices, use them in place of water. Delicious!

Curried Rice with Carrots

~

YIELD: SERVES 6

Do you ever think about all the foods you simply loathe because you were forced to eat them in childhood? High on my list are carrots. I'll only eat them today when they're part of a potpourri of apples, apple juice, curry, ginger (and other spices), sweet vegetables, and rice—as they are in this colorful dish. It's a sweet dish, and had it been served to me as a child I think I would have loved it. If your child can't stomach carrots, why not serve curried rice with carrots instead, and listen joyfully to those cries for more? Adults are likely to behave the same way, too.

Per serving
Calories: 112
Carbohydrate: 22 g
Protein: 2 g
Fat: 2 g
Saturated fat: trace
Cholesterol: 1 mg
Dietary fiber: 2.0 g
Sodium: 29 mg
Exchanges: 1 starch/bread
           1 vegetable

3   medium carrots, peeled and diced

2   teaspoons Italian olive oil

2   tablespoons each minced sweet red pepper and celery

2   large cloves garlic, minced

1   medium onion, minced

½   cup enriched rice

⅔   cup Easy Chicken Stock (page 216)

⅓   cup apple juice (no sugar added)

1   tablespoon fresh lemon juice

½   cup water

1½   teaspoons mild curry powder

½   teaspoon each ground ginger and thyme leaves, crushed

2   sprigs parsley

1   small crisp sweet apple (such as Washington State), peeled, cored, and coarsely chopped

1. Cook carrots in rapidly boiling water for 10 minutes. Drain. Set aside. Preheat oven to 375°F.

2. Heat oil over medium heat in non-stick skillet until hot. Sauté sweet red pepper, celery, garlic, and onion until softened (do not brown). Add rice. Sauté for 2 minutes, stirring to coat.

3. Add stock, apple juice, lemon juice, water, spices, and thyme. Bring to simmering point. Transfer to 1½-quart ovenproof casserole. Add parsley. Cover and bake for 15 minutes.

4. Stir in carrots and chopped apple. Return covered casserole to oven and bake for 10 minutes. Remove from oven. Let stand, covered, for 5 to 10 minutes. Discard parsley and serve.

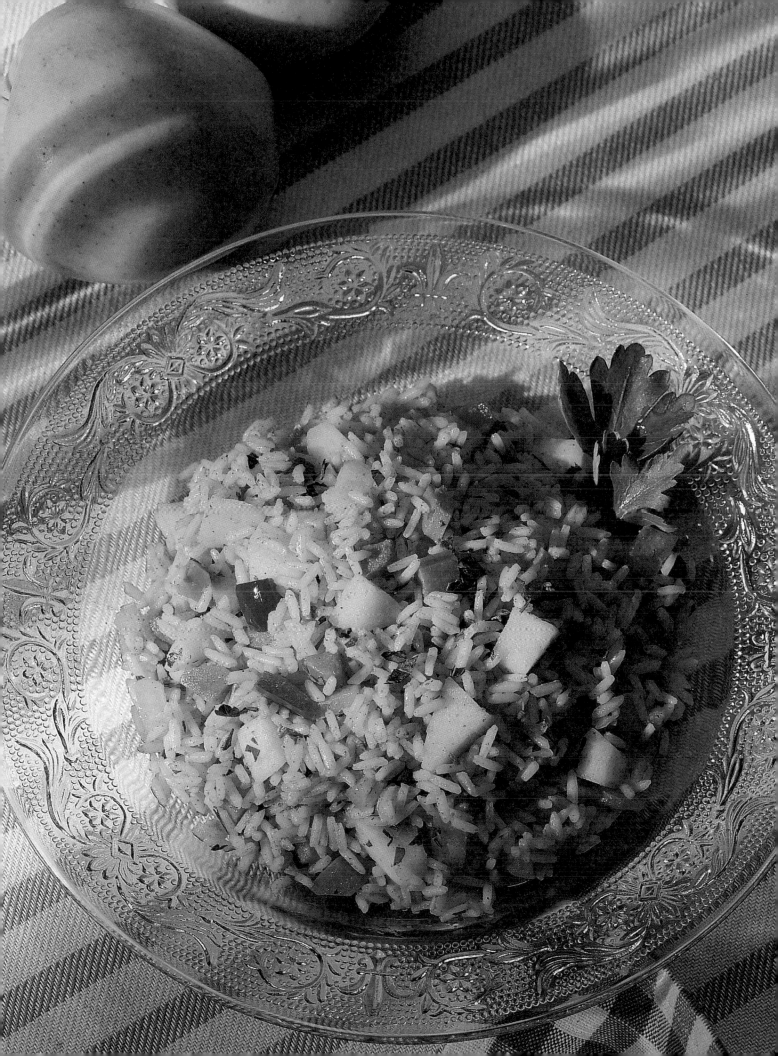

Delicious Wild Rice I
~

YIELD: SERVES 4

Rice is the staff of life in Asia, and the principal food of at least half the people in the world. But not wild rice. That's a different plant entirely, and it's purely American, flourishing in Canada and in the northern part of the USA (but not in Alaska). It was a favorite food of the Indians of that area, and your taste buds will tell you why. Don't expect a ricy taste; you won't get it. But do expect a grain taste of an unusual nature. Since the unusual deserves unusual care in preparation, Delicious Wild Rice I is simmered here in an amalgam of stock, apple juice, vermouth, and herbs; and Wild Rice II is enriched by mushrooms and a soupçon of oil. Both are elegant dishes.

¾ cup raw wild rice

1¼ cups each Easy Chicken Stock (page 216) and water

¼ cup each dry vermouth and apple juice (no sugar added)

1 tablespoon peeled and minced yellow turnip (rutabaga)

1 teaspoon minced dried onion

1 sprig each fresh dill and parsley

6 dashes ground red (cayenne) pepper

½ teaspoon dried tarragon, crumbled

1 tablespoon minced fresh tarragon, mint, or any fresh herb of your choice

1. Pour rice into strainer. Rinse under cold running water. Transfer to stainless steel pot or waterless cooker. Add stock and water. Let soak for 1 hour.

2. Add balance of ingredients except minced herb. Bring to boil. Reduce heat to simmering. Partially cover and simmer gently for 35 to 40 minutes, stirring from time to time. All water will be absorbed and rice will be tender and crunchy. (If you prefer it softer, add ¼ cup water or stock and continue cooking to desired consistency.) Discard dill and parsley sprigs, pressing out juices. Keep rice warm over simmering water until ready to serve.

3. Turn into warmed serving bowl. Sprinkle with fresh herb of your choice and serve.

Per serving
Calories: 74
Carbohydrate: 14 g
Protein: 2 g
Fat: 1 g
Saturated fat: trace
Cholesterol: 3 mg
Dietary fiber: 0.4 g
Sodium: 239 mg
Exchanges: 1 starch/bread

Delicious Wild Rice II

YIELD: SERVES 4

Per serving
Calories: 104
Carbohydrate: 18 g
Protein: 2 g
Fat: 2 g
Saturated fat: trace
Cholesterol: 1 mg
Dietary fiber: 1.1 g
Sodium: 214 mg
Exchanges: 1 starch/bread
1 vegetable

¾ cup raw wild rice

2 cups water

½ cup apple juice (no sugar added)

¼ cup dry vermouth

1 sprig each fresh dill and parsley

2 teaspoons Italian olive oil

1 large green onion, cut into ¼-inch slices

1 teaspoon peeled and minced fresh ginger

2 tablespoons minced sweet red pepper

¼ pound fresh snow-white mushrooms, washed, dried, and thinly sliced

½ teaspoon each smoked yeast (see page 297) and chili con carne seasoning

6 dashes ground red (cayenne) pepper

¼ cup Easy Chicken Stock (page 216)

1 tablespoon minced fresh mint

1. Pour rice into strainer. Rinse under cold running water. Transfer to stainless steel pot of waterless cooker. Add water. Let soak for 1 hour.

2. Add apple juice, vermouth, and herb sprigs. Bring to boil. Reduce heat to simmering. Partially cover and simmer gently for 35 to 40 minutes, stirring from time to time. Remove from heat and discard dill and parsley sprigs, pressing out juices.

3. In nonstick skillet, heat oil until hot. Sauté green onion, ginger, sweet red pepper, and mushrooms over medium-high heat, stirring constantly until lightly browned (about 5 minutes).

4. Add rice and combine with sautéed ingredients. Sprinkle with smoked yeast, chili con carne seasoning, and ground red pepper. Stir to combine.

5. Add stock and mint. Cook until well heated. Serve immediately.

NOTE: If fresh mint isn't available, substitute 2 tablespoons minced fresh basil or tarragon.

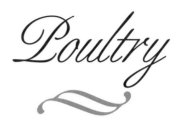

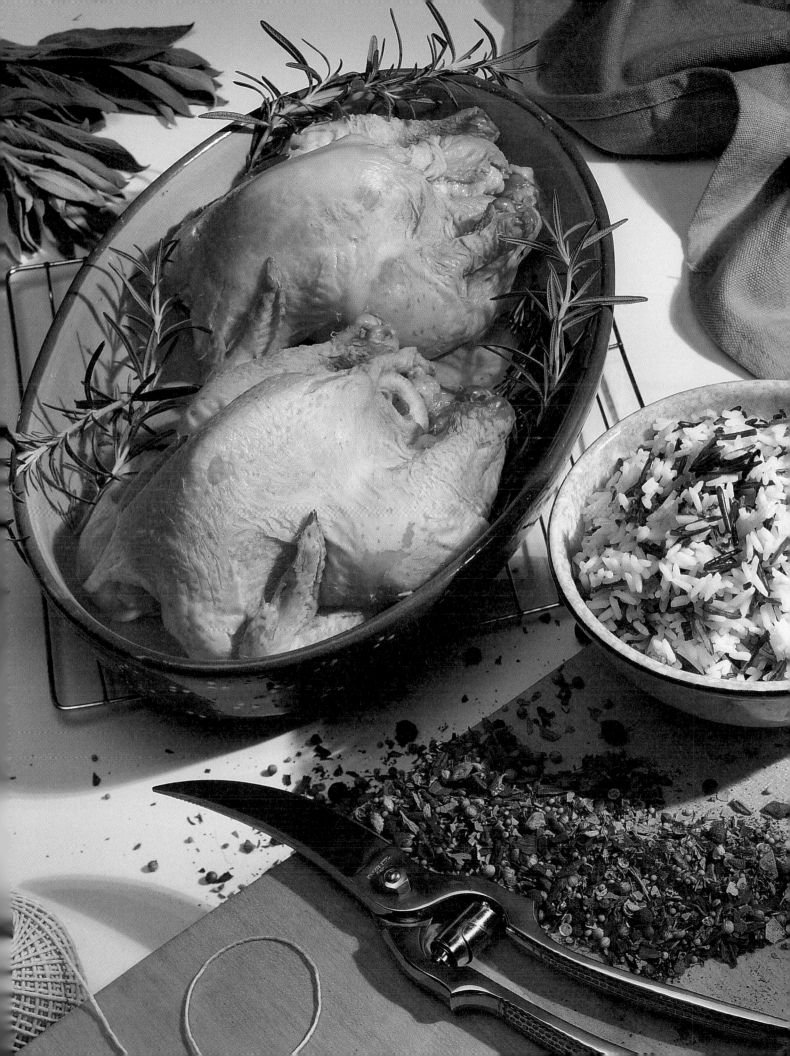

Chicken and Ham Paillards with Madeira Glaze

~

YIELD: SERVES 4

Elegantly served in fine restaurants, this many-textured dish can now be made in your kitchen quickly and deliciously. Butterflied breasts of chicken envelop lean slices of ham. The packages are coated with a light breading, sautéed on a moist bed of minced shallots, garlic, and ginger (which do wonders to the taste) and browned; then a sweet, fruity wine is poured around the sides of the skillet. Most of the wine evaporates, leaving an enticing glazed residue on the packages. Surprise: The chicken tastes more like veal. Caveat: Don't wander too far from the stove; the packages need frequent turning to retain their tender succulence.

Per serving
Calories: 270
Carbohydrate: 9 g
Protein: 34 g
Fat: 10 g
Saturated fat: 3 g
Cholesterol: 98 mg
Dietary fiber: 1.0 g
Sodium: 405 mg
Exchanges: ½ starch/bread
          4 lean meat

4   **small chicken breasts (about 1¼ pounds), boned and skinned**

2   **teaspoons oregano**

1   **teaspoon mild curry powder**

4   **ounces boiled ham (preferably low-sodium)**

5   **tablespoons unbleached flour**

3   **tablespoons regular wheat germ**

2   **tablespoons freshly grated Parmesan cheese**

1   **teaspoon finely minced lemon zest**

1   **egg, lightly beaten with 1 tablespoon water**

4½   **teaspoons Italian olive oil**

¼   **cup minced shallot**

2   **teaspoons minced garlic**

1   **teaspoon minced fresh ginger**

½   **cup sweet Madeira (Malmsey)**

   Minced parsley or fresh coriander

   Lemon or lime wedges

---

1. Wash chicken and pat dry with paper toweling. Butterfly by slicing horizontally through each breast, cutting almost to the edge. Open out.

2. In a cup, combine the oregano and half the curry. Sprinkle and rub all over the chicken. Place equal amounts of ham on one side of each butterfly. Fold over uncovered side to make a sandwich. Secure openings with toothpicks.

3. Prepare a coating by combining flour with wheat germ, cheese, lemon zest, and remaining ½ teaspoon curry powder. Sprinkle half the mixture across a sheet of wax paper.

4. Put egg mixture into a bowl. Dip chicken packages in it, draining off excess, then arranging each piece over coating. Sprinkle balance of coating over chicken packages and press with palm of hand to ensure adherence. Chill for 15 minutes.

5. Heat 2¼ teaspoons oil in a large, well-seasoned iron skillet (or non-stick skillet) over medium heat. Sauté shallots, garlic, and ginger over medium-high heat for 1½ minutes. Spread evenly across pan. Arrange chicken packages over mixture and cook until lightly browned on each side, adding remaining 2¼ teaspoons oil just before turning (total cooking time about 5 minutes). Turn again. Cover, reduce heat slightly, and cook for 5 minutes longer.

6. Uncover. Pour wine around sides of pan, tilting pan from side to side to distribute liquid evenly. Adjust heat to medium. Cook for 2 minutes. Scoop up with spatula, turn, and cook for 2 minutes longer. Most of liquid will evaporate. Serve at once, sprinkled with parsley and garnished with lemon or lime wedges.

VARIATION: Add 4 ounces thin-sliced snow-white fresh mushrooms (ends trimmed) that have been damp-wiped, and sauté for 2 minutes after wine is added in step 6.

Aromatic Chicken
~

YIELD: SERVES 4

Here's a step-by-step guide for eating in—fast, easy, and as delightfully as eating out. Just follow the numbers.

Per serving
Calories: 266
Carbohydrate: 7 g
Protein: 30 g
Fat: 12 g
Saturated fat: 3 g
Cholesterol: 97 mg
Dietary fiber: 1.4 g
Sodium: 322 mg
Exchanges: 4 lean meat
1 vegetable

With 1 Cup Pasta
Per serving
Calories: 421
Carbohydrate: 39 g
Protein: 35 g
Fat: 12 g
Saturated fat: 3 g
Cholesterol: 97 mg
Dietary fiber: 2.5 g
Sodium: 323 mg
Exchanges: 2 starch/bread
4 lean meat
1 vegetable

1½ teaspoons each dried oregano and mild curry powder

¼ teaspoon dried thyme leaves, crushed

4 small chicken legs with thighs (about 1¾ pounds), skinned, disjointed

1 tablespoon Italian olive oil

2 teaspoons each, peeled and minced, fresh ginger and garlic

½ cup minced shallot, or a combination of shallot and onion

1 small red bell pepper, seeded, cut into 1-inch strips

3 tablespoons apple cider vinegar

1 cup tomato juice (preferably without salt)

3 tablespoons Italian-style tomato paste

2 large sprigs fresh parsley tied together with white cotton thread

Minced fresh parsley or fresh oregano

1. In a cup, combine oregano, curry and thyme. Wash chicken and dry well with paper toweling. Prick all over with a sharp-pronged fork. Sprinkle and rub with seasonings. (Taste is enhanced if seasoned chicken is covered and refrigerated for several hours before proceeding with step 2.)

2. Heat oil over medium heat in a large nonstick skillet until hot. Spread ginger, garlic, and shallot across pan. Over medium-high heat, sauté until mixture wilts but does not brown. Arrange chicken pieces over mixture. Cook until lightly brown (about 3 minutes). Scoop up with spatula and turn. Add red pepper to skillet. Cook for 3 minutes longer.

3. Spoon vinegar around sides of skillet. Cook for 1 minute. Turn chicken.

4. In a small bowl, whisk tomato juice with tomato paste until smooth. Pour around sides of pan. Bring sauce to a boil. Add herb bundle. Reduce heat to simmering. Cover and cook for 40 minutes, spooning with sauce and turning once midway.

5. Uncover. Raise heat and cook until sauce lightly thickens, taking care not to scorch (about 5 minutes). Discard herb bundle after pressing out juices. Spoon sauce over chicken. Cover and let stand for 10 minutes. Arrange on warmed serving platter, sprinkled with fresh herb of your choice.

SERVING SUGGESTION: Pasta or basmati rice (imported from India and available in gourmet specialty shops).

VARIATION: For a totally different taste, substitute dried dill weed for oregano, green bell pepper for red pepper, and 2 tablespoons balsamic vinegar for 3 tablespoons cider vinegar.

Broiled Spicy Chicken

YIELD: SERVES 4

Working men and women: Do you crave a healthful, delicious, simple-to-make alternative to store-bought rotisseried chicken? Here it is.

Per serving
Calories: 205
Carbohydrate: 0 g
Protein: 29 g
Fat: 10 g
Saturated fat: 3 g
Cholesterol: 78 mg
Dietary fiber: 0 g
Sodium: 98 mg
Exchanges: 4 lean meat

1   3-pound broiling chicken, skinned, wing tips removed, cut into serving pieces

3   large cloves garlic, minced

½   teaspoon ground ginger

2   teaspoons chili con carne seasoning

½   teaspoon dry mustard

1   teaspoon dried oregano leaves, crushed

¼   cup wine vinegar

1   tablespoon Italian olive oil

1–2 teaspoons freshly grated Parmesan cheese

Minced fresh parsley

Parsley sprigs

1. Wash chicken and pat dry with paper toweling. Place in small bowl.

2. Prepare quick marinade by combining balance of ingredients except Parmesan cheese and parsley in jar. Shake to blend. Pour over chicken, turning to coat.

3. Drain chicken, reserving marinade. Place in shallow broiling pan. Sprinkle with Parmesan cheese. Broil 4 inches from heat for 7 minutes. Turn, spoon with marinade, and broil for 7 minutes. Continue broiling, turning, and spooning with marinade until chicken is done (about 25 to 30 minutes). Chicken should be crispy when done.

4. Arrange on serving platter. Sprinkle with parsley. Garnish with parsley sprigs and serve.

NOTE: If you have the time and the foresight, chicken may be prepared the night before through step 2 and popped under the broiler any time next day.

Sautéed Indian-Spiced Chicken

~

YIELD: SERVES 4

This recipe and the one that follows are inspired by the cuisine of India, but they're American originals—subtly flavored to please everybody's palate. Moreover, they're two of the simplest dishes you'll ever prepare; and they're as fast to cook as TV dinners—or faster.

2	whole chicken breasts, boned and skinned (1¼ pounds boned weight), each breast cut in half
½	teaspoon each ground cinnamon, coriander, cardamom, and mild curry powder
6	dashes ground red (cayenne) pepper
¼	teaspoon ground sage

2	teaspoons Italian olive oil
2	large shallots, minced
2	large cloves garlic, minced
¼	cup each Easy Chicken Stock (page 216) and dry vermouth
3	tablespoons currants
	Minced fresh parsley

Per serving
Calories: 161
Carbohydrate: 5 g
Protein: 24 g
Fat: 5 g
Saturated fat: 1 g
Cholesterol: 57 mg
Dietary fiber: 0.7 g
Sodium: 54 mg
Exchanges: 3 lean meat

With Bulgur
Per serving
Calories: 330
Carbohydrate: 41 g
Protein: 30 g
Fat: 5 g
Saturated fat: 1 g
Cholesterol: 57 mg
Dietary fiber: 5.2 g
Sodium: 59 mg
Exchanges: 2 starch/bread
3 lean meat

1. Wash chicken. Dry thoroughly with paper toweling. Combine spices, ground red pepper, and sage. Sprinkle and rub into chicken.

2. Heat oil in nonstick skillet until hot. Spread shallots and garlic across skillet. Sauté for 1 minute. Lay spiced chicken on top of mixture and cook for 3 minutes on each side. Chicken should be lightly browned.

3. Add stock, vermouth, and currants. Bring to simmering point. Turn chicken several times to coat. Reduce heat, cover, and simmer gently for 25 minutes, turning once midway.

4. Uncover. Turn heat up to medium-high, and reduce liquid by one-third, turning chicken every 30 seconds. Finished chicken will be a lovely chestnut brown and sauce will be syrupy. Serve at once, sprinkled liberally with minced parsley.

SERVING SUGGESTION: Delicious served over a bed of cooked bulgur.

VARIATION: Blend in 1 tablespoon low-fat plain yogurt at end of step 4.

Roast Indian-Spiced Chicken

YIELD: SERVES 4

Per serving
Calories: 229
Carbohydrate: 2 g
Protein: 32 g
Fat: 10 g
Saturated fat: 3 g
Cholesterol: 90 mg
Dietary fiber: 0.1 g
Sodium: 91 mg
Exchanges: 4 lean meat

1 3-pound broiling chicken, skinned, wing tips removed

½ teaspoon each ground cardamom, turmeric, dry mustard, ginger, and mild curry powder

1 tablespoon each fresh lemon and lime juice

2 tablespoons grated onion

1 clove garlic, minced (optional)

¼ cup buttermilk, preferably without salt

1 teaspoon grated orange zest

1. Wash chicken inside and out under cold running water. Dry with paper toweling. Place in large bowl.

2. In small bowl, combine balance of ingredients. Whisk to blend. Mixture will be thick. Spread evenly over chicken, spooning and spreading small amount into cavity. Let stand at room temperature for 30 minutes or well covered in refrigerator overnight.

3. Lay bird on its side on rack in roasting pan. Cover loosely with aluminum foil. Roast in preheated 375°F oven for 30 minutes. Turn chicken on other side, re-cover, and roast for 30 minutes. Roast, uncovered, on each side for 5 minutes. Cut into serving pieces and serve immediately.

Sophisticated Chicken
~

YIELD: SERVES 4

What makes a chicken dish sophisticated? High originality. Super taste. Swiftness and simplicity of preparation. All specifications are met when you tenderly marinate the bird in an innovative combination of savory herbs and spices, then sauté to a butternut-brown gastronomic triumph in just 20 minutes. But you don't have to be a sophisticated cook to make a sophisticated chicken; even if you've never cooked before, all you have to do is follow this recipe.

Per serving
Calories: 233
Carbohydrate: 4 g
Protein: 33 g
Fat: 9 g
Saturated fat: 2 g
Cholesterol: 96 mg
Dietary fiber: 0.2 g
Sodium: 88 mg
Exchanges: 4 lean meat

1 whole chicken breast, skinned and boned (¾ pound boned weight), cut into 4 pieces

2 chicken legs with thighs (1 pound), skinned and disjointed

⅓ cup fresh orange juice

2 tablespoons dry vermouth

½ teaspoon each ground marjoram, sage, and mild curry powder

3 dashes ground red (cayenne) pepper

2 teaspoons Italian olive oil

2 tablespoons each minced garlic, shallot, and sweet green pepper

¼ cup Easy Chicken Stock (page 216)

1. Wash chicken and dry with paper toweling. Place in a bowl.

2. Combine orange juice, vermouth, and seasonings, blending well with fork. Pour over chicken, turning to coat. Let stand for 30 minutes, turning twice. (Chicken may also marinate overnight if you choose.) Drain on paper toweling, reserving marinade.

3. Heat oil over medium heat in well-seasoned, large, iron skillet (see Note) until hot. Spread minced mixture across skillet and sauté over medium heat for 1 minute. Lay chicken parts on top of mixture. Sauté on both sides until lightly browned (about 5 minutes).

4. Add reserved marinade and stock. Bring to simmering point, turning several times to coat. Cover and simmer gently for 25 minutes, turning twice.

5. Remove cover. Turn up heat slightly and reduce liquid by two-thirds (it will take 3 to 4 minutes to do this), taking care not to cook too rapidly or skinned chicken will stick to skillet. Turn chicken every 30 seconds, piggybacking white meat on top of dark meat after 2 minutes. Finished chicken will be a beautiful butternut brown and small amount of sauce will be thick.

6. Serve on individual warmed plates.

NOTE: To keep your iron skillet well seasoned, wash in soapy water (do not soak). Dry thoroughly. Rub sparingly with oil. Place skillet over medium heat for 3 minutes, then let cool. Wipe out with paper toweling. Your skillet is now ready to use. After use, wash in soapy water with sponge or cloth (do not use steel wool). Repeat seasoning process whenever skillet looks dry.

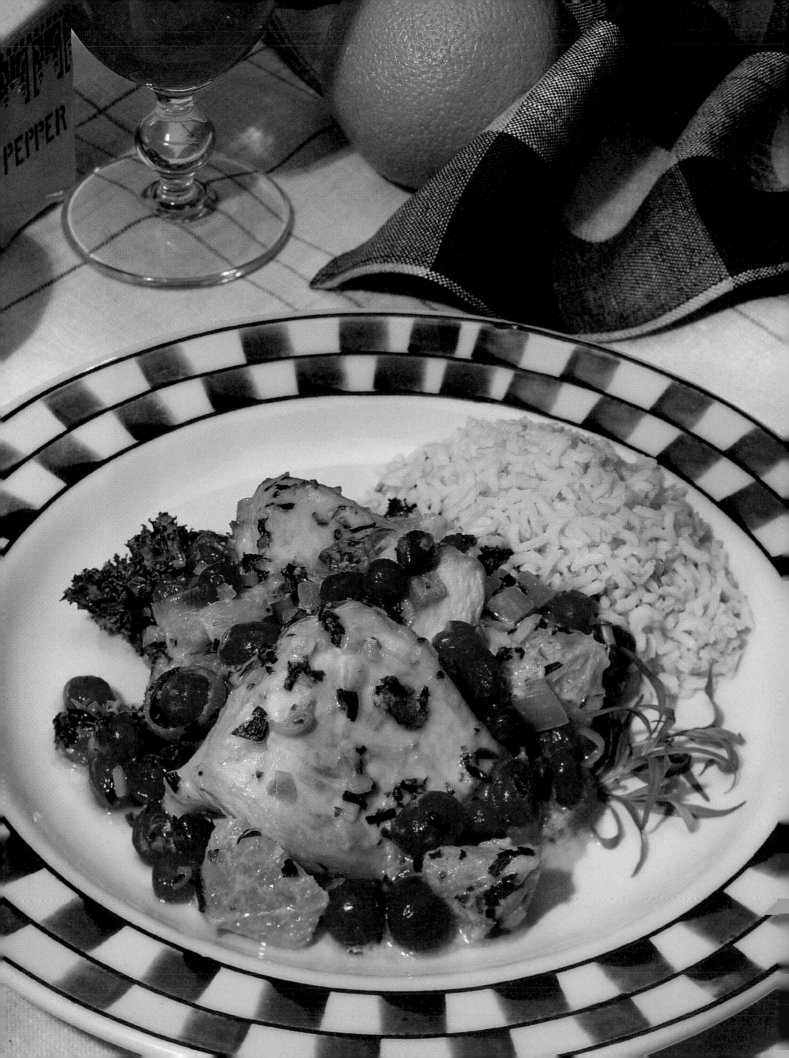

Orange-Cranberry Chicken

~

YIELD: SERVES 4

I've extolled the virtues of cranberries elsewhere in this book (see pages 156 and 159). Those tart wonders are the theme for this symphony of flavors. Serve it to your guests and they'll sing your praises for weeks on end.

Per serving
Calories: 233
Carbohydrate: 10 g
Protein: 31 g
Fat: 7 g
Saturated fat: 1 g
Cholesterol: 74 mg
Dietary fiber: 2.0 g
Sodium: 92 mg
Exchanges: 4 lean meat
              ½ fruit

2   whole chicken breasts, boned and skinned (1¼ pounds boned weight), each breast cut in half

1   teaspoon dried tarragon leaves, crushed

⅛   teaspoon ground red (cayenne) pepper

4½ teaspoons Italian olive oil

1   small leek, white part only, well washed and minced

2   cloves garlic, minced

1   small rib celery, minced

1   tablespoon tarragon vinegar (see Note 2)

¼   cup fresh orange juice

½   cup fresh cranberries, rinsed and picked over

2   tablespoons minced fresh parsley

1   medium navel orange, peeled, cut into 1-inch chunks

¼   cup evaporated skim milk

1. Wash chicken. Dry with paper toweling. Sprinkle and rub on both sides with tarragon and ground red pepper.

2. Heat 3 teaspoons oil in nonstick skillet until hot. Sauté chicken on both sides until lightly browned (about 6 minutes). Transfer to dish.

3. Heat balance of oil (1½ teaspoons) in skillet. Sauté leek, garlic, and celery until wilted but not brown.

4. Add vinegar. Stir and cook for 1 minute.

5. Add orange juice, cranberries, and parsley. Bring to simmering point. Return chicken to skillet. Spoon with sauce. Add orange chunks. Cover tightly and simmer for 25 minutes, basting with sauce twice and turning once.

6. Transfer chicken to heated serving plate. Cover to keep warm. Pour balance of ingredients in skillet into food blender. Blend until smooth. Pour back into skillet. Reheat to simmering point. Gradually add skim milk. Stir and heat until just under simmering point. Pour over chicken and serve immediately.

NOTES:

1. I like the tart flavor of the naturally sweetened sauce. If you prefer a sweeter taste, sprinkle in 1 teaspoon granulated fructose (see page 297) during blending process.

2. Bottled tarragon vinegar is available in supermarkets. It's much more economical though to make your own. Here's how: Bring 1 cup white wine or apple cider vinegar to simmering point. Place 4 teaspoons dried, crushed tarragon leaves in jar. Pour hot vinegar over herbs, stirring vigorously. Strain and use immediately. For stronger-tasting tarragon vinegar, tightly cover jar with vinegar and herb leaves and let stand at room temperature for a week or more, turning upside down once a day. Strain into sterile bottle.

Broccoli and Chicken
~

YIELD: SERVES 4

One of the quickest, easiest, most delicious chicken recipes ever!

Per serving
Calories: 273
Carbohydrate: 4 g
Protein: 33 g
Fat: 13 g
Saturated fat: 3 g
Cholesterol: 104 mg
Dietary fiber: 1.7 g
Sodium: 116 mg
Exchanges: 4 lean meat
            1 vegetable
            ½ fat

4   small chicken legs with thighs (about 1¾ pounds), skinned and disjointed

1   teaspoon dried fine herbs

1   tablespoon Italian olive oil

1   tablespoon each minced garlic, shallots, green pepper, and peeled fresh ginger

⅓   cup Easy Chicken Stock (page 216)

½   teaspoon dry mustard

2   teaspoons tomato paste (no salt added)

½   pound (1 small bunch) broccoli florets

1. Wash chicken. Dry with paper toweling. Sprinkle and rub with fine herbs.

2. Heat 1½ teaspoons oil in well-seasoned iron skillet until hot. Sauté chicken on all sides until lightly browned (about 8 minutes). Transfer to plate.

3. Heat balance of oil (1½ teaspoons) in skillet. Sauté minced ingredients, stirring constantly, until lightly browned (about 2 minutes).

4. Combine stock, mustard, and tomato paste. Add to skillet. Cook over medium-high heat for 30 seconds. Return chicken to skillet, turning to coat. Reduce heat to simmering. Cover and simmer for 20 minutes, turning once midway.

5. Add broccoli, spooning with sauce. Bring to simmering point. Re-cover and cook for 10 minutes, spooning with sauce twice. Serve immediately to preserve the bright green color and crunchy texture of broccoli.

Cilantro Chicken

~

YIELD: SERVES 4

Cilantro, also known as coriander or Chinese parsley, is a highly aromatic green herb with broad, flat, serrated leaves. I've used it freely here to set this chicken dish apart from any other. It's quick to make, too.

Per serving
Calories: 216
Carbohydrate: 3 g
Protein: 31 g
Fat: 9 g
Saturated fat: 2 g
Cholesterol: 93 mg
Dietary fiber: 0.1 g
Sodium: 124 mg
Exchanges: 4 lean meat

1   whole chicken breast, skinned and boned (¾ pound boned weight), cut into 4 pieces

2   chicken legs with thighs (1 pound), skinned and disjointed

1½ teaspoons dried tarragon leaves, crushed

⅛   teaspoon ground red (cayenne) pepper

2   teaspoons Italian olive oil

1   teaspoon peeled and minced fresh ginger

2   large cloves garlic, minced

2   large shallots, minced

1   tablespoon coarsely chopped sweet green pepper

⅓   cup Easy Chicken Stock (page 216)

¼   cup dry vermouth

¼   cup minced fresh cilantro (Chinese parsley; also called coriander)

1. Wash chicken and dry with paper toweling. Rub with tarragon and ground red pepper. Let stand for 10 minutes.

2. Heat oil over medium heat in non-stick skillet until hot. Spread ginger, garlic, shallots, and green pepper across skillet. Sauté for 1 minute (do not stir). Lay chicken pieces on top of mixture and lightly brown on both sides, stirring minced ingredients when turning.

3. Add stock and vermouth. Bring liquid to simmering point, turning chicken to coat. Sprinkle with cilantro. Reduce heat. Cover and simmer for 25 minutes, turning once. Uncover.

4. Turn up heat under skillet and cook chicken for about 6 minutes, turning every 2 minutes. Most of sauce will be reduced and chicken will be moist and delicious.

5. Serve immediately on individual warmed plates. This one won't wait.

SERVING SUGGESTION: A fine accompaniment to this dish would be a combination of simply steamed cauliflower, broccoli, and carrots.

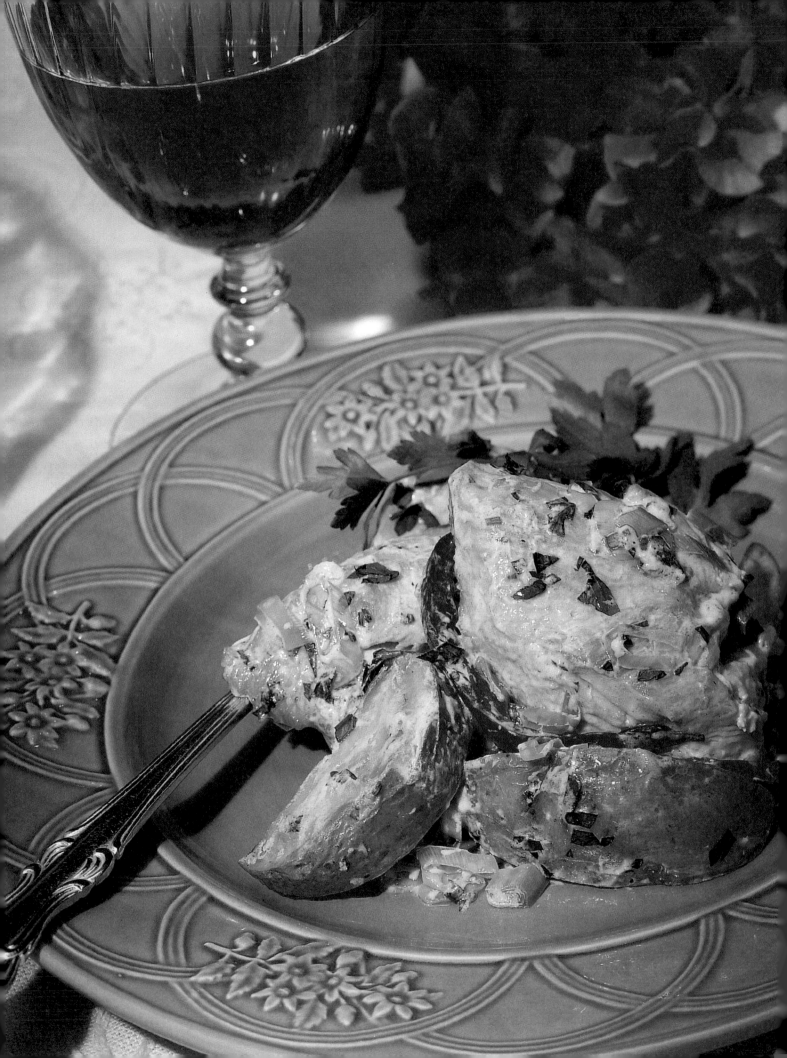

Chicken Stroganoff with Potatoes

~

YIELD: SERVES 4

My version of Stroganoff has all the delightful taste of the original, but is created from only healthful ingredients. What more could any food lover ask for?

Per serving
Calories: 295
Carbohydrate: 27 g
Protein: 32 g
Fat: 6 g
Saturated fat: 1 g
Cholesterol: 74 mg
Dietary fiber: 2.7 g
Sodium: 78 mg
Exchanges: 1 starch/bread
     4 lean meat
     1 vegetable

2	whole chicken breasts, boned and skinned (1¼ pounds boned weight), each breast cut in half
½	teaspoon each dry mustard, ground coriander, ginger, and dried sage leaves, crushed
3	teaspoons Italian olive oil
3	cloves garlic, minced
1	medium leek, white part only, well washed and thinly sliced

⅓	cup thinly slivered sweet red pepper
¼	cup each apple juice (no sugar added) and dry vermouth
4	red-skinned potatoes (1 pound), cooked, skin left on
¼	cup low-fat plain yogurt

1. Wash chicken. Dry with paper toweling. Sprinkle and rub on both sides with mustard, coriander, ginger, and sage. Slice into ⅜-inch strips.

2. Heat 2 teaspoons oil over medium heat in well-seasoned iron skillet until hot. Sauté chicken until lightly browned, taking care that it doesn't stick to skillet. If so, reduce heat. Transfer to plate.

3. Spread balance of oil (1 teaspoon) across skillet with spatula. Sauté garlic, leek, and sweet red pepper, stirring often, until lightly browned. Return chicken to skillet.

4. Combine apple juice and vermouth in a bowl. Add to skillet. Bring to simmering point. Turn chicken to coat. Cover and simmer gently for 15 minutes, turning chicken and spooning with sauce twice.

5. Skin potatoes, if desired, and add to skillet. Cover and cook for 5 minutes.

6. Reduce heat, stir in yogurt. Blend and cook briefly, just under boiling point, stirring constantly. Serve immediately.

Unusual Roast Chicken

YIELD: SERVES 4

What else but unusual would you call a mixture of orange juice, raisins, herbs, and spices? You'll also find the taste unusual, the speed of preparation unusual, and the simplicity of the recipe unusual. Unusual!

Per serving
Calories: 211
Carbohydrate: 5 g
Protein: 31 g
Fat: 7 g
Saturated fat: 2 g
Cholesterol: 84 mg
Dietary fiber: 0.4 g
Sodium: 94 mg
Exchanges: 4 lean meat

1	3-pound broiling chicken, skinned, wing tips removed
2	tablespoons wine vinegar
1	tablespoon orange juice concentrate
5	tablespoons low-fat plain yogurt
½	teaspoon crushed dried rosemary leaves
⅛	teaspoon crushed red (cayenne) pepper
4	whole cloves, crushed
1	tablespoon juniper berries, crushed
2	tablespoons dark seedless raisins

1. Wash chicken inside and out under cold running water; dry with paper toweling.

2. In small bowl, combine vinegar, orange juice concentrate, 3 tablespoons yogurt, rosemary, crushed red pepper, and cloves. Beat with fork to blend. Stir in juniper berries and raisins.

3. Spread thick mixture evenly over bird, spreading a teaspoon inside cavity. Truss bird. Place bird on its side on a rack in roasting pan. Cover with aluminum foil. Roast in preheated 350°F oven for 35 minutes.

4. Turn bird on other side. Recover and roast for 30 minutes. Uncover. Spread balance of yogurt on chicken. Baste with any exuded juices in pan. Turn chicken on other side (it won't lie on its back anymore), and roast uncovered for 10 minutes. Cut into serving pieces and serve immediately.

Moist Baked Chicken Legs

~

YIELD: SERVES 4

Chicken legs rank high on the favorites list of most fast-food-loving Americans. These finger-licking goodies with skin intact are usually rolled in flour, doused with salt and pepper, and deep-fried. When I point out that chicken legs prepared this way are fattening and might pose a threat to blood pressure, astonished chicken-leg lovers exclaim, "But ma'am, what other way is there to cook them?" My way. No skin, no flour, no salt, no pepper, no deep frying. But, what a mouth-watering medley of herbs and spices! They taste, and they believe (The skin is removed before cooking because it contains at least 25 percent of the bird's fat.)

Per serving
Calories: 235
Carbohydrate: 4 g
Protein: 31 g
Fat: 10 g
Saturated fat: 3 g
Cholesterol: 104 mg
Dietary fiber: 0.2 g
Sodium: 106 mg
Exchanges: 4 lean meat

4   **small chicken legs with thighs (about 1¾ pounds), skinned and disjointed**

1   **tablespoon fresh lime juice**

¼   **cup apple juice (no sugar added)**

2   **tablespoons low-fat plain yogurt**

2   **large cloves garlic, minced**

1   **large shallot, minced**

½   **teaspoon each dry mustard, ground cumin seed, ginger, and coriander**

1   **tablespoon minced fresh parsley**

1. Wash chicken. Dry with paper toweling. Place in small bowl.

2. In another bowl, whisk together balance of ingredients. Pour mixture over chicken, turning to coat. Preheat oven to 375°F.

3. Drain chicken, reserving marinade. Lay on rack in shallow roasting pan. Bake uncovered for 20 minutes. Turn. Spoon with half of marinade. Return to oven and bake for 15 minutes. Turn again.

4. Spoon with balance of marinade. Turn oven heat up to 425°F and bake chicken for 15 minutes. Delicious served hot or cold.

COOKING SUGGESTION: If you like to cook outdoors with a barbecue, prepare chicken through step 1; then lay a sheet of heavy-duty aluminum foil over barbecue grill. Cook chicken for 30 to 35 minutes, turning often, and spooning with marinade each time it's turned. Then remove foil with chicken. Roll pieces in cooking juices then lay them directly on grill. Broil until done (15 to 20 minutes), spooning with marinade and turning often. They'll be browned and crunchy—delicious! (For more delicious marinade suggestions, see recipes starting on page 200.)

Sautéed Lime Chicken

YIELD: SERVES 4

Add a touch of lime, balance it with a trace of naturally sweet apple juice, embellish with an array of herbs and spices, and humdrum chicken becomes an adventure in eating.

Per serving
Calories: 232
Carbohydrate: 4 g
Protein: 31 g
Fat: 10 g
Saturated fat: 2 g
Cholesterol: 92 mg
Dietary fiber: 0.2 g
Sodium: 85 mg
Exchanges: 4 lean meat

1   whole chicken breast, skinned and boned (¾ pound boned weight), cut into 4 pieces

2   chicken legs with thighs (1 pound), skinned and disjointed

2   slices fresh lime plus several slices for garnish

½   teaspoon each ground marjoram and sage

8   dashes ground red (cayenne) pepper

1   tablespoon Italian olive oil

2   large shallots, minced

2   large cloves garlic, minced

¼   cup apple juice (no sugar added)

⅓   cup dry vermouth

2   teaspoons tomato paste (no salt added)

1. Wash chicken and dry with paper toweling. Lay chicken on plate. Rub all over with 1 lime slice. Let stand at room temperature for 15 to 20 minutes. Pat dry with paper toweling. Sprinkle and rub with herbs and ground red pepper.

2. Heat in well-seasoned iron skillet until hot. Sprinkle minced shallots and garlic across skillet. Lay herbed chicken pieces on top of mixture. Sauté over medium heat until lightly browned on both sides, taking care that chicken doesn't stick to skillet.

3. In a bowl, combine apple juice, vermouth, and tomato paste. Pour around sides of skillet. Spoon over chicken. Bring to simmering point. Add lime slice to liquid. Cover and simmer over very low heat for 30 minutes, turning 3 times and piggybacking smaller pieces over larger pieces during last 10 minutes. Transfer to warmed serving plate. Discard lime slice.

4. Turn up heat slightly. Reduce liquid by half. Spoon over chicken. Garnish serving plate with lime slices and serve.

Tomatoey Chicken
~

YIELD: SERVES 4

Why not just tomato chicken? Why tomatoey? Answer: When tomatoes and tomato paste are blended with rosemary—that fragrant cousin of the mints—you get a taste that can only be described as tomatoey. The "ey" stands for new, exciting, and wonderful.

Per serving
Calories: 228
Carbohydrate: 4 g
Protein: 31 g
Fat: 9 g
Saturated fat: 2 g
Cholesterol: 83 mg
Dietary fiber: 1.6 g
Sodium: 88 mg
Exchanges: 4 lean meat
1 vegetable

1	3-pound broiling chicken, skinned, wing tips removed, cut into serving pieces
½	teaspoon ground ginger
8	dashes ground red (cayenne) pepper
2	teaspoons minced fresh rosemary leaves, or 1 teaspoon dried rosemary leaves, crushed
½	teaspoon dried thyme leaves, crushed
3	teaspoons Italian olive oil
1	tablespoon minced sweet green pepper

3	cloves garlic, minced
1	small onion, minced
1	cup canned Italian plum tomatoes (no salt added), chopped
1	tablespoon tomato paste (no salt added)
2	tablespoons Easy Chicken Stock (page 216) (optional)
2	tablespoons minced fresh parsley

1. Wash chicken and dry thoroughly with paper toweling. In a small bowl, combine spices and dried herbs. Sprinkle and rub on both sides of chicken.

2. Heat 2 teaspoons oil in nonstick skillet until hot. Sauté chicken on both sides until golden brown (6 to 7 minutes). Transfer to plate.

3. Heat balance of oil (1 teaspoon) in skillet. Sauté green pepper, garlic, and onion until lightly browned, stirring often.

4. Combine tomatoes with tomato paste and stock. Add to skillet. Bring to simmering point. Return browned chicken to skillet, turning and coating well with sauce. Cover and simmer for 35 minutes, turning twice.

5. Uncover. Sprinkle with parsley. Raise heat under skillet and cook until most of sauce is reduced, turning often. Serve immediately.

Brown and Beautiful Chicken

~

YIELD: SERVES 4

The ingredients are familiar, but the techniques are excitingly new—and so is the taste of this eye-appealing dish.

Per serving
Calories: 262
Carbohydrate: 2 g
Protein: 30 g
Fat: 13 g
Saturated fat: 4 g
Cholesterol: 219 mg
Dietary fiber: 0.6 g
Sodium: 102 mg
Exchanges: 4 lean meat
1 fat

8	small chicken thighs or legs (1¼ pounds), boned and skinned
2	tablespoons fresh lemon juice
½	teaspoon each ground marjoram and sage
⅛	teaspoon ground red (cayenne) pepper
3	teaspoons Italian olive oil
2	teaspoons peeled and minced fresh ginger
2	large cloves garlic, minced
¼	cup minced sweet green pepper
⅓	cup Easy Chicken Stock (page 216)
¼	pound fresh mushrooms, washed, dried, trimmed, and sliced
1	teaspoon ground coriander

1. Wash chicken. Pat dry with paper toweling. Place in bowl. Sprinkle with lemon juice, turning to coat. Let stand at room temperature for 30 minutes. Pat dry with paper toweling.

2. Sprinkle and rub with marjoram, sage, and ground red pepper.

3. Heat 2 teaspoons oil in well-seasoned iron skillet over medium heat until hot. Sauté chicken until lightly browned, turning often with spatula and adjusting heat so that chicken doesn't stick to skillet. Transfer to a plate.

4. Heat balance of oil (1 teaspoon) in skillet. Sauté ginger, garlic, and green pepper, turning often, until lightly browned (about 3 minutes). Return chicken to skillet. Combine with minced ingredients and cook for 1 minute.

5. Add stock, mushrooms, and coriander. Bring to simmering point. Reduce heat, cover, and simmer for 30 minutes, spooning with sauce and turning twice.

6. Uncover, raise heat under skillet, and cook for 10 minutes, turning often and adjusting heat when necessary to avoid sticking. Finished sauce should be reduced by two-thirds. Serve immediately.

Sweet and Sassy Chicken

~

YIELD: SERVES 4

Sweet as the herbs and spices I've selected and sassy as lemon juice and vermouth, this chicken is a taste experience you'll long remember.

Per serving
Calories: 192
Carbohydrate: 4 g
Protein: 30 g
Fat: 6 g
Saturated fat: 1 g
Cholesterol: 73 mg
Dietary fiber: 0.2 g
Sodium: 63 mg
Exchanges: 4 lean meat

2	whole chicken breasts, boned and skinned (1¼ pounds boned weight)
3	teaspoons Italian olive oil
2	tablespoons each fresh lemon juice and dry vermouth
½	teaspoon each dried sage and mint leaves, crushed, and ground cinnamon
6	dashes ground red (cayenne) pepper

1	medium leek, tough ends discarded, well washed, dried, and minced
2	cloves garlic, minced
⅓	cup pineapple juice (no sugar added)
2	tablespoons Easy Chicken Stock (page 216)
2	tablespoons minced fresh parsley

1. Wash chicken. Pat dry with paper toweling. Place in bowl. Combine 1 teaspoon oil, lemon juice, and vermouth in jar, shaking to blend. Pour over chicken and let marinate for at least 30 minutes. Drain, reserving marinade. Pat dry.

2. Combine dried herbs and spices. Sprinkle and rub over chicken.

3. Heat balance of oil (2 teaspoons) in nonstick skillet over medium heat until hot. Spread minced leek and garlic across skillet. Cook for 1 minute. Lay chicken on top of mixture and sauté until lightly brown on both sides (about 4 minutes).

4. Combine reserved marinade, pineapple juice, and stock. Pour over chicken, turning to coat. Bring to simmering point. Cover and simmer for 20 minutes, turning twice.

5. Uncover. Raise heat slightly under skillet and cook for 5 minutes, turning often. Transfer to serving platter. Cover to keep warm. Raise heat again, and cook sauce until reduced to ¼ cup. Spoon over chicken. Sprinkle with minced parsley.

Chicken Paupiettes with Satiny Sauce

~

YIELD: SERVES 4

This recipe and the following one are remarkably simple yet elegant examples of how chicken can be prepared in many delicious variations. Both recipes make lovely party dishes. They can be prepared in advance and reheated without loss of flavor. Serve with broccoli, asparagus, and carrots quickly steamed to retain their exquisite tones of green and orange. Your guests will applaud the bright, fresh combination of colors and textures. Or serve them along with this dish on your regular menu and turn your family meal into a party.

Per serving
Calories: 223
Carbohydrate: 8 g
Protein: 32 g
Fat: 7 g
Saturated fat: 2 g
Cholesterol: 74 mg
Dietary fiber: 0.3 g
Sodium: 93 mg
Exchanges: ½ starch/bread
4 lean meat

FOR THE PAUPIETTES:

2 whole chicken breasts, boned and skinned (1¼ pounds boned weight), each breast cut in half lengthwise

1 teaspoon each minced fresh rosemary and cilantro (Chinese parsley; also called coriander)

¼ teaspoon ground cumin seed

4 dashes ground red (cayenne) pepper

2 large cloves garlic, minced

2 large shallots, minced

1 teaspoon freshly grated Parmesan cheese

2 tablespoons Easy Chicken Stock (page 216)

FOR THE SAUCE:

⅓ cup Easy Chicken Stock (page 216)

1 tablespoon orange or apple juice concentrate

1 tablespoon dry vermouth (optional)

3 dashes ground red (cayenne) pepper

1½ teaspoons minced fresh tarragon or fresh rosemary

2 tablespoons arrowroot flour (or cornstarch) dissolved in 2 tablespoons water

3 tablespoons evaporated skim milk

1. Wash chicken. Dry thoroughly with paper toweling. Place between 2 sheets of waxed paper. Flatten to ⅜-inch thickness. Preheat oven to 375°F.

2. Sprinkle and rub on one side with herbs and spices. Sprinkle with equal amounts of minced garlic and shallots. Sprinkle with Parmesan.

3. Roll up. Place seam side down in 1¾-quart heatproof casserole. Sprinkle with stock. Cover and bake for 25 minutes.

4. To prepare sauce, combine stock, concentrate, and vermouth in heavy-bottom saucepan. Bring to simmering point. Add ground red pepper and tarragon. Simmer for 2 minutes. Whisk in flour mixture. Simmer until lightly thickened. Remove from heat. Whisk in milk.

5. Serve paupiettes on individual warmed serving plates. Spoon with hot sauce and serve.

VARIATION: If fresh rosemary and cilantro aren't available, substitute ½ teaspoon each dried rosemary and cilantro, crushed; for the sauce, substitute ¾ teaspoon crushed dried tarragon.

Chicken à la Emperor

~

YIELD: SERVES 4

*T*his dish is so superior to Chicken à la King that it deserves the "Emperor" designation.

Per serving
Calories: 303
Carbohydrate: 23 g
Protein: 27 g
Fat: 10 g
Saturated fat: 2 g
Cholesterol: 67 mg
Dietary fiber: 1.0 mg
Sodium: 110 mg
Exchanges: 1½ starch/bread
　　　　　3 lean meat
　　　　　1 fat

¼ pound fresh mushrooms, washed, trimmed, and sliced

¾ cup water

4 teaspoons Italian olive oil

2 cloves garlic, minced

1 large shallot, minced

2 tablespoons unbleached flour

¾ cup Easy Chicken Stock (page 216) or Thirty-Minute Chicken Broth (page 215)

½ teaspoon each ground coriander and ground sage

⅛ teaspoon ground red (cayenne) pepper

1 tablespoon minced fresh parsley

1 teaspoon freshly grated Parmesan cheese

2½ cups cooked chicken

3 tablespoons evaporated skim milk

2 cups hot cooked rice

1. Combine mushrooms and water in a small, heavy-bottom saucepan. Bring to simmering point. Partially cover and simmer for 3 minutes. Drain, reserving liquid.

2. Heat oil in nonstick skillet until hot. Sauté garlic and shallot over medium heat until wilted (about 3 minutes), stirring constantly. Sprinkle flour into skillet. Stir and cook for 1 minute.

3. Add reserved mushroom liquid and stock or broth. Cook over medium heat, whisking until thickened.

4. Add coriander, sage, ground red pepper, parsley, and Parmesan. Whisk until well blended.

5. Stir in drained mushrooms and chicken. Simmer for 3 minutes. Remove from heat. Stir in skim milk.

6. Spread ½ cup per portion of just-cooked rice on 4 warmed serving plates. Pour equal amounts of hot mixture over rice. Serve immediately.

Chicken-Veal Birds

~

YIELD: SERVES 4

Here's a sumptuous yet simple dish, subtly accented with delicate tarragon and mild mozzarella, then enrobed in a velvety, fresh-tasting, one-step sauce. As with the preceding recipes, this, too, is a party dish, whether you're inviting guests or just cooking for yourself and your family.

Per serving
Calories: 193
Carbohydrate: 4 g
Protein: 27 g
Fat: 7 g
Saturated fat: 4 g
Cholesterol: 74 mg
Dietary fiber: 0.2 g
Sodium: 125 mg
Exchanges: 3½ lean meat

FOR THE PAUPIETTES:

2   small whole chicken breasts (¾ pound), boned and skinned, pounded thin

2   slices veal scallopini, cut from the leg (about 4 ounces), each slice cut in half, pounded thin

½   teaspoon each dried tarragon and chervil leaves, crushed

¼   teaspoon dried thyme leaves, crushed

8   dashes ground red (cayenne) pepper

1   large shallot, minced

4   slices (2 ounces) part-skim mozzarella cheese

1   tablespoon apple juice (no sugar added)

FOR THE SAUCE:

2   tablespoons minced fresh parsley

⅓   cup Easy Chicken Stock (page 216) or Thirty-Minute Chicken Broth (page 215)

2   tablespoons dry vermouth or sherry

1   clove garlic, minced

1   tablespoon minced celery

½   teaspoon dried tarragon, crushed

2   tablespoons arrowroot flour (or cornstarch) dissolved in 2 tablespoons water

1. Wipe chicken and veal with paper toweling. Cut each chicken breast into 2 pieces. Lay chicken slices on board. Combine tarragon and chervil. Sprinkle with half of mixture and ground red pepper. Lay one slice of veal over each slice of chicken. Sprinkle with balance of dried herbs and red pepper. Preheat oven to 350°F.

2. Sprinkle each set of paupiettes with shallot, then cover with cheese slices. Roll up.

3. Carefully arrange, seam side down, in ovenproof casserole. Sprinkle with apple juice. Cover and bake for 25 minutes. Transfer to warmed serving plate. Cover to keep warm. Pour exuded juices into heavy-bottom saucepan.

4. To saucepan add 2 teaspoons parsley and balance of sauce ingredients, except arrowroot mixture. Bring to boil. Cook over medium heat until liquid is reduced to ½ cup. Slowly add arrowroot mixture to sauce, using only enough to thicken slightly. Pour over paupiettes, sprinkle with balance of parsley, and serve.

NOTE: Dish may be prepared ahead of time through step 2, then arranged in casserole and refrigerated until ready to bake. Allow 30 minutes to complete recipe.

VARIATION: Remove saucepan from heat after liquid is reduced to ½ cup (step 4) and stir in 2 tablespoons evaporated skim milk.

Chili Chicken Breasts

~

YIELD: SERVES 4

When tasting time comes, you'll ask in astonishment, "How can white meat taste so different?" The secret is not only my unique array of ingredients, but the special techniques I've developed over the years for locking in flavor. You can master those techniques easily by following this recipe or the other white meat recipes in this book.

Per serving
Calories: 184
Carbohydrate: 5 g
Protein: 30 g
Fat: 5 g
Saturated fat: 1 g
Cholesterol: 73 mg
Dietary fiber: 0.9 g
Sodium: 76 mg
Exchanges: 4 lean meat

2   teaspoons Italian olive oil

1   small rib celery, minced

3   cloves garlic, minced

1   teaspoon peeled and minced fresh ginger

1   tablespoon minced sweet green pepper

1   small leek, white part and 2 inches of adjacent green part, minced

2   whole chicken breasts, boned and skinned (1¼ pounds boned weight), each cut in half, flattened to uniform thickness

1   teaspoon chili con carne seasoning

¼   teaspoon dried thyme leaves, crushed

½   teaspoon smoked yeast (see page 297)

3   tablespoons each dry vermouth and apple juice (no sugar added)

4   dashes ground red (cayenne) pepper (optional)

1. Heat oil in nonstick skillet over medium heat until hot. Spread the 5 minced ingredients across skillet. Cook for 1 minute. Wash chicken and pat dry with paper toweling. Lay on top of minced mixture.

2. Sprinkle uncooked side of chicken with chili con carne seasoning, thyme, and smoked yeast. Let first side brown lightly, about 3 minutes. Turn and sauté on second side until lightly browned.

3. Add vermouth and apple juice. Turn chicken to coat. Bring to simmering point. Cover and simmer gently for 25 minutes, turning twice.

4. Uncover and cook for 2 minutes, turning every 30 seconds and spooning with small amount of sauce. Taste. If you prefer a spicier sauce, sprinkle with ground red pepper to taste. Finished chicken will be moist and tender.

Apple-Mint Chicken Paupiettes

YIELD: SERVES 4

Per serving
Calories: 197
Carbohydrate: 8 g
Protein: 30 g
Fat: 5 g
Saturated fat: 1 g
Cholesterol: 73 mg
Dietary fiber: 1.2 g
Sodium: 60 mg
Exchanges: 4 lean meat
　　　　　½ fruit

2　whole chicken breasts, boned and skinned (1½ pounds boned weight), each breast cut in half lengthwise

1　teaspoon ground coriander

⅛　teaspoon ground red (cayenne) pepper

1　teaspoon dried tarragon leaves, crushed

2　teaspoons Italian olive oil

3　cloves garlic, minced

1　medium onion, minced

3　tablespoons minced sweet red pepper

1　crisp, tart apple (such as Granny Smith), peeled, cored, and coarsely chopped

2　tablespoons minced fresh mint leaves (See Note)

¼　cup each dry vermouth and apple juice (no sugar added)

1. Wash chicken. Dry thoroughly with paper toweling. Place between 2 sheets of waxed paper. Flatten to ⅜-inch thickness.

2. Sprinkle and rub on one side with coriander, ground red pepper, and tarragon.

3. Heat oil in nonstick skillet over medium heat until hot. Sauté garlic, onion, and sweet red pepper for 2 minutes. Do not brown. Preheat oven to 375°F.

4. Spoon equal amounts of sautéed mixture over each chicken breast. Then sprinkle with chopped apple and 1 tablespoon mint. Roll up. Place seam side down in ovenproof casserole.

5. Heat vermouth and apple juice to boiling point. Pour over paupiettes. Cover and bake for 25 minutes. Drain bundles and transfer to serving casserole. Cover to keep warm.

6. Pour liquids and solids from casserole into heavy-bottom saucepan. Reduce over medium-high heat until almost all liquid evaporates. Pour into food blender and puree until smooth. Spoon over chicken. Sprinkle with balance of mint and serve.

NOTE: This recipe tastes best with fresh mint. If fresh mint isn't available, use fresh tarragon or rosemary, reducing fresh herb measurement to 4 teaspoons.

Skillet Chicken Dinner

~

YIELD: SERVES 4

It's quick and easy. Prepare the vegetables the night before and refrigerate. Next day add them to your savory cooked chicken and enjoy a complete meal in less than 30 minutes.

Per serving
Calories: 332
Carbohydrate: 26 g
Protein: 34 g
Fat: 9 g
Saturated fat: 2 g
Cholesterol: 125 mg
Dietary fiber: 3.0 g
Sodium: 112 mg
Exchanges: 1 starch/bread
           4 lean meat
           1 vegetable

4   red-skinned potatoes (1 pound)

2   medium carrots, peeled, cut into 1-inch slices

1   whole chicken breast, skinned and boned (¾ pound boned weight), cut into 4 pieces

2   chicken legs with thighs (1 pound), skinned and disjointed

½   teaspoon each ground marjoram, mild curry powder, and chili con carne seasoning

2   teaspoons Italian olive oil

2   cloves garlic, minced

1   tablespoon each minced sweet green pepper and shallot

1   teaspoon peeled and minced fresh ginger

¼   cup pineapple juice (no sugar added)

⅓   cup Easy Chicken Stock (page 216)

1. Cut each potato in half. Combine with carrots in saucepan. Cover with water and boil for 12 minutes or steam in steamer until almost done. Drain and set aside.

2. Wash chicken and dry with paper toweling. Rub all over with marjoram, curry, and chili seasoning.

3. Heat oil in well-seasoned iron skillet over medium heat until hot. Spread garlic, green pepper, shallot, and ginger across skillet. Sauté for 1 minute, taking care not to scorch. Lay chicken pieces on top of minced mixture. Brown lightly (about 5 minutes).

4. Pour pineapple juice and stock over chicken. Bring to simmering point. Cover and simmer for 25 minutes, turning once midway.

5. Skin potatoes, if desired. Add to skillet with carrots. Raise heat slightly under skillet. Cook for 10 minutes, turning chicken and vegetables every 2 minutes, taking care that skinned chicken doesn't stick to skillet. (Piggyback white meat on top of dark meat after 2 minutes.) Sauce will be reduced and syrupy. Chicken and vegetables will take on a golden hue.

Cumin Chicken

~

YIELD: SERVES 4

Cumin, so the legend has it, possesses the power to bind a person to a place. So don't be surprised when your family and guests take one bite of your Cumin Chicken and exclaim, "We never want to eat anyplace else."

Per serving
Calories: 261
Carbohydrate: 4 g
Protein: 32 g
Fat: 11 g
Saturated fat: 3 g
Cholesterol: 104 mg
Dietary fiber: 1.0 g
Sodium: 110 mg
Exchanges: 4 lean meat
1 fat

4 small chicken legs with thighs (1¾ pounds), skinned and disjointed

½ teaspoon dried thyme leaves, crushed

⅛ teaspoon crushed red (cayenne) pepper

½ teaspoon ground coriander

2 teaspoons Italian olive oil

1 tablespoon minced sweet green pepper

2 cloves garlic, minced

2 shallots, minced

1 tablespoon grated carrot

⅓ cup Easy Chicken Stock (page 216)

2 tablespoons dry vermouth

1 teaspoon cumin seed, crushed

Minced fresh parsley

4 orange slices for garnish

1. Wash chicken and dry thoroughly with paper toweling. Sprinkle and rub with thyme, crushed red pepper, and coriander.

2. Heat oil in nonstick skillet until hot. Brown legs lightly all around. Transfer to plate.

3. Add minced green pepper, garlic, shallots, and carrot to skillet. Cook until slightly softened, turning constantly (about 4 minutes); do not add any more oil to skillet.

4. In a bowl, combine stock and vermouth. Add to skillet. Sprinkle with cumin seed. Bring to simmering point. Return chicken to skillet, turning and spooning with liquid to coat. Cover tightly and simmer for 35 minutes, turning twice.

5. Uncover, spoon with sauce. Recover and let stand for 10 minutes.

6. Uncover. Turn up heat under skillet and cook for 2 minutes, turning chicken often.

7. Serve chicken on individual warmed serving plates. Spoon with sauce. Sprinkle with parsley and garnish with orange slices.

Juicy Broiled Cornish Hens with Cilantro Sauce

~

YIELD: SERVES 4

A Rock Cornish hen is a breed of small fowl developed by crossing White Plymouth Rock and Cornish strains of chicken. The Cornish hen has a striking culinary advantage over its large barnyard relative. It can be stuffed and served as a single portion, as it is in most restaurants. Or, for the calorie-conscious food lover, it can be split down the middle, and half the bird served as a single portion. That's the way I serve it—but broiled, filled with mixed rice, and moistened with a cilantro-seasoned sauce. It makes a dish as satisfying as it is delectable.

Per serving
Calories: 227
Carbohydrate: 22 g
Protein: 26 g
Fat: 5 g
Saturated fat: 2 g
Cholesterol: 64 mg
Dietary fiber: 0.8 g
Sodium: 459 mg
Exchanges: 1 starch/bread
   3 lean meat

2   1½-pound Cornish hens (fresh if possible), skinned, split in half

1   tablespoon each fresh lemon juice and pineapple juice (no suagar added)

¾   teaspoon each ground marjoram and rosemary leaves, crushed

6   dashes ground red (cayenne) pepper

¾   cup each cooked wild rice and cooked enriched white rice combined

¾   cup Easy Chicken Stock (page 216)

¼   cup pineapple juice (no sugar added)

1   tablespoon minced cilantro (Chinese parsley; also called coriander), or 1 teaspoon dried cilantro leaves, crushed

2   tablespoons arrowroot flour (or cornstarch) dissolved in 2 tablespoons water

½   teaspoon finely grated lemon zest

1. Wash hens under cold running water. Dry well with paper toweling. Lay in shallow dish. Preheat oven to 350°F.

2. Combine next 4 listed ingredients in jar. Shake well to blend. Pour over hens, turning to coat. Let marinate for 30 minutes, turning once. Drain, reserving marinade.

3. Place hens meaty side up in shallow roasting pan. Roast for 15 minutes, brushing with reserved marinade once.

4. Reduce heat to 350°F. Brush hens with marinade, sprinkling a small amount over rice. Spoon equal amounts of rice mixture into cavities. Return hens to oven and roast until done (about 45 minutes).

If you're using frozen hens, cooking time may be 10 to 15 minutes longer.

5. While hens are roasting, combine stock, pineapple juice, and cilantro in heavy-bottom saucepan. Bring to simmering point and cook for 5 minutes. Liquid will reduce slightly. Dribble in only enough arrowroot mixture to make a slightly thickened gravy. Stir in lemon zest.

6. Remove hens from oven. Scoop out rice mixture. Place equal portions on individual warmed serving plates. Place hen halves over rice. Spoon with hot gravy. Serve balance of gravy on the side in sauceboat.

Roast Stuffed Turkey—The Most Sumptuous Ever

~

YIELD: TURKEY SERVES 6

GRAVY ABOUT 1 CUP (ALLOW 2 TABLESPOONS PER PERSON)

STUFFING SERVES 10

What more wonderful holiday gift can you give anybody than an introduction to the delights of this cuisine? And what better way to do that than with a turkey-and-stuffing holiday dinner? But don't tell anybody in advance that what you're serving is healthful food. Only when your dining room rings with cheers for the cook, reveal that your sumptuous dish is low in calories, fat, and cholesterol, is high in fiber, and contains no sugar or salt.

Sumptuous means a sensationally herb-seasoned bird with extravagant veal-and-wild-rice stuffing and a mouth-watering minty gravy. Naturally, leftovers make sumptuous hors d'oeuvres; you can find out how to concoct them by turning to the chapter "Hors d'Oeuvres and Condiments."

FOR THE GRAVY:

Skinned neck and trimmed gizzard from turkey

3 cups water

1 rib celery, sliced

2 fresh mushrooms, washed, trimmed, and sliced

1 small onion, sliced

1 small leek, white part plus 3 inches green part, trimmed, well washed, and sliced

1 small carrot, peeled and sliced

2 large cloves garlic, minced

3 sprigs fresh dill and/or parsley

2 tablespoons minced fresh mint, basil, or dill

2 tablespoons arrowroot flour (or cornstarch) dissolved in 2 tablespoons cold water

FOR THE STUFFING:

½ cup raw wild rice, well washed and drained

2 cups water

1 cup apple juice (no sugar added)

2 cups lightly toasted cubed rye bread (preferably unsalted) or my Magnificent Rye Bread (page 232)

½ teaspoon each dried thyme and sage leaves, crushed

½ teaspoon each ground cumin seed, ginger, and crushed fennel seed

½ cup stock from giblets

1 tablespoon Italian olive oil

1 rib celery, coarsely chopped

1 medium onion, minced

2 cloves garlic, minced

½ pound lean stewing veal, cut into ½-inch cubes (optional)

1 tablespoon apple cider vinegar

FOR THE TURKEY:

1 fresh 8-pound turkey

1 teaspoon Italian olive oil

½ teaspoon each ground sage and dried thyme leaves, crushed

6 dashes ground red (cayenne) pepper

⅓ cup defatted stock from giblets

For the gravy (2 tablespoons)
Calories: 8
Carbohydrate: 1 g
Protein: 1 g
Fat: trace
Saturated fat: trace
Cholesterol: 2 mg
Dietary fiber: 0 g
Sodium: 8 mg
Exchanges: free

For the stuffing without veal
(about ½ cup)
Calories: 82
Carbohydrate: 13 g
Protein: 2 g
Fat: 2 g
Saturated fat: trace
Cholesterol: trace
Dietary fiber: 1.0 g
Sodium: 50 mg
Exchanges: 1 starch/bread

For the stuffing with veal
(about ⅔ cup)
Calories: 117
Carbohydrate: 13 g
Protein: 7 g
Fat: 4 g
Saturated fat: 1 g
Cholesterol: 15 mg
Dietary fiber: 1.0 g
Sodium: 57 mg
Exchanges: 1 starch/bread
　　　　　½ lean meat

For the turkey (3 ounces)
Calories: 122
Carbohydrate: 0 g
Protein: 22 g
Fat: 4 g
Saturated fat: 1 g
Cholesterol: 15 mg
Dietary fiber: 1.0 g
Sodium: 57 mg
Exchanges: 3 lean meat

1. Prepare the stock for gravy a day ahead. Place neck and gizzard in small waterless cooker for 3 minutes, removing any scum that rises to the top. Add balance of ingredients except mint (or basil or dill) and arrowroot mixture. Lower heat to simmering, partially cover, and simmer for 1½ hours. Let cool in pot. Remove meat from neck. Refrigerate, well covered. Strain stock through fine mesh strainer or chinois (see Note) with bowl underneath. Then strain through washed cotton cheesecloth. Refrigerate overnight. Next day discard any hardened fat that rises to top.

2. To prepare stuffing, combine rice, water, and apple juice in saucepan. Bring to boil. Reduce heat to simmering and cook rice, uncovered, for 30 minutes. Drain. Rice will be slightly undercooked. Turn into bowl. Add bread cubes, herbs, spices, and stock.

3. Heat oil in well-seasoned iron skillet until hot. Sauté celery, onion, garlic, and veal over medium-high heat until lightly browned, stirring often (about 4 minutes). Add vinegar. Cook for 30 seconds. Combine and blend with rice mixture. Preheat oven to 350°F.

4. Trim any fat from turkey. Wash inside and out. Wipe dry with paper toweling. Fill body and neck cavities with stuffing. Sew up openings. Truss turkey. Prick skin every inch with sharp-pronged fork. Combine oil with herbs and ground red pepper. Mixture will be thick. Spread over turkey.

5. Place bird on rack in large roasting pan. Cover loosely with aluminum foil. Roast for 1 hour. Spoon half of stock over bird. Baste with pan juices. Re-cover. Raise oven heat to 375°F, and roast for 1 hour. Pour balance of stock over turkey, basting with pan juices. Re-cover loosely with aluminum foil, and roast for 1½ hours (total cooking time is about 3½ hours). Remove from oven. Pour pan juices into heavy-bottom saucepan. Cover turkey loosely with foil and let stand for 20 minutes before carving.

6. Meanwhile, finish gravy preparation. Pour balance of defatted stock into saucepan with pan juices. Add minced mint, basil, or dill. Bring to slow boil and cook until reduced to ¾ cup. Chop reserved meat from neck. Stir into gravy. Dribble in only enough arrowroot flour mixture to lightly thicken. Serve in sauceboat along with stuffing and turkey.

CAUTION: Do not use frozen, seasoned, butter-injected turkeys. If you do, the nutrition statistics will not apply.

NOTE: A chinois is a conical-shaped fine-meshed metal sieve. It's a superb accessory for straining stocks and sauces.

SERVING SUGGESTION: Brussels Sprouts with Mushrooms (page 102) makes a fine accompaniment to this dish.

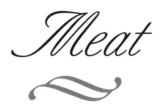

Meat

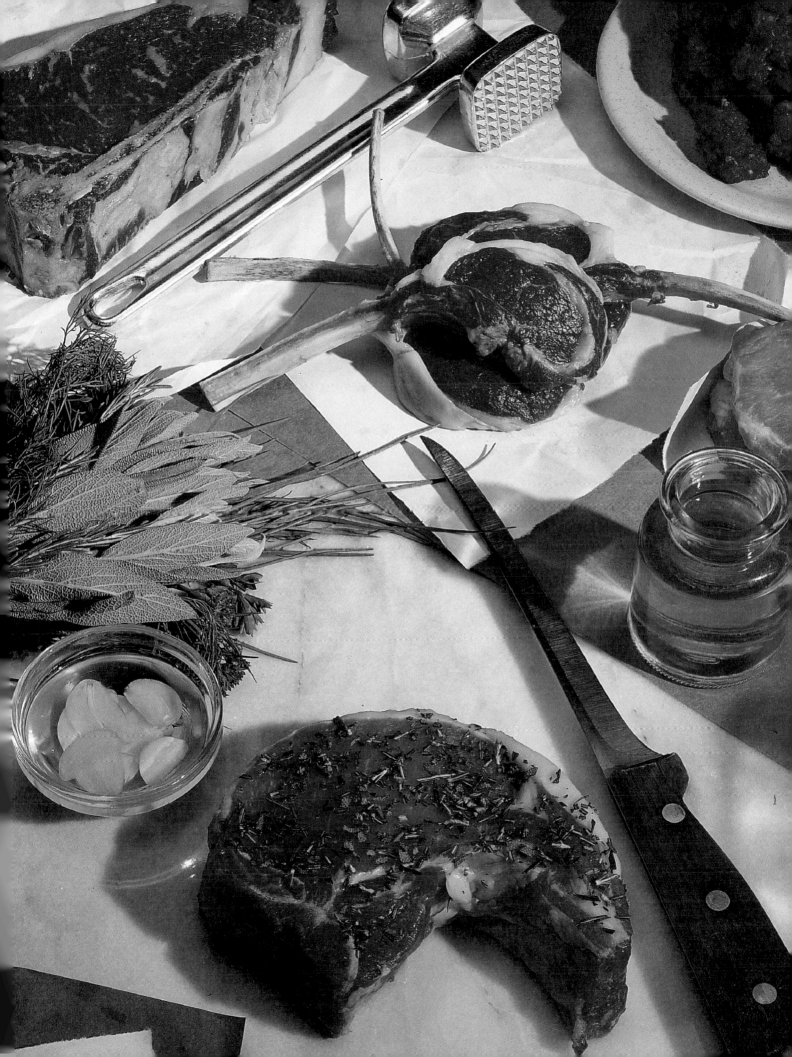

Romantic Filet Mignon

YIELD: SERVES 4

There are dishes so romantic they conjure visions of candlelight, Strauss waltzes, and two hearts beating as one. Among our favorites of this kind is this voluptuously prepared filet mignon—a cherished experience that will touch your heart.

Per serving
Calories: 208
Carbohydrate: 3 g
Protein: 26 g
Fat: 10 g
Saturated fat: 3 g
Cholesterol: 64 mg
Dietary fiber: 0.6 g
Sodium: 59 mg
Exchanges: 3½ lean meat
          ½ fat

4	small filet mignon steaks, well trimmed, cut 1 inch thick (total trimmed weight 1 pound)
½	teaspoon each dried tarragon and savory leaves, crushed
4	dashes ground red (cayenne) pepper
3	teaspoons Italian olive oil
2	large fresh mushrooms, washed, dried, trimmed, and coarsely chopped
1	teaspoon peeled and minced fresh ginger
2	large cloves garlic, minced
2	shallots, minced
3	tablespoons minced sweet green pepper
¼	cup each dry red wine and Easy Chicken Stock (page 216)
1	tablespoon tomato paste (no salt added)
2	tablespoons minced fresh parsley

1. Wipe steaks well with paper toweling. Sprinkle and rub on both sides with dried herbs and ground red pepper.

2. Heat 1½ teaspoons oil in well-seasoned iron skillet until hot. Sauté steaks for 5 minutes over medium heat on each side. Turn twice more and sauté for 2 minutes on each side. (Do not overcook; steak should be medium rare.) Transfer to warmed plate. Cover to keep warm.

3. Add balance of oil (1½ teaspoons) to skillet. (It will heat instantaneously.) Add mushrooms and minced ingredients and sauté until lightly browned, stirring constantly (about 3 minutes).

4. Combine wine, stock, tomato paste, and parsley. Pour into skillet. Bring to medium boil. Stir and cook until reduced by one-half. Pour any exuded juices from steak into skillet. Finished sauce will be thick.

5. Arrange steaks on warmed individual serving plates. Spoon with sauce, and serve immediately.

Macho Sirloin

YIELD: SERVES 4

For steak aficionados who demand a sauce that's aggressive and self-assertive, and who are sick and tired of that stuff that comes out of a bottle. The secret is the perfect blending of feisty ginger and brassy mustard with a team of tongue-tingling ingredients. As original as it's unforgettable.

Per serving
Calories: 228
Carbohydrate: 2 g
Protein: 30 g
Fat: 11 g
Saturated fat: 4 g
Cholesterol: 74 mg
Dietary fiber: 0.3 g
Sodium: 74 mg
Exchanges: 4 lean meat

1¼ pounds lean boneless sirloin, well-trimmed, cut 1 inch thick

1 teaspoon dried rosemary leaves, crushed

6 dashes ground red (cayenne) pepper

3 teaspoons Italian olive oil

2 large cloves garlic, minced

2 tablespoons minced sweet green pepper

2 large shallots, minced

1 teaspoon peeled and minced fresh ginger

⅓ cup dry vermouth

1 tablespoon tomato paste (no salt added)

½ teaspoon prepared Dijon mustard

1. Wipe steaks well with paper toweling. Sprinkle and rub on both sides with rosemary and ground red pepper.

2. Heat 1½ teaspoons oil in well-seasoned iron skillet until hot. Sauté steaks for 5 minutes over medium heat on each side. Turn twice more and sauté for 2 minutes on each side. Your steak should be medium rare. Transfer to warmed serving plate. Cover to keep warm.

3. Add balance of oil (1½ teaspoons) to skillet. Sauté minced ingredients until lightly browned, stirring constantly so that mixture doesn't stick to skillet (about 3 minutes).

4. Combine vermouth, tomato paste, and mustard. Add to skillet. Bring to medium boil. Stir and cook until reduced by half. Pour any exuded juices from steak into skillet. Finished sauce will be thick.

5. Transfer steak to carving board. Cut thinly at an angle. Serve portions on warmed individual plates spooned with hot sauce.

Braised Beef with Cranberries

YIELD: SERVES 6

Did you know that these bright red berries were probably the first native American fruit enjoyed by Europeans? They're such good keepers that, centuries before sophisticated preservation technology, they made the transatlantic journey packed in nothing but water. They're rife in vitamin C, rate "free" on the exchange list, and, properly prepared, are irresistible. Here, their unique tartness combines with fork-tender beef to create a dish as original as it is enticing.

Per serving
Calories: 242
Carbohydrate: 10 g
Protein: 29 g
Fat: 10 g
Saturated fat: 3 g
Cholesterol: 81 mg
Dietary fiber: 1.6 g
Sodium: 59 mg
Exchanges: 4 lean meat
         1 vegetable

1   2-pound slice top-round beef, well trimmed, or very lean center-cut shoulder steak, cut 1¼ inches thick

1   tablespoon ground coriander

½   teaspoon crushed red (cayenne) pepper

1   tablespoon Italian olive oil

½   cup peeled and diced yellow turnip

1   medium onion, coarsely chopped

1   sweet green pepper, seeded and coarsely chopped

1   medium carrot, peeled and coarsely chopped

1   rib celery, coarsely chopped

4   large cloves garlic, minced

1   tablespoon peeled and shredded fresh ginger

1   cup apple juice (no sugar added)

1   cup fresh cranberries

1   tablespoon medium-dry sherry

Bouquet garni (1 sprig parsley, 1 bay leaf, tied together with white thread)

1. Wipe meat with paper toweling. Rub on both sides with coriander and crushed red pepper. Set aside. Preheat oven to 350°F.

2. On top of stove, heat oil in heavy casserole until hot. Add next 7 ingredients. Sauté over medium-high heat until just softened and lightly browned, stirring often (about 10 minutes).

3. Transfer half of mixture to plate. Spread balance of mixture across casserole. Lay meat over mixture in casserole. Spread reserved mixture over meat.

4. Add apple juice, cranberries, sherry, and bouquet garni. Bring to simmering point, spooning sauce over meat. Cover. Bake for 1½ to 1¾ hours, basting and turning after 45 minutes and twice thereafter at equal intervals. Finished meat should be fork-tender. Remove from oven and let meat rest for 10 minutes.

5. Place meat on carving board. Slice thinly. Serve on warmed individual serving plates spooned with thick sauce.

Magic Skillet Swiss Steak

YIELD: SERVES 4

The magic is turnip. What? Turnip? Yes, turnip. And herbs and spices never used before with Swiss steak, and just the right amount of smoked yeast. The magic that transforms any ordinary dish into an extraordinary one is the unusual. But try this unusual dish, and it will become a usual item on your family's menu.

Per serving
Calories: 230
Carbohydrate: 4 g
Protein: 28 g
Fat: 11 g
Saturated fat: 3 g
Cholesterol: 56 mg
Dietary fiber: 0.7 g
Sodium: 47 mg
Exchanges: 4 lean meat

1¼ pounds top round of beef, well trimmed, cut ½ inch thick, or flattened to ½-inch thickness

1 tablespoon unbleached flour

1 teaspoon dried savory leaves, crushed

6 dashes ground red (cayenne) pepper

½ teaspoon smoked yeast (see page 297)

4 teaspoons Italian olive oil

1 teaspoon peeled and minced fresh ginger

1 tablespoon minced sweet green pepper

1 leek, white part plus 1 inch green part, well washed and minced

2 tablespoons peeled and minced yellow turnip (rutabaga)

2 cloves garlic, minced

⅓ cup dry red wine

Watercress sprigs for garnish

1. Wipe meat with paper toweling. Combine flour with savory, ground red pepper, and smoked yeast. Sprinkle over both sides of meat; then press into meat.

2. Heat 1½ teaspoons oil over medium heat in well-seasoned iron skillet until hot. Brown meat lightly on one side. Add 1½ teaspoons oil. Turn meat and lightly brown on second side. Transfer to dish. Cover to keep warm.

3. Add balance of oil (1 teaspoon) to skillet. Sauté ginger, green pepper, leek, turnip, and garlic until lightly browned, stirring continuously.

4. Add wine. Scrape skillet to remove any browned particles. Bring to simmering point. Return browned meat to skillet, spooning with sauce. Cover and simmer gently for 45 to 50 minutes until fork-tender, turning and spooning with sauce at 15-minute intervals.

5. Transfer meat to carving board. Slice thinly at an angle. Serve on hot serving plate, spooned with sauce that has been reheated to simmering point. Garnish with watercress sprigs.

Indian-Style Meatballs

YIELD: SERVES 4

*M*ild Indian spices marry with good old-fashioned American ingredients to produce meatballs such as you've never tasted before. They're intriguing conversation pieces, whether they're served as a main dish with rice or bulgur, or with steamed, crunchy vegetables such as broccoli, Brussels sprouts, or carrots.

Per serving
Calories: 275
Carbohydrate: 9 g
Protein: 25 g
Fat: 15 g
Saturated fat: 6 g
Cholesterol: 105 mg
Dietary fiber: 1.4 g
Sodium: 102 mg
Exchanges: ½ starch/bread
          3 lean meat
          1 fat

2   tablespoons dark seedless raisins

¼   cup evaporated skim milk

1   pound extra-lean ground beef

2   tablespoons each toasted whole-wheat bread crumbs (preferably unsalted) or my Coriander Whole-Wheat Bread (page 224), and unprocessed bran

½   teaspoon each ground coriander, cinnamon, and cumin seed

⅛   teaspoon ground red (cayenne) pepper

3   teaspoons Italian olive oil

2   cloves garlic, minced

1   scallion, minced

1   teaspoon peeled and minced fresh ginger

1   egg (use ½ egg yolk, all egg white), lightly beaten

4   teaspoons tomato paste (no salt added)

½   cup dry red wine

1. Combine raisins with milk in small bowl. Let soak for 10 minutes.

2. In a separate bowl, place meat, crumbs, bran, spices, and ground red pepper. Blend well.

3. Heat 2 teaspoons oil over medium heat in nonstick skillet until hot. Sauté garlic, scallion, and ginger until wilted but not brown (about 3 minutes). Turn into bowl with meat. Blend.

4. Combine egg with 1 teaspoon tomato paste. Add to bowl. Then add raisin mixture and blend well. Shape into 16 balls.

5. Heat balance of oil (1 teaspoon) in skillet until hot. Add meatballs and brown over medium-high heat on all sides.

6. In a cup, beat wine and balance of tomato paste (3 teaspoons) with fork. Add to skillet. Bring to simmering point. Cover and simmer for 20 minutes, turning meatballs and spooning with sauce, every 5 minutes. Sauce will be reduced and slightly thickened, and meatballs will be a luscious bronze color. Serve immediately.

Cranberry Meat Loaf

~

YIELD: SERVES 4

No, you don't taste the cranberries as such. But sweetened with apple juice and sweet spices, this incomparably tart berry adds such an exquisite new taste to this dish that your family will never again protest, "What? Meat loaf again?" As the cranberry season comes to an end, why not, as I do, scoop up a dozen or more packages into your shopping cart, then freeze them for all-season enjoyment.

Per serving
Calories: 246
Carbohydrate: 10 g
Protein: 23 g
Fat: 13 g
Saturated fat: 5 g
Cholesterol: 70 mg
Dietary fiber: 1.3 g
Sodium: 74 mg
Exchanges: 3 lean meat
         ½ fruit
         1 fat

1	pound extra-lean ground beef from tenderloin
¼	cup soft Coriander Whole-Wheat Bread crumbs (page 224) (see also Note 1 below)
¼	cup cooked brown rice or buckwheat groats (kasha)
½	teaspoon each ground coriander, mild curry powder, cinnamon, and crushed dried thyme leaves
6	dashes ground red (cayenne) pepper
1½	teaspoons Italian olive oil

1	leek, white part plus 1 inch green part, well washed and minced
2	tablespoons minced sweet green pepper
2	cloves garlic, minced
⅓	cup fresh cranberries, rinsed, picked over, and coarsely chopped (see Note 2)
½	sweet crisp apple, peeled, cored, and coarsely chopped
½	cup apple juice (no sugar added)
¼	teaspoon sweet soft corn oil margarine

1. Place first 5 listed ingredients in bowl. Blend well (fingers will do the best job).

2. Heat oil in nonstick skillet until hot. Sauté leek, green pepper, and garlic until wilted but not brown. Stir into meat mixture.

3. Add cranberries, apple, and apple juice, blending well.

4. Shape meat into an 8" × 4" loaf. Place in margarine-greased baking pan. (Do not use loaf pan.) Bake in preheated 350°F oven for 20 minutes. Skim off any fat. Then spoon loaf with sauce. Return to oven uncovered, and bake for 25 minutes. Most of sauce will evaporate.

5. Transfer to hot serving plate. Spoon with remaining sauce, and serve.

NOTES:

1. Commercial low-sodium whole-wheat bread may be substituted for Coriander Whole-Wheat Bread.

2. The food processor chops cranberries in seconds.

VARIATION: Substitute 4 tablespoons each unsweetened grape juice and unsweetened pineapple juice for apple juice. Lovely!

Curried Steakburger with Onions and Mushrooms

~

YIELD: SERVES 4

There's generally no salt added to curry powder. It's a tongue-tingling blend of cardamom, coriander, cumin seed, fenugreek, turmeric, and, sometimes, ginger, allspice, and mustard. Here it's used so subtly that you never taste the curry as such. You just know that you've never tasted a burger like this before. But you'll want to taste it again and again and again.

Per serving
Calories: 243
Carbohydrate: 5 g
Protein: 23 g
Fat: 15 g
Saturated fat: 5 g
Cholesterol: 70 mg
Dietary fiber: 0.9 g
Sodium: 78 mg
Exchanges: 3 lean meat
　　　　　　1 vegetable
　　　　　　1 fat

1　pound extra-lean ground beef

3　teaspoons tomato paste (no salt added)

4　tablespoons dry red wine

2　teaspoons mild curry powder

6　dashes ground red (cayenne) pepper

½　teaspoon dried thyme leaves, crushed

2　tablespoons minced fresh parsley

½　teaspoon caraway seed, partially crushed

¼　cup rye bread crumbs (preferably unsalted) or my Magnificent Rye Bread (page 232)

3　teaspoons Italian olive oil

1　large onion, thinly sliced, separated into rings

2　large cloves garlic, minced

¼　pound fresh mushrooms, washed, dried, trimmed, and thinly sliced

1. Place beef in bowl. Combine 2 teaspoons tomato paste with 3 tablespoons wine. Stir into meat.

2. Combine curry powder with 2 dashes ground red pepper, thyme, 1 tablespoon parsley, and caraway seed. Add to meat mixture, blending well with spoon. Then add crumbs and blend. (Your fingers will do the most efficient job here.) Shape into 8 burgers, ½ inch thick. Set aside.

3. Heat 1½ teaspoons oil over medium heat in well-seasoned iron skillet until moderately hot. Sauté onion rings and garlic for 1 minute. Add mushrooms and sauté until lightly browned, stirring often (about 4 minutes). Sprinkle with 2 dashes ground red pepper. Transfer to dish. Cover to keep warm.

4. Spread balance of oil (1½ teaspoons) across skillet with spatula. Heat for 30 seconds. Add burgers and sauté until browned on both

sides, taking care that skillet doesn't get too hot. If meat appears to be sticking, loosen with spatula and lower heat. Do not overcook. (Fifty percent of nutritive value of meat is destroyed by overcooking.) Transfer to warmed individual plates. Cover to keep warm.

5. Return sautéed onion mixture to skillet. Combine balance of tomato paste (1 teaspoon) with balance of wine (1 tablespoon) and parsley (1 tablespoon). Add to skillet. Sprinkle with balance of ground red pepper (2 dashes), stirring to combine. Sauté briefly until heated through. Spoon over burgers, and serve immediately.

NOTE: Commercial good quality rye bread may be substituted for Magnificent Rye Bread.

VARIATION: Substitute 4 tablespoons Easy Chicken Stock (page 216) for wine and add 1 teaspoon wine vinegar to skillet in step 5.

Sautéed Veal Cutlets with Watercress

YIELD: SERVES 4

Did you ever dream of being a food critic? It's easy. First, build up a vocabulary: succulent, regal, delightful, fork-tender, perfumed. Then weave the words together: "This delightful dish of succulent fork-tender veal perfumed with herbs and spices makes a regal repast." And that's what you would write after tasting Sautéed Veal Cutlets with Watercress.

Per serving
Calories: 249
Carbohydrate: 4 g
Protein: 24 g
Fat: 14 g
Saturated fat: 6 g
Cholesterol: 89 mg
Dietary fiber: 0.2 g
Sodium: 66 mg
Exchanges: 4 lean meat
          1 fat

4	veal cutlets, cut from the leg, ¾ inch thick (1¼ pounds)
1	tablespoon fresh lemon juice
1	teaspoon dried rosemary leaves, well-crushed
½	teaspoon chili con carne seasoning
1	tablespoon Italian olive oil
3	cloves garlic, minced
2	large shallots, minced
1	teaspoon peeled and minced fresh ginger
1	tablespoon coarsely grated carrot
¼	cup each Easy Chicken Stock (page 216) and fresh orange juice
4	dashes ground red (cayenne) pepper
2	tablespoons finely minced watercress (leaves only)

1. Wipe cutlets with paper toweling. Place in flat dish. Sprinkle with lemon juice on both sides, rubbing juice into meat. Let stand at room temperature for 10 minutes. Then drain on paper toweling.

2. Rub cutlets with rosemary and chili con carne seasoning. Heat oil over medium heat in well-seasoned iron skillet until hot. Sauté cutlets over medium heat until lightly browned on one side (about 4 minutes). Turn.

3. Add garlic, shallots, ginger, and carrot. Sauté with meat until all ingredients are lightly browned (about 5 minutes).

4. Add stock and orange juice to skillet. Sprinkle cutlets with ground red pepper. Bring liquid to simmering point, spooning over cutlets. Cover and simmer gently for 10 minutes. Turn, spoon with sauce. Re-cover and simmer for 10 minutes. Repeat sequence twice. Total cooking time will be about 40 minutes.

5. Transfer meat to warmed serving plate. Cover to keep warm. Add watercress to skillet. Turn up heat under skillet and cook for 1 minute. Spoon sauce over cutlets, and serve immediately.

Miracle Veal Chops

YIELD: SERVES 4

Do you ever play "What's in That Dish?" with your family? The object is to identify all the ingredients. When I played the game with this dish, my husband exclaimed, "I don't care what's in it—it's a miracle!" Hence, the title. P.S. The miracle gets a little help from chopped eggplant and pineapple juice.

Per serving
Calories: 252
Carbohydrate: 7 g
Protein: 23 g
Fat: 14 g
Saturated fat: 6 g
Cholesterol: 79 mg
Dietary fiber: 13 g
Sodium: 62 mg
Exchanges: 3 lean meat
      1 vegetable
      1 fat

4	loin veal chops (1½ pounds), well trimmed
½	teaspoon each ground sage, marjoram, and chili con carne seasoning
6	dashes ground red (cayenne) pepper
4	teaspoons Italian olive oil
2	cups peeled and coarsely chopped eggplant (½ pound)
1	large shallot, minced
2	large cloves garlic, minced
2	tablespoons minced onion
1	teaspoon apple cider vinegar
¼	cup each Easy Chicken Stock (page 216) and pineapple juice (no sugar added)
1	tablespoon tomato paste (no salt added)

1. Wipe chops with paper toweling. Rub both sides with herbs and seasonings.

2. Heat 2 teaspoons oil over medium heat in well-seasoned iron skillet until hot. Sauté chops until lightly browned. Transfer to plate.

3. Heat balance (2 teaspoons) of oil in skillet. Sauté eggplant, shallot, garlic, and onion until lightly browned, stirring constantly (about 3 minutes). Add vinegar. Stir and cook for 1 minute.

4. Combine stock, pineapple juice, and tomato paste. Add to skillet, stirring to blend. Return chops to skillet, turning and spooning with sauce. Bring to simmering point. Cover and simmer for 5 minutes, turning and spooning with sauce twice.

5. Uncover. Reduce sauce over medium heat for 5 minutes, turning chops and stirring eggplant often. Serve on individual warmed serving plates, spooned with thick sauce.

SERVING SUGGESTION: Steamed fresh corn removed from the cob makes a colorful and high-fiber accompaniment to this unusual dish.

Two-Way Savory Veal Chops: Broiled and Sautéed

~

YIELD: SERVES 4

You use the same ingredients in both ways but not quite the same way, which proves once again it's not always what you do but the way you do it that counts. Either way, you can look forward to an easy-to-make delight, as sophisticated as it is novel.

4	loin or rib veal chops (1½ pounds), well trimmed
½	teaspoon each dried savory and rosemary leaves, crushed
½	teaspoon each ground ginger and chili con carne seasoning
1	teaspoon Italian olive oil
2	large cloves garlic, minced

2	shallots, minced
1	tablespoon wine vinegar or balsamic vinegar
1	tablespoon pineapple juice (no sugar added)
1	tablespoon minced fresh parsley
	Lemon wedges

Per serving
Calories: 196
Carbohydrate: 1 g
Protein: 22 g
Fat: 11 g
Saturated fat: 5 g
Cholesterol: 78 mg
Dietary fiber: 0.1 g
Sodium: 51 mg
Exchanges: 3 lean meat
⅓ fat

BROILED:

1. To prepare broiled chops, wipe with paper toweling. Combine balance of ingredients, except lemon wedges, in small bowl, blending with fork. Mixture will be thick.

2. Spread half of mixture over one side of chops. Place on rack in shallow broiling pan and broil 4 inches from heat, coated side up, for 8 to 10 minutes, or until lightly browned. (Cooking time will vary with thickness of chops.) Turn, spread with balance of mixture and broil for 8 to 10 minutes, or until lightly browned. For greatest taste and nutrition, finished chops should be delicately pink inside and lightly browned on both sides. Garnish with lemon wedges and serve.

SAUTÉED:

1. To prepare sautéed chops, wipe meat with paper toweling. Combine dried herbs, ginger, and chili seasoning. Sprinkle and rub over meat on both sides.

2. Heat 2 teaspoons Italian olive oil over medium heat in well-seasoned iron skillet until hot. Spread garlic and shallots across skillet. Sauté for 1 minute. Lay chops on minced ingredients. Brown lightly on both sides (about 8 minutes).

3. Add vinegar. Cook for 30 seconds. Increase pineapple juice measurement to ¼ cup. Add to skillet, spooning chops with juice. Bring to simmering point. Reduce heat, cover, and simmer gently for 30 to 35 minutes. Do not overcook. Serve chops on warmed individual plates, sprinkled with parsley and garnished with lemon wedges.

Veal and Meatballs with Peppers

~

YIELD: SERVES 5

These tender veal chunks and meatballs enrobed in a delicately herbed-and-spiced tomato sauce deserve a Tiffany presentation. So serve in your most elegant tureen and delight the eyes of the beholders as well as their palates.

Per serving
Calories: 274
Carbohydrate: 9 g
Protein: 25 g
Fat: 14 g
Saturated fat: 6 g
Cholesterol: 83 mg
Dietary fiber: 2.4 g
Sodium: 67 mg
Exchanges: 3 lean meat
2 vegetable
1 fat

2   tablespoons unbleached flour

½   teaspoon ground ginger

1   teaspoon freshly grated Parmesan cheese

1   pound lean veal (cut from the leg) cut into ½-inch chunks

½   pound lean ground veal

1   large shallot, minced

4½ teaspoons Italian olive oil

3   medium sweet red or green peppers, cored, seeded, and cut into ⅜-inch slivers

2   large cloves garlic, minced

1   large onion, minced

½   teaspoon each dried savory leaves, crushed, and ground cumin seed

1   teaspoon mild curry powder

2   tablespoons dry vermouth

1   cup canned Italian plum tomatoes (no salt added), chopped

1   teaspoon fresh lemon juice

1   tablespoon minced fresh parsley

¼   pound fresh mushrooms, washed, dried, trimmed, and sliced

1. In small bowl, combine flour, ginger, and Parmesan cheese.

2. Dry meat thoroughly with paper toweling. Combine ground meat with shallot. Shape into 8 balls. Dredge veal chunks with meatballs in flour mixture, shaking off excess.

3. Heat 1½ teaspoons of oil over medium heat in well-seasoned iron skillet until hot. Sauté meats until very lightly browned, turning often (about 5 minutes). Transfer to plate.

4. Heat 1½ teaspoons of oil in skillet until hot (do not let skillet smoke). Sauté green peppers, garlic, and onion for 2 minutes, turning frequently. Sprinkle with savory and spices. Stir and sauté for 2 more minutes.

5. Add vermouth. Cook and stir for 1 minute, scraping skillet to loosen any browned particles. Add tomatoes, lemon juice, and parsley. Bring to simmering point. Return browned meats to skillet. Spoon with sauce. Cover and simmer over very low heat for 40 minutes, stirring twice.

6. Five minutes before meat is done, heat balance of oil (1½ teaspoons) over medium heat in nonstick skillet until hot. Sauté mushrooms for 3 minutes, stirring continually. They will not brown. Remove skillet from heat. Stir mushrooms into meat mixture. Cover and let stand for 10 minutes. Reheat, if necessary, and serve.

SERVING SUGGESTION:
Wonderful served over a bed of cooked brown or wild rice. Or, if you're adventurous, try whole wheat couscous for the most luxurious bed that any meat could rest on.

Veal Shanks in Imperial Sauce

YIELD: SERVES 4

If you're like me, there comes a time when you get the irresistible urge to dazzle family and friends with a specialty of awesome lavishness. That's why I dreamed up my Imperial Sauce to glorify one of the most luscious cuts of veal.

Per serving
Calories: 334
Carbohydrate: 11 g
Protein: 30 g
Fat: 17 g
Saturated fat: 7 g
Cholesterol: 105 mg
Dietary fiber: 1.6 g
Sodium: 107 mg
Exchanges: 4 lean meat
2 vegetable
1 fat

4	2-inch meaty slices veal shank (about 1½ pounds), well trimmed
⅛	teaspoon ground red (cayenne) pepper
½	teaspoon each ground sage, dried thyme, and savory leaves, crushed
2	tablespoons unbleached flour
4	teaspoons Italian olive oil
1	large onion, minced
3	large cloves garlic, minced
2	tablespoons coarsely chopped sweet green pepper
1	rib celery, coarsely chopped
⅓	cup coarsely chopped yellow turnip (rutabaga)
2	large fresh mushrooms, washed, dried, trimmed, and coarsely chopped (optional)
½	cup each dry vermouth, Easy Chicken Stock (page 216), and apple juice (no sugar added)
2	tablespoons tomato paste (no salt added)
1	teaspoon dried mint leaves, crumbled
1	teaspoon finely grated lemon zest

1. Wipe meat with damp cloth. Dry with paper toweling. Rub with ground red pepper and herbs. Then sprinkle with flour, smoothing a thin film over meat so that herbs adhere to veal.

2. Heat 2 teaspoons oil over medium-high heat in Dutch oven until hot. Brown shanks on all sides. Transfer to plate.

3. Heat balance of oil (2 teaspoons) in Dutch oven until hot. Brown onion, garlic, green pepper, celery, turnip, and mushrooms until lightly browned, stirring constantly (about 3 minutes).

4. In a bowl, combine and blend vermouth, stock, apple juice, and tomato paste. Pour around meat.

Bring to boil, scraping to loosen browned particles. Return meat to pot. Spoon with sauce. Sprinkle with mint. Cover tightly and simmer for 2 hours, spooning with sauce every ½ hour and turning 3 times. Finished meat should be fork tender and come away from bone.

5. Serve on individual warmed plates, spooned with thick sauce and sprinkled with lemon zest. Serve any leftover sauce along with meat in sauceboat.

SERVING SUGGESTION: Wild rice and green salad are sumptuous accompaniments to this luxurious dish.

Exotic Leg of Lamb

YIELD: SERVES 8

*L*amb has long been a favorite in my kitchen because you can do so many things with it. The leg is the leanest of lamb cuts, and, naturally, it's high on my recommended list. Don't pass up leg of lamb because it's a bit on the expensive side, or because your family is too small to consume all that meat in one meal. Buy a half leg instead of a whole one, or ask your butcher for lamb steaks cut from the leg; either way your purchase becomes affordable, and there's no excess to worry about.

If you've never tried leg of lamb before, there's a wonderful new experience ahead of you; and if you have tried it—well, there's still a wonderful new experience ahead of you.

Per serving
Calories: 296
Carbohydrate: trace
Protein: 34 g
Fat: 17 g
Saturated fat: 10 g
Cholesterol: 103 mg
Dietary fiber: 0.1 g
Sodium: 84 mg
Exchanges: 4 medium-fat
  meat

½ leg of lamb (3½ pounds), prefer-ably shank end, well trimmed

3 large cloves garlic, minced

½ teaspoon dry mustard

1 teaspoon each ground coriander and dried rosemary leaves, crushed

¼ teaspoon ground ginger

2 teaspoons juniper berries, well crushed

¼ cup sweet Madeira wine (also called Malmsey)

2 teaspoons tomato paste (no salt added)

1 teaspoon fresh lemon juice

2 teaspoons Italian olive oil

1 tablespoon minced fresh parsley

¼ cup Easy Chicken Stock (page 216)

1. Wipe meat with damp paper tow-eling, then again with dry paper toweling. Place on large sheet of heavy-duty aluminum foil.

2. In a bowl, combine balance of ingredients, except stock, blending well. (Mixture will be thick.) Spoon over meat, turning to coat. Close foil tightly. Let marinate at room temperature for 1 hour, turn-ing foil bundle upside down several times. Drain liquid from bundle into measuring cup with stock. Set stock mixture aside. Preheat oven to 400°F.

3. Place meat on rack in roasting pan. Roast, uncovered, for 15 minutes. Baste with stock mixture. Reduce heat to 350°F. Roast for 45 to 50 minutes, basting twice more with balance of stock at 15-minute intervals. Remove from oven. Cover loosely with aluminum foil and let meat rest for 10 minutes. Meat will be medium rare.

4. Slice thin and serve, spooned with pan juices.

NOTE: Roasting time may vary slightly with thickness of meat and bone.

SERVING SUGGESTION: In step 4, serve with pan juices and Delicate Juniper Berry Sauce (page 211) on the side.

Tangy Roast Leg of Lamb

YIELD: SERVES 6

Per serving
Calories: 303
Carbohydrate: 2 g
Protein: 32 g
Fat: 17 g
Saturated fat: 10 g
Cholesterol: 92 mg
Dietary fiber: 0.3 g
Sodium: 77 mg
Exchanges: 4 medium-fat
        meat

¼   cup wine vinegar

2   tablespoons Italian olive oil

½   teaspoon dried fine herbs

2   teaspoons chili con carne seasoning

2   large cloves garlic, minced

1   large shallot, minced

3   tablespoons tomato juice (no salt added)

6   dashes ground red (cayenne) pepper

1   tablespoon grated orange zest (preferably from navel orange)

2   pounds well-trimmed boned and rolled leg of lamb, preferably from shank end (see Note)

1. Prepare marinade by combining all ingredients except lamb in a jar, shaking to blend.

2. Wipe meat with damp paper toweling, then again with dry paper toweling. Tear off large sheet of heavy-duty aluminum foil. Lay lamb on foil. Spoon half of marinade over meat, turning to coat. Reserve balance of marinade. Close foil tightly. Let marinate at room temperature for 2 hours. Preheat oven to 400°F.

3. Drain meat. Place on rack in shallow roasting pan. Combine marinade remaining in aluminum foil with reserved marinade. Set aside. Roast meat, uncovered, for 15 minutes. Baste with marinade. Reduce heat to 350°F. Roast for 30 to 40 minutes, basting every 10 minutes with marinade and turning after 20 minutes. Meat will be medium to medium rare. Cover loosely with aluminum foil and let meat rest for 10 minutes.

4. Slice thin with very sharp knife and serve immediately.

NOTE: Have your butcher trim meat well before rolling.

SERVING SUGGESTION: Delicate Juniper Berry Sauce (page 211) may be served on the side, if desired, and Rich Puree of Broccoli (page 96) makes an extraordinary vegetable accompaniment to this luxurious dish.

Curried Lamb Kabobs

YIELD: SERVES 4

Kabobs, which may have originated over campfires in the Fertile Crescent, are now a favorite the world around. They're simple to prepare, and serving them is a form of theater. Here, lean lamb is tenderly cosseted in an exotic fruit-spice marinade, then skewered alternately with slivers of bright red pepper and deep-green unpeeled zucchini to produce a dish as colorful as it is desirable.

1   pound lean boneless lamb, cut from leg into 1-inch cubes

¾   cup fresh orange juice

¼   cup wine vinegar

1   tablespoon fresh lemon juice

1   teaspoon granulated fructose (see page 297)

½   teaspoon each ground coriander and cinnamon

1   tablespoon mild curry powder

⅛   teaspoon ground red (cayenne) pepper

1   onion, coarsely chopped

2   medium zucchini, well scrubbed, cut into 1-inch slices

1   medium sweet red pepper, seeded, cut into 1-inch pieces

1   large sweet onion, cut into ¼-inch slices

1   large navel orange, cut into 8 slices

Per serving
Calories: 284
Carbohydrate: 18 g
Protein: 24 g
Fat: 13 g
Saturated fat: 7 g
Cholesterol: 69 mg
Dietary fiber: 3.2 g
Sodium: 58 mg
Exchanges: 3 medium-fat
         meat
         1 vegetable
         1 fruit

1. Wipe meat dry with paper toweling. Place in bowl.

2. In a saucepan, combine orange juice, vinegar, lemon juice, fructose, coriander, cinnamon, curry, ground red pepper, and onion. Bring to boil. Reduce heat and simmer for 1 minute. Pour over meat. Cover and let stand for 6 hours or overnight, refrigerated.

3. Drain meat, reserving marinade. On each of 4 long skewers thread meat, zucchini, sweet red pepper, and onion slice, alternating ingredients in an attractive pattern.

4. Lay skewers on rack in shallow broiling pan. Brush with marinade. Broil under preheated broiler for 15 to 20 minutes, turning and brushing with marinade every 4 or 5 minutes. Meat should be delicately pink on inside and browned on outside.

5. Serve kabobs on skewers, or remove with fork to individual hot serving plates. Garnish each portion with 2 orange slices. Reheat remaining marinade and serve in sauceboat along with meat.

SERVING SUGGESTION: Wild rice makes a sumptuous accompaniment to this sophisticated dish. Try Delicious Wild Rice I or II (pages 120 and 121).

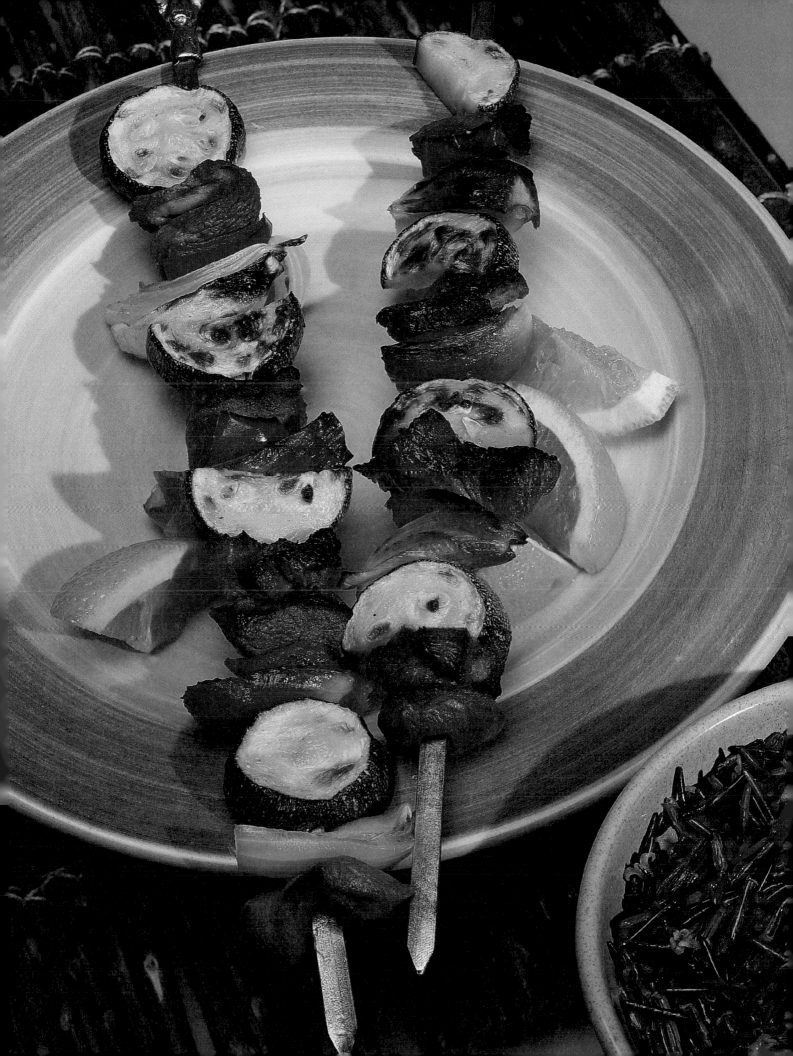

Baked Lamb Steaks—Skillet to Oven

YIELD: SERVES 4

Per serving
Calories: 312
Carbohydrate: 3 g
Protein: 32 g
Fat: 19 g
Saturated fat: 10 g
Cholesterol: 101 mg
Dietary fiber: 0.1 g
Sodium: 85 mg
Exchanges: 4 medium-fat
meat

2   lamb steaks cut from leg, ½ inch thick (1¼ pounds), each steak cut in half

1½ teaspoons dried rosemary leaves, crushed

1   teaspoon chili con carne seasoning

1   tablespoon Italian olive oil

3   large cloves garlic, minced

2   teaspoons peeled and minced fresh ginger

2   scallions, trimmed and sliced

1   tablespoon frozen orange juice concentrate

¼   cup Easy Chicken Stock (page 216)

2   tablespoons balsamic vinegar

3   sprigs fresh parsley

Orange slices

1. Trim meat of all visible fat. Wipe with damp paper toweling. Sprinkle and rub with rosemary and chili con carne seasoning. Preheat oven to 375°F.

2. Heat oil over medium-high heat in well-seasoned iron skillet. Add garlic, ginger, and scallions, and spread across skillet. Sauté for 1 minute. Lay meat on sautéed ingredients and sauté for 2 minutes on each side. (Meat will lose its pink color.)

3. Combine orange juice concentrate with stock and vinegar. Pour around sides of skillet. Add pars-ley. Bring to simmering point, turning meat several times to coat. Cover tightly. Bake for 45 minutes, turning once midway. Check skillet after 30 minutes to be certain meat isn't sticking. If skillet looks dry, add a little more stock, stirring to blend. Re-cover and continue baking. Finished lamb will be a deep mahogany brown and sauce will be reduced to a coating.

4. Serve immediately, garnished with orange slices.

Herbed-and-Spiced Lamb Chops

~

YIELD: SERVES 4

*E*nglish lamb, noted for its delicate texture and natural sweet taste, needs no seasoning to point up its exquisite flavor. But, alas, the same is not true of our American counterpart, which needs all the help it can get. My unusual mixture of dill and spices fills this need with little effort and great success.

Per serving
Calories: 262
Carbohydrate: 1 g
Protein: 23 g
Fat: 14 g
Saturated fat: 7 g
Cholesterol: 82 mg
Dietary fiber: 0.2 g
Sodium: 54 mg
Exchanges: 3 medium-fat
          meat

4   baby lamb chops, cut from rib, well trimmed, ends of bone removed (1½ pounds trimmed weight)

3   tablespoons wine vinegar

2   large cloves garlic, minced

2   large shallots, minced

2   tablespoons minced fresh dill

½   teaspoon each crushed dried tarragon and mild curry powder

⅛   teaspoon ground red (cayenne) pepper

1   teaspoon tomato paste (no salt added)

Minced fresh parsley

1. Wipe chops with paper toweling. Lay in shallow dish in one layer.

2. Combine balance of ingredients except parsley in small bowl, whisking to blend. Mixture will be thick. Spread on both sides of chops. Cover with waxed paper and let stand at room temperature for 15 minutes or longer.

3. Transfer chops to rack in shallow broiling pan. Broil 2 to 3 inches from heat for 8 minutes on each side. (Broiling time will vary with thickness of meat.) For the sweetest flavor and juiciest texture, do not overcook.

4. Serve immediately, sprinkled with minced fresh parsley.

VARIATION: If fresh dill is not available, substitute fresh basil, or 2 teaspoons fresh rosemary.

Pork Fillets with Apples and Yams

~

YIELD: SERVES 4

Pork is one of the tastiest of all meats, but only when it's fork-tender. The fillets I use come from the leg and are as lean and sweet-tasting as pork can be. Taking a lesson from classical Chinese cooking, which seldom offers desserts per se but rather intermixes sweets in the main courses, I've enriched this sophisticated herbed dish with apples and yams. In the next pork recipe, utterly delicious figlets supply the sweetness. For the first time in your life, you can skip your dessert and have it, too.

Per serving
Calories: 325
Carbohydrate: 24 g
Protein: 24 g
Fat: 14 g
Saturated fat: 6 g
Cholesterol: 83 mg
Dietary fiber: 2.5 g
Sodium: 72 mg
Exchanges: 1 starch/bread
           3 lean meat
           ½ fruit
           1 fat

4   lean pork fillets (cut from the leg), cut ½ inch thick (1 pound), well trimmed

½   teaspoon each dried sage and thyme leaves, crushed, and ground ginger

6   dashes ground red (cayenne) pepper

3   teaspoons Italian olive oil

3   large cloves garlic, minced

2   large shallots, minced

2   tablespoons minced sweet red pepper

1   tablespoon apple cider vinegar or balsamic vinegar

½   cup Easy Chicken Stock (page 216)

2   tablespoons orange juice concentrate

1   yam (½ pound), peeled and cut into ¼-inch slices

1   large, crisp sweet apple (such as Washington State), peeled, cored, and cut into ½-inch slices

1   tablespoon minced fresh parsley

1. Wipe meat with paper toweling. In a small bowl, combine sage, thyme, ginger, and ground red pepper. Sprinkle and rub meat on both sides with mixture. Let stand for 10 minutes.

2. Heat 2 teaspoons oil over medium heat in large well-seasoned iron skillet until hot. Add fillets and sauté for 2 minutes on each side until lightly browned. Transfer to plate.

3. Add remaining teaspoon oil to skillet. Sauté garlic, shallots, and sweet pepper until lightly browned, stirring constantly. Add vinegar. Cook for 30 seconds.

4. Combine stock with orange juice concentrate. Add to skillet, stirring to blend. Return browned fillets to skillet, turning to coat. Bring sauce to simmering point. Cover and simmer gently for 20 minutes, turning once midway.

5. Add yam slices, making sure that they are immersed in liquid. Re-cover and simmer for 15 minutes.

6. Add sliced apple. Re-cover and simmer for 10 minutes.

7. Arrange meat on warmed individual serving plates. Sprinkle with parsley, and serve.

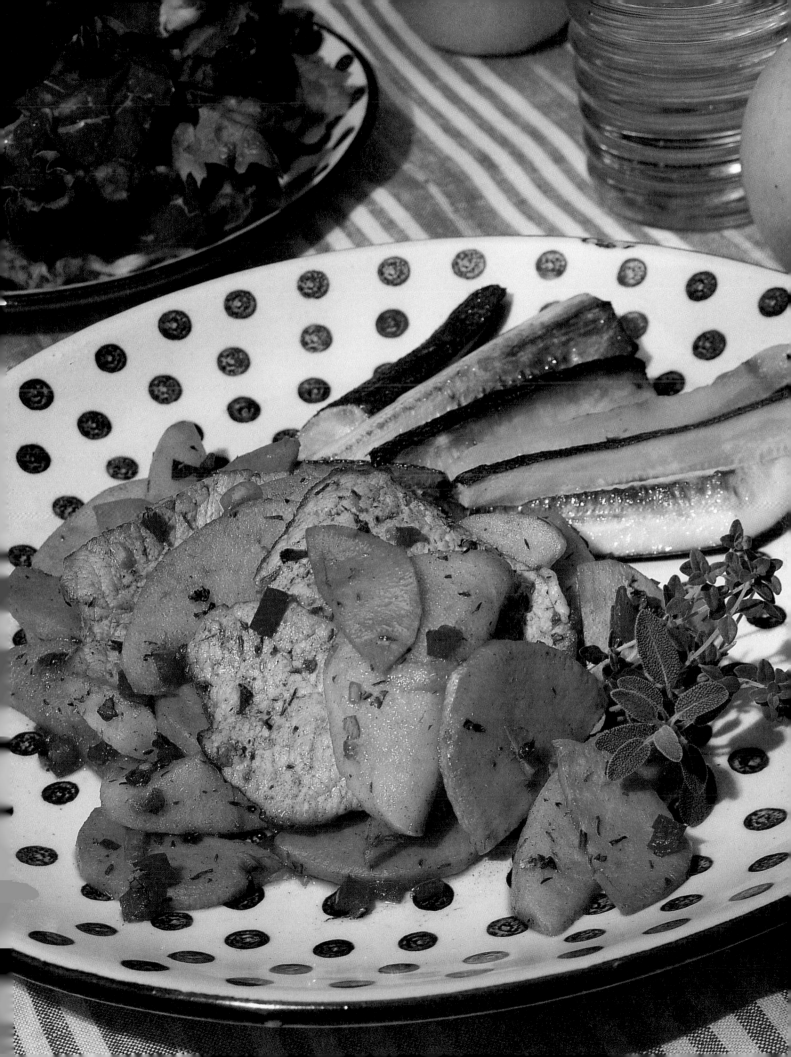

$\mathcal{P}$ork Chops with Fruit

YIELD: SERVES 4

Per serving
Calories: 240
Carbohydrate: 8 g
Protein: 25 g
Fat: 11 g
Saturated fat: 4 g
Cholesterol: 76 mg
Dietary fiber: 1.7 g
Sodium: 83 mg
Exchanges: 3 lean meat
           1 vegetable
           1 fat

4   loin or rib pork chops, ½ inch thick (1½ pounds), well trimmed

½   teaspoon each dried savory and sage leaves, crushed

1   teaspoon ground ginger

⅛   teaspoon ground red (cayenne) pepper

4   teaspoons Italian olive oil

1   small rib celery, minced

1   small onion, minced

3   large cloves garlic, minced

2   large fresh mushrooms, washed, dried, trimmed, and sliced

2   teaspoons wine vinegar

⅓   cup Easy Chicken Stock (page 216)

¼   cup apple juice (no sugar added)

⅓   cup coarsely chopped figlets, stems removed (see Note)

1   tablespoon minced fresh parsley

1. Wipe chops with paper toweling. Rub on both sides with dried herbs and spices.

2. Heat 2 teaspoons oil over medium heat in well-seasoned iron skillet until hot. Add chops and brown lightly on both sides. Transfer to plate.

3. Add balance of oil (2 teaspoons). Sauté celery, onion, garlic, and mushrooms until lightly browned, stirring continually (about 4 minutes). Return chops to skillet.

4. Add vinegar. Cook for 30 seconds. Add stock, apple juice, and figlets, stirring to blend, turning chops several times to coat. Bring to simmering point. Cover and simmer for 50 minutes to 1 hour, basting and turning chops at 15-minute intervals.

5. Uncover. Turn up heat under skillet. Add parsley. Cook chops for 5 minutes, turning and stirring sauce every minute, taking care that mixture doesn't stick. Finished chops will be dark brown and sauce will be thick. Serve on warmed individual plates.

NOTE: Figlets are small black mission figs that are generally available in supermarkets.

SERVING SUGGESTIONS:
Browned Cabbage with Caraway (page 99), Pan-Fried Escarole (page 98), or Brussels Sprouts with Mushrooms (page 102) are marvelous companions to this unusual dish.

Roast Fresh Ham with Savory Sauce

YIELD: SERVES 16

F resh ham is the leanest of all pork cuts. Get the most flavor from an economical six-pound piece by roasting it with a fruity basting sauce until tender and delicious. Then capture the exceptional flavor in another dish by using the bone as a base for a luxurious Hearty Soup (page 90).

Per serving
(about 3 ounces each)
Calories: 150
Carbohydrate: 2 g
Protein: 24 g
Fat: 5 g
Saturated fat: 2 g
Cholesterol: 50 g
Dietary fiber: trace
Sodium: 118 mg
Exchanges: 3 lean meat

FOR THE HAM:

½ fresh ham with bone (6 pounds), well trimmed

1 cup fresh orange juice

⅓ cup apple cider vinegar

2 teaspoons each ground ginger and coriander

⅛ teaspoon ground red (cayenne) pepper

6 whole cloves, crushed

2 tablespoons juniper berries, crushed

4 large cloves garlic, minced

2 teaspoons grated orange zest (preferably from navel orange)

FOR THE SAUCE:

¼ cup reserved marinade

⅔ cup Easy Chicken Stock (page 216)

3 tablespoons apple juice (no sugar added)

½ teaspoon ground coriander

Ground red (cayenne) pepper (3–4 dashes or to taste)

2 teaspoons arrowroot flour (or cornstarch) dissolved in 1 tablespoon water

Minced fresh parsley

1. Wipe ham with damp paper toweling. Prick all over with sharp-pronged fork. Place in large bowl.

2. Combine ¾ cup orange juice and balance of ingredients in jar, shaking to blend. Pour over ham, turning to coat. Cover tightly, refrigerate, and marinate for at least 6 hours or overnight. Remove from refrigerator 1 hour before roasting. Measure out ¼ cup marinade for sauce. Balance of marinade will be used to baste roasting meat.

3. Place meat on rack in roasting pan. Cover with aluminum foil and roast in center section of preheated 350°F oven for 40 minutes. Baste with one-third of marinade. Re-cover and roast for 30 minutes. Turn meat. Repeat basting, re-covering, and roasting procedure twice more.

4. Reduce oven heat to 325°F. Pour balance of orange juice (¼ cup) into roasting pan. Baste meat with pan juices. Return ham to oven and roast, uncovered, for about 1¼ hours (cooking time for ham, bone in, is 25 minutes per pound). Remove from oven. Cover loosely with aluminum foil to keep warm.

5. Prepare sauce by combining first 5 ingredients in heavy-bottom saucepan. Bring to simmering point and simmer for 3 minutes. Strain. Pour back into saucepan. Add only enough arrowroot flour mixture to lightly thicken sauce.

6. Slice meat thinly. Arrange portions on warmed individual plates, spooned with hot sauce. Sprinkle with parsley and serve.

SERVING SUGGESTION: Beet Relish (page 56) is a delicious condiment for this dish.

Fish

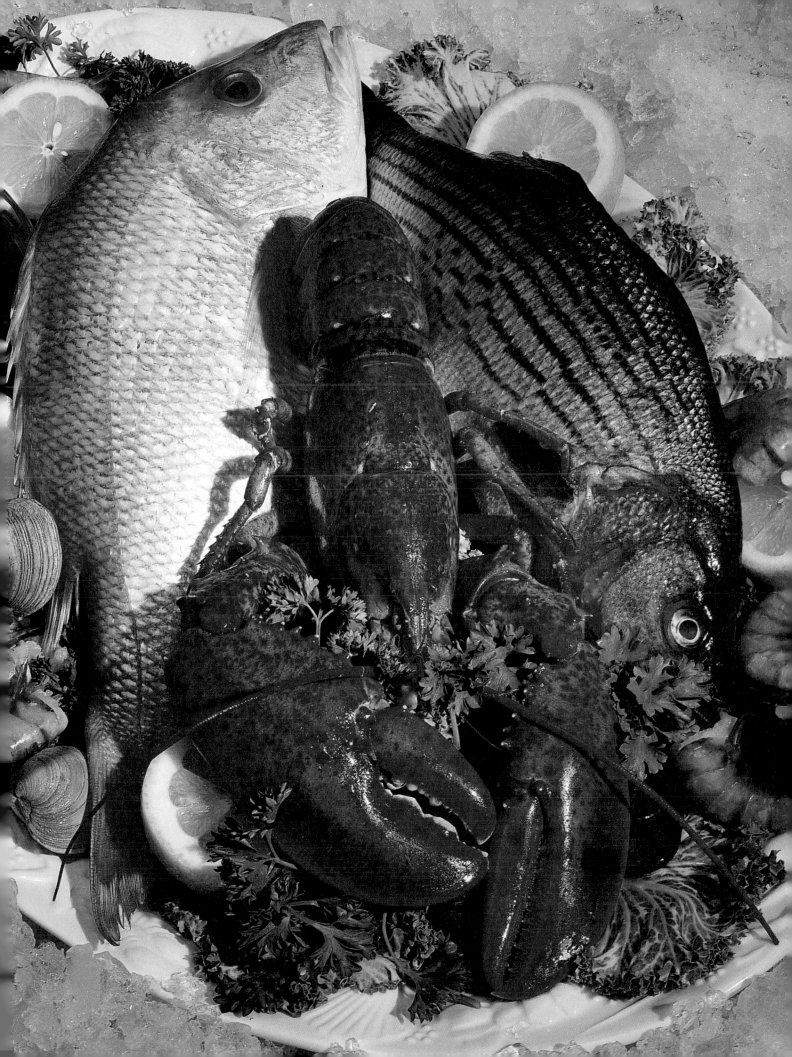

Skillet Halibut

~

YIELD: SERVES 4

Per serving

Calories: 149

Carbohydrate: 2 g

Protein: 26 g

Fat: 4 g

Saturated fat: 1 g

Cholesterol: 38 mg

Dietary fiber: 0.7 g

Sodium: 99 mg

Exchanges: 3 lean meat

2 halibut steaks, cut ½ inch thick (1¼ pounds total weight), each steak cut in half along length of bone

2 tablespoons fresh lemon juice

1½ teaspoons dried tarragon, crushed

8 dashes ground red (cayenne) pepper

¼ cup toasted homemade bread crumbs

1 tablespoon freshly grated Parmesan cheese

1 tablespoon Italian olive oil

1 large shallot, minced

2 cloves garlic, minced

Lemon and lime wedges

Watercress sprigs

1. Wash fish under cold running water. Dry with paper toweling. Lay in shallow dish. Pour lemon juice over fish, turning to coat. Then sprinkle with tarragon and rub into fish.

2. Combine ground red pepper with bread crumbs and cheese. Spread half of mixture across flat plate. Lay fish on top of mixture. Sprinkle with balance of crumb mix, pressing gently into fish.

3. Heat oil over medium-high heat in nonstick skillet until hot. Spread shallot and garlic across skillet. Cook for 30 seconds. Lay fish on top of mixture and sauté about 3 minutes on each side. Fish should be lightly browned on the outside and moist on the inside. Do not overcook.

4. Serve on individual warmed plates garnished with lemon and lime wedges and watercress sprigs.

NOTE: For extra-special results, use crumbs made from any of my breads. See pages 218–235 for bread recipes, and Note, page 235, for crumb recipe.

Delicious Broiled Halibut Steaks

~

YIELD: SERVES 4

Halibut looks like a flounder, but there the resemblance ends. The flesh of this denizen of the saltwater deeps is almost meatlike in taste and texture. In this recipe and in the next, I've enhanced halibut's natural appeal with a modicum of selected ingredients. If you're not yet a fish lover, here's an attractive way to start.

Per serving
Calories: 146
Carbohydrate: 1 g
Protein: 25 g
Fat: 4 g
Saturated fat: 1 g
Cholesterol: 36 mg
Dietary fiber: trace
Sodium: 62 mg
Exchanges: 3 lean meat

2	halibut steaks (1¼ pounds total weight), each steak cut in half along length of bone
¼	cup wine vinegar
1	tablespoon fresh lemon juice
2	teaspoons minced fresh parsley
2	teaspoons Italian olive oil
½	teaspoon dried thyme leaves, crushed
6	dashes ground red (cayenne) pepper
½	teaspoon dry mustard
2	cloves garlic, minced
	Lemon and lime wedges

1. Wash fish under cold running water. Dry with paper toweling. Lay in small shallow broiling pan.

2. Combine balance of ingredients except lemon and lime wedges in jar, shaking to blend. Pour over fish, turning to coat. Let marinate for 15 minutes, turning twice.

3. Drain fish, reserving marinade. Broil 4 inches from heat for 7 to 8 minutes. Spoon with some reserved marinade. Turn and broil 7 to 8 minutes, spooning with marinade once midway. (Cooking time will vary with thickness of fish.)

4. Peel away skin and serve fish on individual warmed plates garnished with lemon and lime wedges.

SERVING SUGGESTION: Plain boiled or steamed small red-skinned potatoes and broccoli or asparagus make a fine accompaniment to this elegant dish.

Sesame Flounder

YIELD: SERVES 4

Flounder is a flat fish in looks and taste. You can't do anything about its looks, but you can give it a taste lift with this recipe and the two that follow. In this recipe, I dip the fillets in fruit juices, pat them with oat flour and sesame seed, then sauté on a bed of fresh leek and garlic. In the next recipe, I dip the fillets in a mixture of bran flatbread and wheat germ (it gives the fillets crunchy skins and moist centers).

And in the third recipe—well, the title Cracked-Wheat Flounder with Mustard speaks for itself. If you're like my husband and me, you'll have a hard time picking your favorite.

Per serving
Calories: 211
Carbohydrate: 17 g
Protein: 26 g
Fat: 4 g
Saturated fat: 1 g
Cholesterol: 60 mg
Dietary fiber: 2.7 g
Sodium: 100 mg
Exchanges: 1 starch/bread
　　　　　 3 lean meat

½ cup old-fashioned rolled oats

2 tablespoons each stone-ground cornmeal and unshelled sesame seed (see page 297)

⅛ teaspoon ground red (cayenne) pepper

2 tablespoons fresh lemon juice

2 teaspoons frozen orange juice concentrate

1 teaspoon ground ginger

1 pound fresh fillet of flounder, cut into 4 serving pieces

4 teaspoons Italian olive oil

1 leek, white part only, well washed and minced

1 large clove garlic, minced

Lemon and lime wedges

1. Pulverize rolled oats in food blender for 30 seconds on high speed. Measure out 2 tablespoons and reserve balance for other recipes. Place in small bowl with cornmeal, sesame seed, and ground red pepper. Pour half of mixture onto flat plate, reserving balance. Set aside.

2. In small bowl, combine lemon juice, orange juice concentrate, and ginger, beating with fork to blend.

3. Wash fish and dry with paper toweling. Lay in shallow dish. Pour lemon juice mixture over fish, turning to coat. Let stand for 15 minutes at room temperature. Drain.

4. Lay fish on top of oatmeal mixture. Sprinkle with reserved oatmeal mixture.

5. Heat 2 teaspoons oil in large non-stick skillet until hot. Spread leek and garlic across skillet and sauté for 1 minute. Lay fish on top of mixture. Sauté over medium-high heat until golden brown (6 minutes). Add balance of oil (2 teaspoons), turn, and sauté until golden brown, adjusting heat if necessary so that crumbs do not burn.

6. Serve immediately on warmed serving platter. Garnish with lemon and lime wedges.

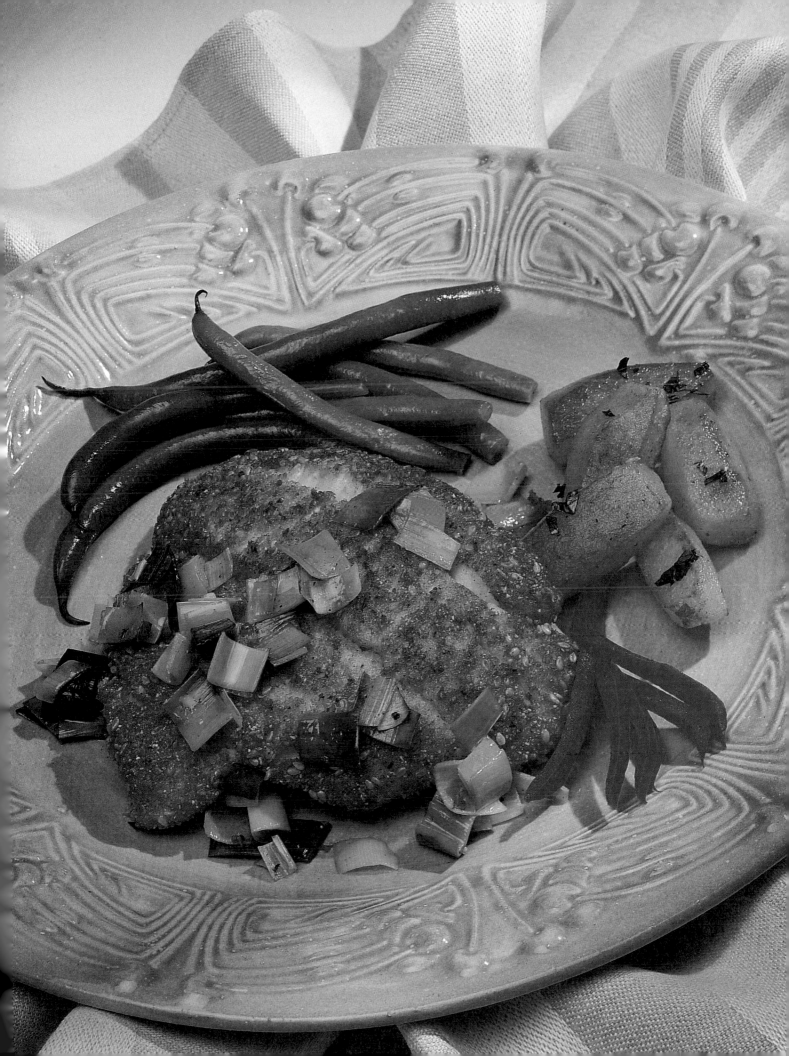

Norwegian Flatbread Flounder

~

YIELD: SERVES 4

Per serving
Calories: 192
Carbohydrate: 9 g
Protein: 26 g
Fat: 5 g
Saturated fat: 1 g
Cholesterol: 61 mg
Dietary fiber: 5.1 g
Sodium: 133 mg
Exchanges: ½ starch/bread
           3 lean meat

1   pound fresh flounder fillets, cut into 4 serving pieces

1   tablespoon each fresh lemon and lime juice

6   bran flatbread wafers (no salt added)

2   tablespoons toasted wheat germ (no sugar added)

1   tablespoon freshly grated Parmesan cheese

⅛   teaspoon each ground red (cayenne) pepper and ginger

½   teaspoon dried savory leaves, crushed

3   teaspoons Italian olive oil

3   large shallots, minced

Lemon and lime wedges

1. Wash fish under cold running water. Dry with paper toweling. Place in shallow dish. Sprinkle with lemon and lime juices, turning to coat. Let stand for 15 minutes.

2. Break up flatbread and combine in food blender with wheat germ. Blend until pulverized. Pour into cup. Add cheese, spices, and savory, blending with fork. Spread half of mixture in flat plate.

3. Lay fillets on top of mixture. Sprinkle balance of mixture over fillets, pressing into fish.

4. Heat 1½ teaspoons oil over medium-high heat in nonstick skillet until hot. Sprinkle shallots across skillet. Sauté for 30 seconds. Lay fish on top of shallots and sauté over medium-high heat until golden brown (5 to 6 minutes). Add balance of oil (1½ teaspoons); turn and sauté until golden brown, adjusting heat if necessary so that crumbs do not burn.

5. Serve immediately on warmed serving platter, garnished with lemon and lime wedges.

Cracked-Wheat Flounder with Mustard

~

YIELD: SERVES 4

Per serving
Calories: 170
Carbohydrate: 4 g
Protein: 25 g
Fat: 5 g
Saturated fat: 1 g
Cholesterol: 61 mg
Dietary fiber: 0.9 g
Sodium: 140 mg
Exchanges: 3 lean meat

¼ cup wine vinegar

1 teaspoon dried savory leaves, crushed

1 tablespoon dry vermouth

1 pound fresh fillet of flounder, cut into 4 serving pieces

¼ cup evaporated skim milk

2 teaspoons prepared Dijon mustard (no salt added)

½ cup No-Fuss Cracked-Wheat Bread Crumbs (page 234 and Note, page 235)

½ teaspoon ground ginger

3 dashes ground red (cayenne) pepper

4 teaspoons Italian olive oil

Lemon and lime wedges

1. In a small bowl, combine vinegar, savory, and vermouth, beating with fork to blend.

2. Wash fish and dry with paper toweling. Lay in shallow dish. Pour vinegar mixture over fish, turning to coat. Let stand for at least 15 minutes at room temperature.

3. While fish is marinating, combine evaporated milk and mustard in bowl, blending with whisk. Let stand until fish is ready to cook.

4. Combine and blend crumbs with ginger and ground red pepper. Lay half of mixture across flat plate.

5. Drain fish. Lay fillets on paper toweling and pat fairly dry (do not wipe). Dip each piece into milk mixture, turning to coat, draining excess. Lay on top of crumbs, pressing fish into mixture. Sprinkle fish with balance of crumbs, making certain that all pieces are well coated.

6. Heat 2 teaspoons oil over medium-high heat in nonstick skillet until hot. Sauté fish until golden brown (about 4 minutes). Add balance of oil (2 teaspoons), turn, and sauté until crispy. Do not overcook. Serve immediately, garnished with lemon and lime wedges.

SERVING SUGGESTION: Mince 4 shallots (about ¼ cup) to sprinkle over fish before serving.

Sole with Roasted Potatoes and Horseradish Sauce

~

YIELD: SERVES 4

Opposite textures attract the discerning food lover in this happy marriage of tender, moist sole fillets (accented with a light horseradish sauce), and crunchy potatoes. A delightful departure from the same old sameness of textures on your plate—and on your palate.

Per serving
Calories: 280
Carbohydrate: 22 g
Protein: 25 g
Fat: 8 g
Saturated fat: 3 g
Cholesterol: 60 mg
Dietary fiber: 3.9 g
Sodium: 477 mg
Exchanges: 1½ starch/
bread
3 lean meat

2	tablespoons each fresh lemon juice and rice wine vinegar
2	teaspoons dried tarragon leaves, crumbled
¼	cup minced shallots
1	dash ground red (cayenne) pepper
4	teaspoons minced parsley
1	pound fillet of lemon sole or flounder

1½	teaspoons prepared white horseradish
2½	tablespoons reduced-fat sour cream
2	tablespoons tomato juice (no salt added)
2	tablespoons Italian olive oil
1¼	pounds Idaho potatoes, peeled
½	teaspoon mild curry powder

1. In a medium glass or earthenware bowl, make a marinade by combining the lemon juice, vinegar, half the tarragon, half the shallots, the cayenne pepper, and half the parsley. Let stand for 5 minutes.

2. Rinse fish under cold running water. Slice and discard the narrow bony section that runs down the center of each fillet. Then cut each piece in half crosswise. Place in marinade, turning several times to coat. Cover and let stand at room temperature for 45 minutes, or several hours in refrigerator, returning to room temperature before cooking.

3. In a small bowl, whisk together the horseradish, sour cream, tomato juice, and remaining 2 teaspoons parsley. Cover and set aside.

4. Preheat oven to 450°F. Pour oil into a 10" × 15" jelly roll pan. Place pan in oven for 8 minutes.

5. While pan is in oven, cut each potato in half lengthwise; then cut into ⅜-inch slices crosswise. Dry on paper toweling. Spread potatoes across hot pan. In cup, combine remaining teaspoon tarragon and the curry powder. Sprinkle over potatoes. Cover with remaining 2 tablespoons shallots. With spatula, turn ingredients over several times. Arrange slices in one layer. Reduce oven heat to 425°F. Bake potatoes for 20 minutes. Turn and return to oven for 15 minutes longer.

6. Drain fish, leaving any clinging ingredients from marinade intact. Arrange pieces over hot potatoes. Bake for 10 to 12 minutes (the thickness of the fillets will affect cooking time). Do not overcook.

7. To serve, scoop up portions from pan with spatula and place on warmed individual dinner plates. Dribble a teaspoon of sauce over each serving; pour remaining sauce into a sauceboat to serve along with dish.

SERVING SUGGESTION: Try this with steamed broccoli, peas, or green beans.

Broiled Fillet of Any Sole

~

YIELD: SERVES 4

I don't know if this practice has spread to your neighborhood, but here in Manhattan fillet of sole often arrives at the fish market packed in brine. To avoid becoming a victim of hidden salt, buy a whole sole and have it filleted. That also prevents fillets of scrod, flounder, and other fish from being palmed off on you as the more expensive sole.

There are many kinds of sole—gray, Dover, lemon, petrale, and so on—and while they differ in flavor and texture, they're so much alike that just one recipe can convert any sole into a piscatorial masterpiece. Here's that recipe.

Per serving
Calories: 136
Carbohydrate: 1 g
Protein: 23 g
Fat: 4 g
Saturated fat: 1 g
Cholesterol: 60 mg
Dietary fiber: 0 g
Sodium: 128 mg
Exchanges: 3 lean meat

1   **pound fresh sole fillets, cut into 4 serving pieces**

½   **teaspoon ground ginger**

⅛   **teaspoon ground red (cayenne) pepper**

1   **teaspoon dried tarragon leaves, crushed**

4   **teaspoons sweet soft corn oil margarine**

2   **tablespoons shallots, minced**

2   **tablespoons toasted homemade bread crumbs, or crumbs made from any of my breads (see Note, page 235)**

3   **tablespoons dry vermouth**

    Lemon and lime wedges

1. Wash fish under cold running water. Dry thoroughly with paper toweling. Rub on both sides with ginger and ground red pepper. Sprinkle with tarragon on both sides.

2. Lightly grease shallow broiling pan with ½ teaspoon margarine. Melt balance of margarine. Lay fish in pan. Sprinkle first with shallots, then with crumbs, and then with melted margarine.

3. Broil close to heat for 6 minutes. Spoon with vermouth. Broil for 4 minutes. (Cooking time will vary with thickness of fillets.)

4. Serve on individual warmed serving plates garnished with lemon and lime wedges.

Baked Gray Sole Paupiettes

YIELD: SERVES 4

Easy enough to prepare at the end of a day's work, yet pretty and festive enough to satisfy any discerning gourmet.

Per serving
Calories: 122
Carbohydrate: 2 g
Protein: 23 g
Fat: 1 g
Saturated fat: 1 g
Cholesterol: 61 mg
Dietary fiber: 0.1 g
Sodium: 111 mg
Exchanges: 3 lean meat

1	pound fresh gray sole fillets, cut into 4 serving pieces
½	teaspoon each ground ginger and cumin seed
2	teaspoons minced fresh tarragon
2	tablespoons minced shallots
4	dashes ground red (cayenne) pepper
¼	cup each Aromatic Fish Stock (page 217) and apple juice (no sugar added)

1	medium fresh tomato, peeled, cored, seeded, and coarsely chopped
1	teaspoon fresh lemon juice
2	teaspoons arrowroot flour or cornstarch dissolved in 1 tablespoon water

1. Wash fish under cold running water. Dry thoroughly with paper toweling. Sprinkle and rub on one side with ginger and cumin seed. Then sprinkle each fillet with 1 teaspoon tarragon. Preheat oven to 400°F.

2. Place equal amounts of minced shallots on top of each fillet. Sprinkle with ground red pepper. Roll up. Place seam side down in 1¾-quart ovenproof casserole.

3. Combine stock, apple juice, and tomato in saucepan. Bring to simmering point, and cook gently for 3 minutes. Pour over paupiettes. Cover and bake for 12 minutes. With slotted spoon, transfer paupiettes to warmed serving plate. Cover with waxed paper to keep warm.

4. Pour cooking juices and solids into food blender. Add lemon juice and blend until smooth. Pour mixture into saucepan. Pour any exuded juice from serving plate into saucepan. Bring to simmering point. Dribble in only enough arrowroot flour mixture to thicken sauce slightly. Stir in balance of fresh tarragon (1 teaspoon). Pour over paupiettes and serve.

NOTE: Only fresh herbs will do here. If fresh tarragon isn't available, substitute fresh mint, rosemary, or 1 teaspoon each minced fresh parsley and dill.

VARIATION: Add 1 tablespoon medium-dry sherry at beginning of step 4.

Delectable Stir-Fried Lemon Sole

~

YIELD: SERVES 4

For millennia, the peoples of the Far East have known the secret of sealing in the flavors of cooked food. Several years ago, the secret spread all over the United States. It's fast, fast cooking—and the utensil that makes it possible is an all-purpose pan in the shape of a sphere cut in half: the wok. Wok cooking is unadulterated fun, and the results are a joy —firm-textured bites of flavors you never imagined familiar foods could possess. With this recipe, you'll flashcook lemon sole and fresh vegetables of contrasting textures. This recipe is not Chinese; it's American —but the taste is strictly exotic.

Per serving
Calories: 222
Carbohydrate: 16 g
Protein: 25 g
Fat: 6 g
Saturated fat: 1 g
Cholesterol: 61 mg
Dietary fiber: 3.8 g
Sodium: 332 mg
Exchanges: ½ starch/bread
            3 lean meat
            1 vegetable

¾ pound potatoes, peeled, cut into 1-inch chunks

3 tablespoons white vinegar

2 whole cloves, crushed

1 pound fresh lemon sole fillets, cut into 2-inch pieces

4 teaspoons Italian olive oil

2 large cloves garlic, minced

1 tablespoon peeled and shredded fresh ginger

¼ pound fresh snow peas, washed, dried, stems and strings removed

1 large green onion, diagonally sliced into ½-inch pieces

1 small sweet red pepper, seeded and cut into ⅜-inch slivers

½ teaspoon each crushed dried oregano leaves and smoked yeast (see page 297)

⅛ teaspoon ground red (cayenne) pepper

½ cup Aromatic Fish Stock (page 297)

2 teaspoons arrowroot flour or cornstarch dissolved in 1 tablespoon water

1. Cook potatoes in rapidly boiling water for 8 minutes. (Potatoes should be half-cooked.) Set aside.

2. Combine vinegar and cloves in shallow dish. Add fish, turning to coat. Marinate for 30 minutes or longer, turning often. Drain on paper toweling. Set aside.

3. Place wok on ring over high heat for 1½ minutes. Pour 2 teaspoons oil around rim of wok. Add half of garlic and ginger. Stir-fry for 30 seconds (see Note 2 for preceding recipe). Add fish in one layer, spreading across wok. Sauté for 1½ minutes without moving pieces. Turn. Sauté for 1½ minutes. Carefully transfer to hot serving plate. Cover with waxed paper to keep warm.

4. Pour balance of oil (2 teaspoons) around rim of wok. Add balance of ginger and garlic. Stir-fry for 30 seconds.

5. Add snow peas, green onion, and sweet red pepper. Stir-fry for 1½ minutes. Add parcooked potatoes. Stir-fry for a few seconds.

6. In a cup, combine and blend oregano, smoked yeast, ground red pepper, and stock. Slowly pour around rim of wok. Reduce heat. Cover and simmer for 1½ minutes.

7. Uncover and pour arrowroot or cornstarch mixture around rim of wok, stirring to blend. Sauce will be lightly thickened and ready to serve within 30 seconds. Do not overcook.

8. Spoon over fish, arranging attractively on platter. Serve immediately.

Sautéed Sea Bass with Vegetables

~

YIELD: SERVES 4

Because sea bass has a strong and distinctive flavor, it thrives heartily when combined with corn and potatoes. Here's an entire meal in a skillet. Serve it in your favorite tureen and watch your family's expression at the first taste. Sheer joy!

Per serving
Calories: 253
Carbohydrate: 25 g
Protein: 24 g
Fat: 6 g
Saturated fat: 1 g
Cholesterol: 91 mg
Dietary fiber: 4.0 g
Sodium: 102 mg
Exchanges: 1 starch/bread
3 lean meat
1 vegetable

1	1½-pound sea bass (black or white), filleted and skinned, cut into 1-inch pieces
1	tablespoon fresh lemon juice
1	tablespoon Italian olive oil
1	tablespoon peeled and minced fresh ginger
2	large cloves garlic, minced
1	large scallion, trimmed, cut diagonally into ½-inch slices
1	small sweet red pepper, seeded, cut into ⅜-inch slivers
1	tablespoon minced fresh tarragon or fresh mint
1	teaspoon prepared Dijon mustard (no salt added)
2	tablespoons dry vermouth
¼	cup tomato juice (no salt added)
1	medium Idaho potato (½ pound), diced and slightly undercooked
2	medium corn, cooked, kernels removed from cob (1 cup)

1. Wash fish and dry thoroughly with paper toweling. Pull out any remaining bones with pliers. Place in bowl. Sprinkle with lemon juice, turning to coat.

2. Heat oil over medium-high heat in large nonstick skillet until hot. Lay ginger, garlic, scallion, and sweet red pepper across skillet. Sauté for 1 minute.

3. Drain fish. Lay on sautéed mixture. Sauté on each side for 2½ minutes.

4. Combine tarragon (or mint), mustard, vermouth, and tomato juice, blending well. Pour over fish. Bring to simmering point. Simmer for 1 minute.

5. Push fish mixture to outer circle of skillet. Add potato and corn to center of skillet, spooning with sauce. Bring to simmering point again. Cover and simmer for 1 minute. Uncover.

6. Gently combine vegetables with fish, spooning with sauce. Cover and simmer for 1 minute until vegetables are heated through. Spoon into warmed tureen or serving plate and serve immediately.

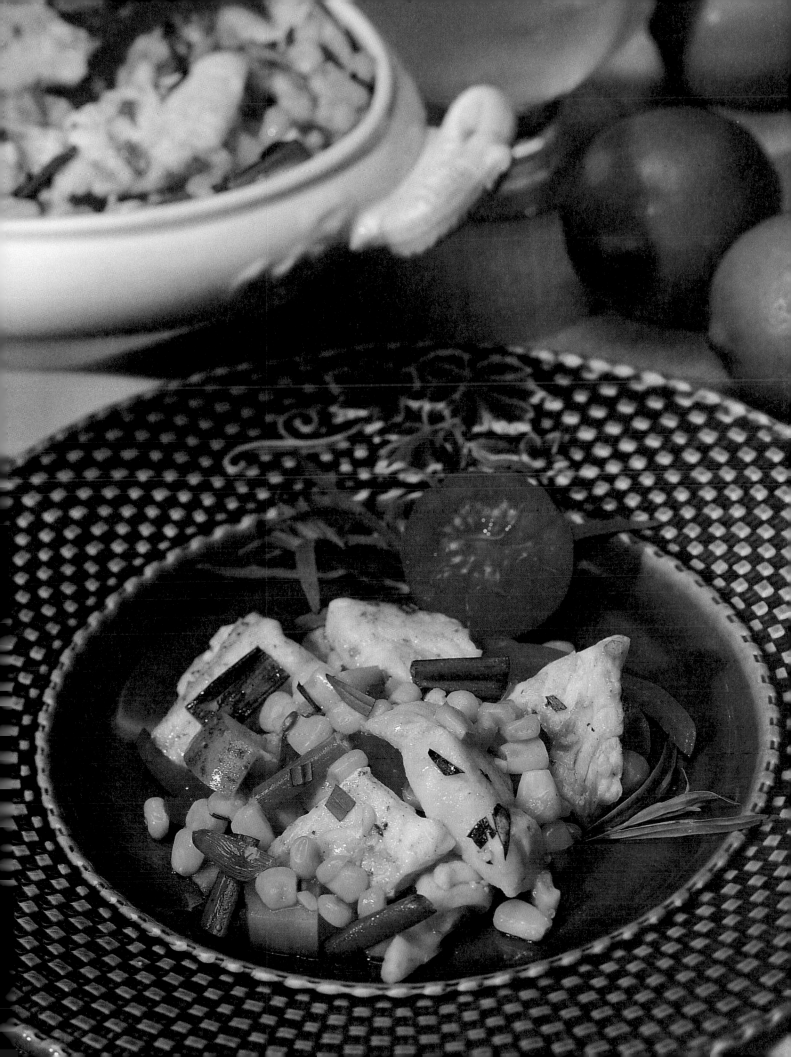

Stir-Fried Sea Bass and Asparagus

~

YIELD: SERVES 4

In this recipe, flash-cooked sea bass (the favorite fish of Chinese-Americans) is accompanied by fresh asparagus, celery, mushrooms, and spices to deliver a homegrown, but exotic, flavor.

1   2½-pound sea bass, filleted and skinned, cut into 1½-inch pieces (reserve bones for stock)

2   tablespoons brown rice flour (see Note 3)

⅛   teaspoon each freshly grated nutmeg and ground red (cayenne) pepper

2   large cloves garlic, minced

2   teaspoons peeled and minced fresh ginger

1   rib celery, cut diagonally into ⅜-inch slices

4   teaspoons Italian olive oil

1   cup freshly sliced asparagus tips (cut diagonally into 1-inch pieces)

¼   pound fresh mushrooms, washed, diced, trimmed, and thinly sliced

½   cup Aromatic Fish Stock (page 217)

2   tablespoons dry vermouth

1   tablespoon minced fresh mint leaves

2   teaspoons arrowroot flour or cornstarch dissolved in 1 tablespoon water

1. Wash fish and dry thoroughly with paper toweling. Pull out any remaining bones with pliers.

2. Dust fish with mixture of flour, nutmeg, and ground red pepper. Set aside. Combine garlic, ginger, and celery in a cup. Set aside.

3. Place wok on ring over high heat for 1½ minutes. Pour 2 teaspoons oil around rim of wok. Add half of garlic-ginger-celery mixture and asparagus. Stir-fry (see Note 2) very gently for 2 minutes. Add mushrooms and stir-fry for 1 minute. Transfer to dish.

4. Pour balance of oil (2 teaspoons) around rim of wok. Add balance of garlic mixture, spreading across

Per serving
Calories: 190
Carbohydrate: 7 g
Protein: 23 g
Fat: 7 g
Saturated fat: 1 g
Cholesterol: 90 mg
Dietary fiber: 1.6 g
Sodium: 107 mg
Exchanges: 3 lean meat
1 vegetable

wok. Lay fish pieces on top of mixture. Stir-fry for 1 minute on each side. Add stock, vermouth, and mint. Bring to simmering point.

5. Return asparagus-mushroom mixture to wok. (Handle very gently so that asparagus doesn't fall apart.) Cover and cook over medium heat for 2 minutes.

6. Pour arrowroot or cornstarch mixture around rim of wok, stirring to blend. Mixture will thicken rapidly. Do not overcook. Serve immediately.

VARIATION: For a creamy sauce, stir in 2 tablespoons evaporated skim milk just before serving.

NOTES:
1. Fresh herbs taste best in this recipe. You can successfully substitute fresh tarragon, rosemary, or dill for mint.

2. Stir-fry means just that—stir while frying. In this instance, you are really sautéing (cooking in a small amount of oil) over a high heat so that all ingredients are cooked rapidly. If you don't have a wok, you can successfully prepare this recipe and the one following in a nonstick skillet, adding the oil directly to the skillet rather than around the rim of the utensil. Cooking time will be longer because a nonstick skillet never reaches a superhigh heat.

3. Brown rice flour (it's slightly sweet) is available in many health food stores. Cornstarch may be substituted for rice flour.

Striped Bass with Fennel

YIELD: SERVES 4

Striped bass is a graceful, beautiful game fish with black, longitudinal stripes. Its flesh is delicately flavored, tender, and very juicy. In this recipe, I've dressed it with minced vegetables, herbs, and aromatic fennel seed. Totally irresistible!

Per serving
Calories: 139
Carbohydrate: 2 g
Protein: 22 g
Fat: 4 g
Saturated fat: 1 g
Cholesterol: 91 mg
Dietary fiber: 0.3 g
Sodium: 93 mg
Exchanges: 3 lean meat

1 pound fillet of striped bass

1 tablespoon fresh lemon juice

1 teaspoon fennel seed, crushed

⅛ teaspoon ground red (cayenne) pepper

2 teaspoons Italian olive oil

2 cloves garlic, minced

1 large shallot, minced

2 tablespoons minced celery

1 tablespoon minced sweet green pepper

1 teaspoon peeled and minced fresh ginger

3 tablespoons each Aromatic Fish Stock (page 217) and dry vermouth, or 6 tablespoons stock or vermouth

1 teaspoon prepared Dijon mustard (no salt added)

Lemon or lime wedges

1. Wash fish under cold running water. Dry thoroughly with paper toweling. Place in shallow dish. Sprinkle with lemon juice, turning several times to coat. Let stand for 15 minutes. Then sprinkle with fennel seed, pressing into fish. Sprinkle with ground red pepper. Set aside.

2. Heat oil over medium-high heat in nonstick skillet until hot. Add garlic, shallot, celery, green pepper, and ginger, spreading across skillet. Sauté over medium-high heat for 1 minute. Lay fish on top of mixture. Sauté for 3 minutes. Turn and sauté for 1 minute.

3. In a cup, combine stock, vermouth, and mustard. Add to skillet. Turn heat up. Spoon fish with sauce and cook until sauce is reduced by half (about 3 minutes).

4. Discard any dark sections from fish. Arrange fillets on warmed individual plates, spooned with sauce, and garnished with lemon or lime wedges.

VARIATION: Substitute Easy Chicken Stock (page 216) for fish stock.

Baked Red Snapper Veronique

~

YIELD: SERVES 4

Red snapper, a delicate saltwater fish, is particularly delicious when baked. Here it is enrobed in a sauce of herbs, stock, and sherry; baked to perfection in a hot oven; then enriched with flour and margarine and sweetened with the fruity flavor of fresh grapes. What could be lovelier?

1	3-pound red snapper, cleaned, head left on	2	large cloves garlic, minced
1	small bay leaf, crumbled	⅓	cup Aromatic Fish Stock (page 217)
2	sprigs fresh parsley	3	tablespoons dry sherry
1	tablespoon fresh lemon juice	1	tablespoon unbleached flour
¾	teaspoon combined dried rosemary and thyme leaves, crushed	1	tablespoon sweet soft corn oil margarine
⅛	teaspoon ground red (cayenne) pepper	1	cup fresh seedless green grapes
3	large shallots, minced		

Per serving
Calories: 183
Carbohydrate: 11 g
Protein: 24 g
Fat: 5 g
Saturated fat: 1 g
Cholesterol: 65 mg
Dietary fiber: 0.7 g
Sodium: 140 mg
Exchanges: 3 lean meat
½ fruit

1. Wash fish under cold running water. Dry thoroughly inside and out with paper toweling. Sprinkle cavity with crumbled bay leaf. Then tuck parsley sprigs into cavity. Secure with toothpicks or skewers. Preheat oven to 400°F.

2. Make several ½-inch gashes on each side of fish. Sprinkle and rub with lemon juice, then with dried herbs and ground red pepper.

3. Combine shallots and garlic. Strew half of mixture across shallow baking pan. Lay fish on top. Sprinkle fish with balance of garlic and shallots.

4. Combine and heat stock and 2 tablespoons sherry to simmering point. Gently pour around and over fish. Cover with aluminum foil and bake for 20 to 25 minutes,

basting once midway. (Cooking time will vary with thickness of fish.) Transfer fish to warmed serving platter. Cover with waxed paper to keep warm.

5. Strain cooking juices through fine sieve into saucepan. Bring to simmering point. Simmer for 1 minute.

6. Combine flour with margarine. Add to saucepan, whisking and cooking for 3 minutes until lightly thickened. Add balance of sherry (1 tablespoon) and grapes. Cook for 2 minutes.

7. Skin fish. Serve portions on warmed individual plates spooned with sauce and grapes.

Spicy Broiled Tilefish

YIELD: SERVES 4

Its skin looks like tile. It feeds on the crustacea at the bottom of the sea, so it tastes somewhat like them. It's low, low, low in fat. And when it's moistened with vinegar and apple juice, and generously showered with herbs and spices, it makes a dish as different as it is delectable.

Per serving
Calories: 147
Carbohydrate: 2 g
Protein: 23 g
Fat: 5 g
Saturated fat: 1 g
Cholesterol: 52 mg
Dietary fiber: 0.1 g
Sodium: 56 mg
Exchanges: 3 lean meat

4   slices tilefish fillets, about ½ inch thick (1 pound)

2   cloves garlic, minced

1   large shallot, minced

2   tablespoons wine vinegar

1   tablespoon apple juice (no sugar added)

1   teaspoon dried tarragon leaves, crushed

8   dashes ground red (cayenne) pepper

1   teaspoon dry mustard

1   teaspoon melted sweet soft corn oil margarine

1   tablespoon soft bread crumbs

Lemon and lime wedges

1. Wash fish under cold running water and dry with paper toweling. Combine next 7 ingredients in bowl, stirring to blend. Add fillets, turning to coat. Let stand for 30 minutes, turning from time to time.

2. Drain fish. Arrange in shallow broiling pan. Pour marinating ingredients into strainer. Spoon solids in strainer onto fillets, distributing evenly and pressing into fish.

3. Broil 4 inches from heat for 4 minutes. Turn. Dribble margarine over fish. Sprinkle with crumbs. Return fish to broiler and broil for 4 minutes or until done. (Cooking time will vary with thickness of fillets.)

4. Serve immediately in warmed individual dishes garnished with lemon and lime wedges.

VARIATION: Add ½ teaspoon chili con carne seasoning in step 1.

Shrimp with Snow Peas

~

YIELD: SERVES 4

Can you improve on perfection? This recipe and the next were originally created for a nonstick skillet, and the consensus of critical comment was "Perfect." Then I adapted them to the wok, and the comment was "Wow!"—which, I should imagine, means better than perfect. Why not try them both ways and taste the difference yourself. When you use the wok, remember: Heat well before using, pour liquid around the rim of the wok, dry vegetables with paper toweling, and insist your family is seated at the table before you start to cook—for the peak enjoyment of the products of the wok, they must be consumed the moment they're finished.

Per serving
Calories: 190
Carbohydrate: 7 g
Protein: 25 g
Fat: 6 g
Saturated fat: 1 g
Cholesterol: 213 mg
Dietary fiber: 3.4 g
Sodium: 115 mg
Exchanges: 3 lean meat
          1 vegetable

1½ pounds fresh, unshelled shrimp (shell and devein before using)

½ teaspoon smoked yeast (see page 297)

6 dashes ground red (cayenne) pepper

4 teaspoons Italian olive oil

2 teaspoons peeled and minced fresh ginger

3 large cloves garlic, minced

¼ pound fresh mushrooms, washed, dried, trimmed, and sliced

¼ pound fresh snow peas, washed, dried

8 water chestnuts, rinsed, dried, and sliced

⅓ cup Easy Chicken Stock (page 216)

1 teaspoon tomato paste (no salt added)

1 tablespoon cornstarch dissolved in 1 tablespoon cold water

1 tablespoon medium-dry sherry

1. Wash shrimp. Dry in paper toweling. Sprinkle with smoked yeast and ground red pepper.

2. Heat 2 teaspoons oil over medium-high heat in nonstick skillet or wok until hot. Add half of ginger and garlic. Spread across skillet or wok. Sauté for 30 seconds. Lay shrimp on mixture. Sauté on each side until lightly pink. Transfer to dish. Do not cover.

3. Heat balance of oil (2 teaspoons) in skillet or wok. Add balance of ginger and garlic. Sauté for 30 seconds. Add mushrooms and sauté until just wilted (about 2 minutes).

4. Add snow peas and water chestnuts to skillet or wok, stirring to combine with mushrooms. Return shrimp to skillet or wok. Stir to combine.

5. Combine stock with tomato paste. Pour around mixture. Stir. Bring to simmering point. Cover and simmer for 30 seconds.

6. Add cornstarch mixture. Stir and cook briefly until liquid thickens. Then stir in sherry. Cook for 30 seconds. Serve immediately.

*L*uscious Sautéed Shrimp and Vegetables

YIELD: SERVES 4

Per serving
Calories: 181
Carbohydrate: 6 g
Protein: 24 g
Fat: 6 g
Saturated fat: 1 g
Cholesterol: 213 mg
Dietary fiber: 1.0 g
Sodium: 112 mg
Exchanges: 3 lean meat
1 vegetable

1½ pounds fresh, unshelled shrimp (shell and devein before using)

1 tablespoon cornstarch

1 teaspoon ground ginger

⅛ teaspoon ground red (cayenne) pepper

4 teaspoons Italian olive oil

2 large cloves garlic, minced

⅓ cup sweet green pepper (¼-inch slivers)

3 green onions or scallions, trimmed and sliced diagonally

¼ pound fresh mushrooms, washed, dried, trimmed, and sliced

½ teaspoon each dried sage leaves, crushed, and mild curry powder

¼ cup Thirty-Minute Chicken Broth (page 215) or Easy Chicken Stock (page 216)

1 teaspoon dry mustard

2 teaspoons grated orange zest (preferably from navel orange)

1 tablespoon medium-dry sherry

1. Wash shrimp under cold running water. Dry thoroughly with paper toweling. Place in bowl.

2. Combine cornstarch, ginger, and ground red pepper in cup. Sprinkle over shrimp.

3. Heat 2 teaspoons oil over medium-high heat in nonstick skillet or wok until hot. Add half each garlic, green pepper, green onions, and mushrooms. Sauté over medium-high heat until softened (about 3 minutes), taking care not to brown. Transfer to dish.

4. Heat balance of oil (2 teaspoons) in skillet or wok. Sauté balance of garlic, green pepper, green onions, and mushrooms for 1 minute. Spread across skillet or wok. Lay shrimp on mixture. Sauté on each side until lightly pink.

5. Return first half of cooked vegetable mixture to skillet or wok. Sprinkle with sage and curry powder. Cook, stirring constantly, for 1 minute.

6. Blend chicken broth or stock with mustard. Pour into skillet or wok. Sprinkle with orange zest. Cook and stir until liquid is thickened (about 1 minute). Then stir in sherry. Cook for 30 seconds. Serve immediately.

NOTE: Cooking time in each step will vary depending upon which cooking utensil you use.

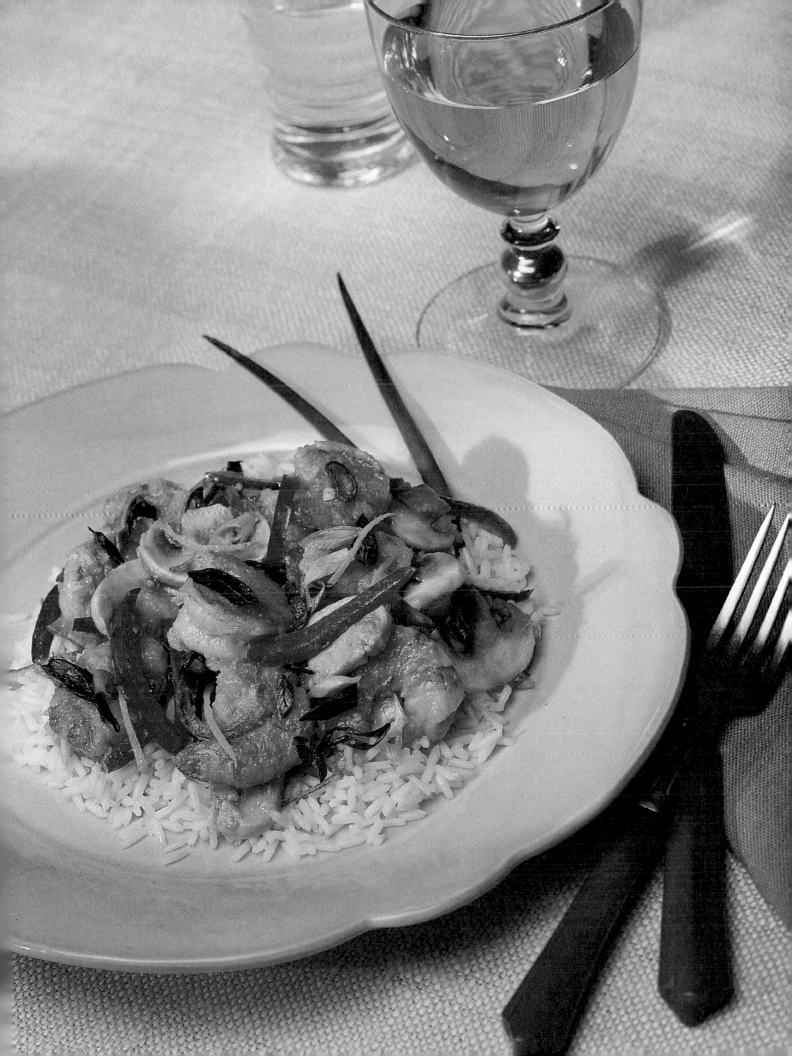

Crisp and Sautéed Codfish Steaks

YIELD: SERVES 4

Take fresh codfish, dip it in an amalgam of sweet and spicy liquids, dress it in a mélange of dry ingredients, and sauté it rapidly on a bed of herbaceous shallots. Result: a fish lover's delight that's crackling crisp on the outside and moist and delicious on the inside. Special bonus: Cod is one of the lowest in fat of all fish.

1¼ pounds codfish steaks (weight with bone), then boned, cut into 4 serving pieces

1 egg white

1 teaspoon prepared Dijon mustard (no salt added)

2 tablespoons evaporated skim milk

1 teaspoon tomato paste (no salt added)

2 tablespoons each toasted wheat germ (no sugar added), unbleached flour, and toasted homemade bread crumbs

4 teaspoons Italian olive oil

2 large shallots, minced

Lemon and lime wedges

Per serving
Calories: 174
Carbohydrate: 6 g
Protein: 25 g
Fat: 5 g
Saturated fat: 1 g
Cholesterol: 49 mg
Dietary fiber: 0.8 g
Sodium: 100 mg
Exchanges: ½ starch/bread
　　　　　 3 lean meat

1. Wash fish under cold running water. Dry thoroughly with paper toweling. Lay in shallow dish.

2. Combine egg white, mustard, milk, and tomato paste in cup. Blend with fork.

3. Combine and blend wheat germ, flour, and bread crumbs. Spread half of mixture across flat plate.

4. Dip fish into egg-white mixture, draining excess, then lay on top of crumb mixture. Sprinkle fish with balance of crumb mixture.

5. Heat 2 teaspoons oil over medium-high heat in nonstick skillet until hot. Spread shallots across skillet. Cook for 30 seconds. Lay fish on top of shallots. Sauté until golden brown (6 to 7 minutes). Add balance of oil. Turn fish. Sauté until done (6 to 7 minutes). Serve immediately, garnished with lemon and lime wedges.

Sautéed Scrod with Fennel and Rye

~

YIELD: SERVES 4

Because it is a bland-textured fish, scrod picks up and absorbs seasonings. Rye crumbs assist in keeping the interior of the fish fresh, moist, and delicious; and fennel, which seems to have been designed by nature to be cooked with fish, adds a warm, sweet taste reminiscent of anise.

1   **pound fresh scrod fillets, gently flattened to uniform thickness between 2 sheets of waxed paper**

2   **teaspoons each apple juice (no sugar added) and apple cider vinegar, combined**

3   **tablespoons soft rye crumbs (see pages 220 and 232, and Note, page 235)**

1   **tablespoon unbleached flour**

¼   **teaspoon each dried rosemary leaves and fennel seed, crushed**

⅛   **teaspoon crushed red pepper**

4   **teaspoons Italian olive oil**

1   **leek, white part only, well washed, dried, and minced**

    Juice from ½ lemon

Per serving
Calories: 164
Carbohydrate: 7 g
Protein: 22 g
Fat: 5 g
Saturated fat: 1 g
Cholesterol: 49 mg
Dietary fiber: 0.9 g
Sodium: 86 mg
Exchanges: ½ starch/bread
          3 lean meat

1. Wash fish under cold running water. Dry with paper toweling. Place in shallow dish. Sprinkle with apple juice and vinegar mixture, turning to coat. Let stand for 15 minutes.

2. In a cup, combine and blend crumbs, flour, rosemary, fennel, and crushed red pepper. Spread half of mixture across plate. Drain fish. Lay on top of crumbs. Sprinkle with balance of crumb mixture, pressing into fish.

3. Heat 2 teaspoons oil over medium-high heat in nonstick skillet until hot. Spread minced leek across skillet. Sauté over medium-high heat for 1 minute. Lay fish on top of leek and sauté until lightly browned (3 to 5 minutes, depending upon thickness of fillets). Turn, add balance of oil (2 teaspoons), and sauté for 2 minutes. Sprinkle with lemon juice, and sauté until done. (Cooking time will vary with thickness of fish.)

Marinades, Sauces, and Stocks

I'm a word detective when it comes to things culinary. That's because the original meaning of a word helps me understand the intent of the cooks who first used that word. Take "marinade." It's derived from the French verb mariner, which means "to put in salt water." So marinating was at first a simple pickling process intended to enhance the flavor of fish and meat. Until relatively recently, high salt content continued to dominate these precooking preparations. In 1979, I introduced my salt-free marinades, drawing on herbs, spices, fruit juices, stock, buttermilk, and low-fat yogurt to create marinades as bursting with flavor as they are with originality. Follow some of the following recipes and see for yourself how easy it is to create cooking magic.

When I traced "sauce" back to its original meaning, I discovered that it derives from the Latin salsa, which means "salted or salty." So there it is again—salt, the ubiquitous seasoning. Can a sauce be a real sauce without salt? Of course, it can. Because a real sauce means "appetizing, piquant, zesty, sometimes even pert, or saucy." And it's easy to make that kind of sauce without salt, as the recipes on the following pages demonstrate.

Stocks, the foundation for all gourmet cooking, are also surprisingly easy to make. Prove it to yourself with the stock recipes in this chapter and capture the essence of chicken and fish flavors in concentrated clear broths. They'll do such wonders for meat, fish, fowl, vegetables, and grains that you'll never be without a supply again.

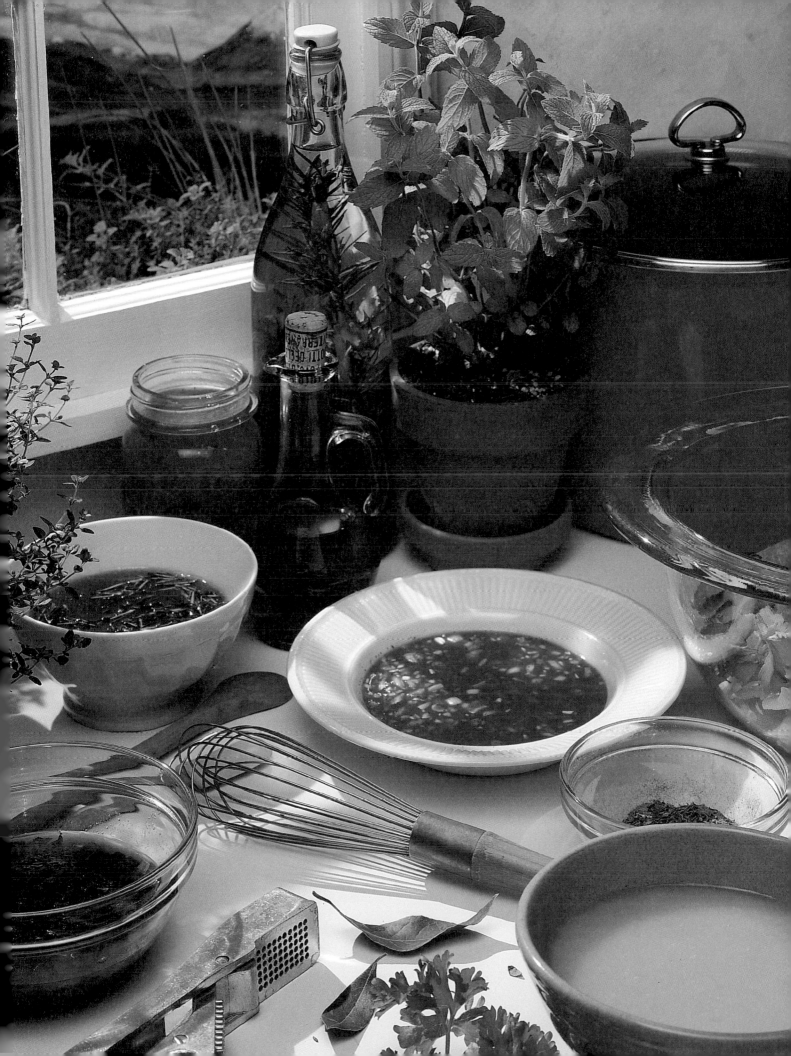

Marinades

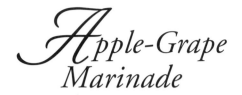

Apple-Grape Marinade

~

YIELD: ABOUT ⅔ CUP

(ENOUGH TO MARINATE A 3-POUND CHICKEN OR
BONED ROAST)

¼   cup each grape and apple juice
(no sugar added)

1   tablespoon fresh lemon juice

1   tablespoon peeled and shredded fresh ginger

2   teaspoons chili con carne seasoning

½   teaspoon cumin seed, crushed

2   large cloves garlic, minced

Combine all ingredients in a jar or bowl. Shake or whisk until well blended.

Per serving when dish serves 4
Calories: 17
Carbohydrate: 4 g
Protein: 0 g
Fat: 0 g
Saturated fat: 0 g
Cholesterol: 0 mg
Dietary fiber: 0.1 g
Sodium: 1 mg
Exchanges: free

Yogurt Marinade

~

YIELD: ABOUT ⅔ CUP

(ENOUGH TO MARINATE A 3-POUND CHICKEN OR
BONED ROAST)

¼ inch slice fresh ginger, peeled and minced

2 tablespoons grated onion

3 large cloves garlic, minced

1 tablespoon fresh lemon juice

⅓ cup tomato juice (no salt added)

1 teaspoon mild curry powder

⅛ teaspoon crushed red pepper

1 teaspoon cumin seed, crushed

¼ cup low-fat plain yogurt

Place all ingredients in a
bowl. Whisk to blend.

Per serving when dish serves 4
Calories: 24
Carbohydrate: 4 g
Protein: 1 g
Fat: trace
Saturated fat: trace
Cholesterol: 1 mg
Dietary fiber: 0.3 g
Sodium: 12 mg
Exchanges: 1 vegetable

Quick and Spicy Marinade

~

YIELD: ABOUT ½ CUP

(ENOUGH TO MARINATE A 3-POUND CHICKEN OR
BONED ROAST)

⅓ cup wine vinegar

2 teaspoons tomato paste (no salt added)

2 large shallots, minced

2 large cloves garlic, minced

1 teaspoon dried basil leaves, crushed

2 tablespoons minced fresh dill

2 teaspoons chili con carne seasoning

1 teaspoon corn oil (optional)

1. In a small bowl,
combine vinegar
with tomato paste.
Blend with whisk.

2. Whisk in balance
of ingredients.

NOTE: This marinade
is particularly deli-
cious with pork or
veal.

Per serving when dish serves 4
Calories: 9
Carbohydrate: 2 g
Protein: trace
Fat: 0 g
Saturated fat: 0 g
Cholesterol: 0 mg
Dietary fiber: 0.3 g
Sodium: 3 mg
Exchanges: free

Ginger-Mint Marinade

~

YIELD: ABOUT ⅔ CUP

(ENOUGH TO MARINATE A 3-POUND CHICKEN OR
BONED ROAST)

1 tablespoon apple juice (no sugar added)

3 tablespoons apple cider vinegar

2 teaspoons Italian olive oil

2 tablespoons dry vermouth

1 teaspoon peeled and minced fresh ginger

2 large cloves garlic, minced

8 dashes ground red (cayenne) pepper

2 tablespoons minced fresh mint

Combine all ingredients in a jar or bowl. Shake or whisk until well blended.

NOTE: This marinade tastes best with fresh ginger and fresh mint.

Per serving when dish serves 4
Calories: 28
Carbohydrate: 2 g
Protein: trace
Fat: 3 g
Saturated fat: trace
Cholesterol: 0 mg
Dietary fiber: 0.1 g
Sodium: 2 mg
Exchanges: ½ fat

Rosemary-Dill Marinade for Fish

~

YIELD: ABOUT ½ CUP

(ENOUGH TO MARINATE A 3-POUND WHOLE FISH OR
1½ POUNDS FILLETS)

1 tablespoon fresh lime juice

2 tablespoons each wine vinegar and apple juice (no sugar added)

2 teaspoons Italian olive oil

1 tablespoon minced fresh dill

½ teaspoon dried rosemary leaves, crushed

1 large clove garlic, minced

1 large shallot, minced

8 dashes ground red (cayenne) pepper

Combine all ingredients in a jar or bowl. Shake or whisk until well blended.

Per serving when dish serves 4
Calories: 29
Carbohydrate: 1 g
Protein: trace
Fat: 3 g
Saturated fat: trace
Cholesterol: 0 mg
Dietary fiber: 0.1 g
Sodium: 1 mg
Exchanges: ½ fat

Orange-Chili Marinade I

~

YIELD: ABOUT ⅔ CUP

(ENOUGH TO MARINATE A 3-POUND CHICKEN OR
BONED ROAST)

⅓ cup frozen orange juice concentrate

¼ cup wine vinegar

1 tablespoon fresh lemon juice

2 large shallots, minced

1 teaspoon chili con carne seasoning

⅛ teaspoon ground red (cayenne) pepper

½ teaspoon ground cinnamon

Combine all ingredients in a jar or bowl. Shake or whisk until well blended.

Per serving when dish serves 4
Calories: 36
Carbohydrate: 7 g
Protein: trace
Fat: 0 g
Saturated fat: 0 g
Cholesterol: 0 mg
Dietary fiber: 0.3 g
Sodium: 6 mg
Exchanges: ½ fruit

Orange-Chili Marinade II

~

YIELD: ABOUT ¾ CUP

(ENOUGH TO MARINATE A 3-POUND CHICKEN OR
BONED ROAST)

2 tablespoons frozen orange juice concentrate

3 tablespoons Easy Chicken Stock (page 216)

3 tablespoons apple cider vinegar

4 cloves garlic, minced

1 teaspoon peeled and minced fresh ginger

1 teaspoon chili con carne seasoning

2 tablespoons minced fresh parsley

Combine all ingredients in a jar or bowl. Shake or whisk until well blended.

Per serving when dish serves 4
Calories: 15
Carbohydrate: 3 g
Protein: trace
Fat: trace
Saturated fat: 0 g
Cholesterol: trace
Dietary fiber: 0 g
Sodium: 8 mg
Exchanges: free

Buttermilk Marinade

~

YIELD: ABOUT ⅞ CUP

(ENOUGH TO MARINATE A 3½-POUND CHICKEN OR BONED ROAST)

2   large cloves garlic, minced

2   tablespoons each minced fresh mint and dill

1   tablespoon fresh lime juice

¼   cup fresh orange juice

2   tablespoons apple cider vinegar

1   tablespoon corn oil

¼   cup low-fat buttermilk (preferably without added salt)

1   teaspoon ground coriander

⅛   teaspoon ground red (cayenne) pepper

Combine all ingredients in a jar or bowl. Shake or whisk to blend.

NOTE: Fresh herbs taste best in this recipe. You may, however, substitute 2 teaspoons crushed dried mint leaves for fresh mint.

Per serving when dish serves 4
Calories: 47
Carbohydrate: 3 g
Protein: 1 g
Fat: 4 g
Saturated fat: 1 g
Cholesterol: 1 mg
Dietary fiber: 0 g
Sodium: 10 mg
Exchanges: 1 fat

Tomato Marinade

~

YIELD: ABOUT ¾ CUP

(ENOUGH TO MARINATE A 3½-POUND CHICKEN OR BONED ROAST)

⅓   cup apple juice (no sugar added)

¼   cup tomato juice (no salt added)

¼   cup apple cider vinegar

1   tablespoon Italian olive oil

3   large cloves garlic, minced

1   tablespoon minced sweet green pepper

2   tablespoons coriander seed, well crushed

1   teaspoon chili con carne seasoning

1   tablespoon minced fresh mint, or 1 teaspoon dried mint leaves, crushed

1   tablespoon granulated fructose (page 297) (optional)

Combine all ingredients in a jar or bowl. Shake or whisk until well blended.

Per serving when dish serves 4
Calories: 52
Carbohydrate: 4 g
Protein: trace
Fat: 4 g
Saturated fat: trace
Cholesterol: 0 mg
Dietary fiber: 0.2 g
Sodium: 2 mg
Exchanges: 1 fat

Unusual Marinade

YIELD: ABOUT ⅔ CUP

(ENOUGH TO MARINATE A 3-POUND CHICKEN OR
BONED ROAST)

Per serving when dish serves 4
Calories: 5
Carbohydrate: 1 g
Protein: trace
Fat: trace
Saturated fat: trace
Cholesterol: 0 mg
Dietary fiber: trace
Sodium: trace
Exchanges: free

2   tablespoons each fresh lime juice,
wine vinegar, and pineapple juice
(no sugar added)

1   teaspoon dry mustard

⅛   teaspoon ground red (cayenne)
pepper

2   teaspoons coffee substitute or
decaffeinated coffee

1   large clove garlic, minced

½   teaspoon each ground ginger and
coriander

1   tablespoon each minced fresh
parsley and mint

1. Combine all ingredients in
saucepan except mint. Bring to
simmering point. Simmer for 1
minute. Let cool for 5 minutes.

2. Pour over uncooked chicken or
meat. Roast, following roasting
directions for Moist Baked
Chicken Legs (page 137).

3. Cut chicken into serving pieces (or
meat into thin slices), then sprinkle
with fresh mint and serve.

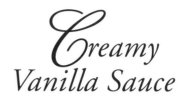

Creamy Vanilla Sauce

~

YIELD: 1 CUP

¼ cup part-skim ricotta cheese

½ cup evaporated skim milk (see page 297)

⅛ teaspoon each ground allspice, cardamom and nutmeg

½ teaspoon granulated fructose (see page 297)

½ teaspoon pure vanilla extract

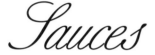

Sauces

1. Place cheese in large mixing bowl. Pour skim milk over cheese. Place bowl and whipping utensils in freezer. Chill until almost frozen.

2. Beat on high speed of mixing machine, sprinkling with spices and fructose, and dribbling with vanilla after mixture starts to thicken (about 1 minute). Continue beating for 2 minutes. Finished sauce will be thickened and creamy in texture. Serve immediately.

Per tablespoon
Calories: 12
Carbohydrate: 1 g
Protein: 1 g
Fat: trace
Saturated fat: trace
Cholesterol: 1 mg
Dietary fiber: 0 g
Sodium: 14 mg
Exchanges: free

$\mathcal{F}$resh Basil Tomato Sauce

~

YIELD: 2 CUPS

Per ¼ cup
Calories: 39
Carbohydrate: 5 g
Protein: 1 g
Fat: 2 g
Saturated fat: trace
Cholesterol: 0 mg
Dietary fiber: 1.5 g
Sodium: 12 mg
Exchanges: 1 vegetable

1 tablespoon Italian olive oil

2 large cloves garlic, minced

1 large onion, minced (about ½ cup)

3 tablespoons minced celery

2 tablespoons minced sweet green pepper

½ teaspoon dried thyme leaves, crushed

4 dashes ground red (cayenne) pepper

3 large ripe fresh tomatoes (1½ pounds), cored, seeded, skinned, and coarsely chopped

½ cup coarsely chopped loosely packed fresh basil leaves

1 tablespoon tomato paste (no salt added)

1 tablespoon apple juice (no sugar added)

1 teaspoon wine vinegar

1. Heat oil over medium heat in non-stick skillet until hot. Add garlic, onion, celery, and green pepper. Sprinkle with thyme and ground red pepper. Sauté until wilted (about 4 minutes), stirring often. Do not brown.

2. Add tomatoes and balance of ingredients. Bring to simmering point. Stir to blend. Cover and simmer for 45 minutes, stirring often.

3. Pour into food mill and puree. You will notice that some of the solids will not puree. Spoon them back into pureed sauce and stir to blend. Sauce will have a combined thick and smooth texture. Reheat, if necessary, and serve.

NOTE: At larger serving sizes, the olive oil begins to matter. For instance, ½ cup (2 servings) is 2 vegetable exchanges and ½ fat exchange.

SERVING SUGGESTIONS:
1. Pour over just-cooked pasta.

2. Pour over steamed fish.

3. Pour over grilled steaks, chops, or chicken.

4. Pour over omelettes (use basic omelette recipes, omitting fillings).

5. Pour over cooked portions of turkey, chicken, meat, or vegetables.

6. Serve as a condiment.

Tomato Sauce with Peppers

YIELD: ABOUT 5 CUPS

Per ½ cup
Calories: 58
Carbohydrate: 7 g
Protein: 1 g
Fat: 3 g
Saturated fat: trace
Cholesterol: trace
Dietary fiber: 1.9 g
Sodium: 9 mg
Exchanges: 1 vegetable
½ fat

2 tablespoons Italian olive oil

2 tablespoons peeled and shredded fresh ginger

4 medium onions, minced

4 large sweet green peppers, minced

4 cloves garlic, minced

¼ pound fresh mushrooms, washed, dried, trimmed, and sliced

2 teaspoons dried rosemary leaves, crushed

1 tablespoon dried mint, crumbled

1 teaspoon chili con carne seasoning

⅛ teaspoon crushed red pepper

2 cups canned Italian plum tomatoes (no salt added)

¼ cup Easy Chicken Stock (page 216)

⅓ cup apple juice (no sugar added)

Large bouquet garni (2 sprigs parsley, 1 bay leaf, tied together with white thread)

1. Heat oil over medium heat in large well-seasoned iron skillet until hot. Sauté ginger, onions, green peppers, garlic, and mushrooms over medium-high heat, stirring often, until softened but not brown.

2. Sprinkle with herbs and seasonings. Stir to blend. Cook for 1 minute.

3. Add remaining ingredients. Bring to simmering point. Cover and simmer for 20 minutes. Uncover. Remove bouquet garni, pressing out juices. Raise heat under skillet to just under boiling point and cook for 10 minutes. Liquid will be reduced and sauce will be thick.

NOTE: It's child's play to prepare this recipe with a food processor. I heat-seal some of it in heavy plastic boilable bags for a quick, fresh-tasting sauce to pour over almost any simply prepared meat, fish, or poultry—and, of course, pasta.

Delicate Juniper Berry Sauce

~

YIELD: 1 CUP

Per tablespoon
Calories: 11
Carbohydrate: 1 g
Protein: trace
Fat: 1 g
Saturated fat: trace
Cholesterol: 1 mg
Dietary fiber: 0.1 g
Sodium: 8 mg
Exchanges: free

2 teaspoons Italian olive oil

2 shallots, minced

2 cloves garlic, minced

1 cup Easy Chicken Stock (page 216)

¼ cup dry red wine

1½ teaspoons tomato paste (no salt added)

¼ teaspoon dried thyme leaves, crushed

1 teaspoon juniper berries, well crushed

1 tablespoon minced fresh parsley

¼ teaspoon Worcestershire sauce

1 tablespoon arrowroot flour (or cornstarch) dissolved in 2 tablespoons water

1. Heat oil in heavy-bottom enameled saucepan until hot. Sauté shallots and garlic over medium-high heat until lightly browned.

2. Combine stock, wine, and tomato paste in a small bowl. Add to saucepan. Cook for 1 minute.

3. Add thyme, juniper berries, parsley, and Worcestershire sauce. Bring to simmering point. Simmer, uncovered, for 5 minutes. Raise heat under saucepan to medium, and cook for 5 minutes.

4. Pour through fine sieve or washed cotton cheesecloth, pressing out juices. Pour back into saucepan, and reheat.

5. Slowly add dissolved arrowroot flour mixture, stirring with wooden spoon. Cook for 2 minutes, stirring constantly. Sauce will be smooth and will thicken to the consistency of heavy cream.

$\mathcal{A}$lmost Instant Orange Sauce
~

YIELD: ABOUT ¾ CUP

Per tablespoon
Calories: 4
Carbohydrate: 1 g
Protein: trace
Fat: 0 g
Saturated fat: 0 g
Cholesterol: 0 mg
Dietary fiber: 0.1 g
Sodium: 5 mg
Exchanges: free

1¾ cups water

1 large rib celery, coarsely chopped

1 tablespoon frozen orange juice concentrate

½ teaspoon fresh lemon juice

1 tablespoon dry vermouth

1 fresh parsley sprig

1 tablespoon arrowroot flour (or cornstarch) dissolved in 4 teaspoons water

1. In heavy-bottom saucepan, combine first 6 ingredients. Bring to simmering point and cook, uncovered, until reduced to ¾ cup.

2. Dribble in only enough arrowroot flour mixture to make a lightly thickened sauce. Then cook for 1 minute more. Remove parsley sprig, and serve immediately.

NOTE: For extra-rich-tasting sauce, replace ¾ cup water with ½ cup Thirty-Minute Chicken Broth (page 215) and ¼ cup water.

Two-Way Blender Sour Cream

(For topping or dip)

~

YIELD: ABOUT 1 CUP

⅔ cup dry curd cottage cheese (no salt added) or well-drained low-fat cottage cheese (no salt added)

⅓ cup low-fat buttermilk (preferably without salt)

2 teaspoons grated onion

½ teaspoon prepared Dijon mustard

1 tablespoon minced fresh dill, basil, rosemary, or tarragon leaves

2 dashes ground red (cayenne) pepper (optional)

Combine all ingredients in food blender and blend until smooth. Chill before serving.

NOTE: At larger serving sizes, the exchanges begin to add up. For instance, 3 tablespoons (3 servings) has ½ lean meat exhange.

SERVING SUGGESTIONS:

1. Serve as topping over steamed vegetables or fish, cold sliced chicken, turkey, or meat.

2. Serve as a dip with whole-grain crackers.

Per tablespoon
Calories: 7
Carbohydrate: trace
Protein: 1 g
Fat: trace
Saturated fat: 0 g
Cholesterol: 1 mg
Dietary fiber: 0 g
Sodium: 3 mg
Exchanges: free

Yogurt Dessert Topping

~

YIELD: ABOUT ¾ CUP

3 tablespoons pineapple juice (no sugar added)

1 teaspoon granulated fructose (see page 297)

½ cup low-fat plain yogurt

½ teaspoon fresh lemon juice

⅛ teaspoon each ground cinnamon and allspice

Dash ground cloves

½ teaspoon finely grated orange zest (preferably from navel orange)

1. Heat pineapple juice in heavy-bottom saucepan until just warm. Remove from heat. Stir in fructose. Let cool.

2. Combine balance of ingredients in bowl, stirring to blend. Add cooled pineapple juice mixture. Gently stir (do not beat).

3. Serve well chilled spooned over fresh fruits, salads, or cakes.

Per tablespoon
Calories: 9
Carbohydrate: 2 g
Protein: 1 g
Fat: trace
Saturated fat: trace
Cholesterol: 1 mg
Dietary fiber: 0 g
Sodium: 7 mg
Exchanges: free

Stocks

Rejuvenated Canned Chicken Broth

~

YIELD: ABOUT 3 CUPS

2   cans unsalted, low-fat, canned chicken broth (about 26 ounces)

¼   cup minced shallot

¼   teaspoon each dried dill weed, thyme, marjoram leaves, and sage leaves

2   whole cloves

3   snow-white fresh mushrooms, trimmed, damp-wiped, and sliced

1   small bay leaf

4   large sprigs parsley or 2 sprigs of fresh dill

*U*nsalted, low-fat, canned chicken broth, you're likely to agree, is taste-less. Tasteless, yes, but not useless. Here's how you can perk it up into a flavorsome stand-in for your homemade chicken stock. Keep 2 cans of unsalted, low-fat chicken broth in your larder, and whenever your own Chicken Stock (page 216) or Thirty-Minute Chicken Broth (page 215) is nearing depletion invigorate the canned broth with this recipe. A wonderful backup until you make the real thing again.

1. Put all ingredients into a 1½-quart heavy-bottom saucepan. Bring to a boil. Reduce heat to simmering. Cover and simmer for 20 minutes. Uncover and cool.

2. Strain contents of pot through a fine sieve (or a cheese-cloth-lined strainer). Store in refrigerator in a tightly closed jar. Stir before using.

NOTE: At larger serving sizes this is no longer a free food. For instance, a ½-cup portion is ½ fat exchange.

Per tablespoon
Calories: 4
Carbohydrate: trace
Protein: trace
Fat: trace
Saturated fat: trace
Cholesterol: 1 mg
Dietary fiber: 0 g
Sodium: 14 mg
Exchanges: free

Thirty-Minute Chicken Broth

~

YIELD: ABOUT 1¾ CUPS

After cooking this recipe, save the chicken breast and use it in any of my recipes calling for cooked chicken; or chill, slice, and serve cold for a low-calorie luncheon treat.

Per tablespoon
Calories: 2
Carbohydrate: 0 g
Protein: trace
Fat: trace
Saturated fat: 0 g
Cholesterol: trace
Dietary fiber: 0 g
Sodium: 7 mg
Exchanges: free

1   whole skinned chicken breast with bone (about 1½ pounds)

1½ cups water

¼   cup each dry vermouth and apple juice (no sugar added)

1   small leek, split, well washed and sliced

1   small carrot, peeled and sliced

2   cloves garlic, minced

½   teaspoon peeled and minced fresh ginger

Bouquet garni (1 sprig each parsley, thyme, and rosemary, and 1 bay leaf, tied together with white thread; see Note 1)

1. Place chicken and water in a 1-quart heavy-bottom saucepan. Bring to boil. Reduce heat to simmering and cook, uncovered, for 3 minutes, removing any scum that rises to top.

2. Add balance of ingredients. Bring to simmering point. Partially cover and simmer for 20 minutes. Uncover and let cool in pot for 10 minutes. Remove chicken.

3. Place fine-meshed strainer or chinois (see Note, page 151) over bowl. Pour broth into strainer, pressing solids to extract juices. Then strain through washed cotton cheesecloth.

4. If you wish to use stock immediately, skim off visible fat from top by using a skimming utensil, or by blotting surface with paper toweling. If you're not planning to use stock until next day, follow step 3 for the following recipe, Easy Chicken Stock.

NOTES:

1. If fresh thyme and rosemary sprigs are not available, substitute ¼ teaspoon each dried thyme and rosemary leaves. Place entire bouquet garni mixture in washed cotton cheesecloth and tie securely with white thread.

2. At larger serving sizes, this is no longer a free food. For instance, the entire recipe (1¾ cups) is 1 fat exchange.

Easy Chicken Stock

~

YIELD: ABOUT 6 CUPS

Per tablespoon
Calories: 2
Carbohydrate: 0 g
Protein: trace
Fat: trace
Saturated fat: 0 g
Cholesterol: trace
Dietary fiber: 0 g
Sodium: 7 mg
Exchanges: free

4 pounds skinned chicken giblets (excluding liver), backs and wings, or 2 small broiling chickens, skinned and well trimmed

7 cups water

1 large onion, peeled and quartered

3 ribs celery with leaves, cut up

2 medium carrots, peeled and sliced

4 cloves garlic, coarsely chopped

2 scallions or green onions, trimmed and coarsely chopped

3 whole cloves

1 teaspoon minced fresh ginger

½ teaspoon dried thyme

Large bouquet garni (3 dill sprigs, 1 parsley sprig, and 1 bay leaf, tied together with white thread)

1. Combine chicken and water in a large stainless steel pot or waterless cooker. Bring to rolling boil. Turn heat down to slow-boil and cook, uncovered, for 5 minutes, removing scum that rises to top.

2. Add balance of ingredients. Bring to boil again. Cover partially and simmer for 2½ hours. Remove whole pieces of chicken for salad or sandwiches.

3. Place fine-meshed strainer or chinois (see Note, page 151) over bowl. Pour stock into strainer, pressing solids to extract juices. Then strain through washed cotton cheesecloth.

4. Transfer to small freezeproof containers. Cover tightly and refrigerate until jelled. Cut away hardened fat that rises to top. Stock is now ready to use.

NOTE: At larger serving sizes, exchanges begin to add up. At 1¾ cups, for instance, this stock has ½ lean meat exhange and 1 fat exchange.

STORING SUGGESTION: Fill each cube of large ice-cube trays with 2 tablespoons stock; freeze. Remove cubes from trays and store in double plastic bags for easy access whenever a recipe calls for 2 tablespoons or more of stock.

Aromatic Fish Stock

YIELD: 2½ CUPS

Per tablespoon
Calories: 2
Carbohydrate: trace
Protein: 1 g
Fat: trace
Saturated fat: trace
Cholesterol: 0 mg
Dietary fiber: trace
Sodium: 29 mg
Exchanges: free

2 pounds bones and heads of any white-fleshed fish, cut into 3-inch pieces (see Note)

1 small leek, well washed, trimmed, and sliced

2 large cloves garlic, coarsely chopped

1 tablespoon grated carrot

2 whole cloves

2 cups water

¾ cup dry white wine

2 sprigs fresh cilantro (Chinese parsley; also called coriander) or ½ teaspoon dried cilantro, crushed

1. Wash bones and heads under cold running water. Place in heavy-bottom saucepan. Add balance of ingredients (except cilantro). Bring to boil and cook over moderate heat for 3 minutes, removing scum that rises to top. Add cilantro.

2. Cover and simmer for 30 minutes. Let stock cool, uncovered, in pot for 15 minutes.

3. Strain through fine sieve or chinois (see Note, page 151), placing bowl underneath, and pressing solids to remove all stock. Then strain through washed cotton cheese-cloth.

4. Pour into freezeproof containers and freeze.

NOTES:
1. Recipe for Stir-Fried Sea Bass and Asparagus (page 190) calls for ½ cup of fish stock. Here's your chance to prepare two recipes at one time and have stock left over for another fabulous dish from the sea. Hint: Try substituting equal amounts of fish stock (in fish recipes only) whenever recipe calls for dry vermouth.

2. At larger serving sizes, this is no longer a free food. At 1¾ cups, for instance, this fish stock is 1 lean meat exchange.

Breads

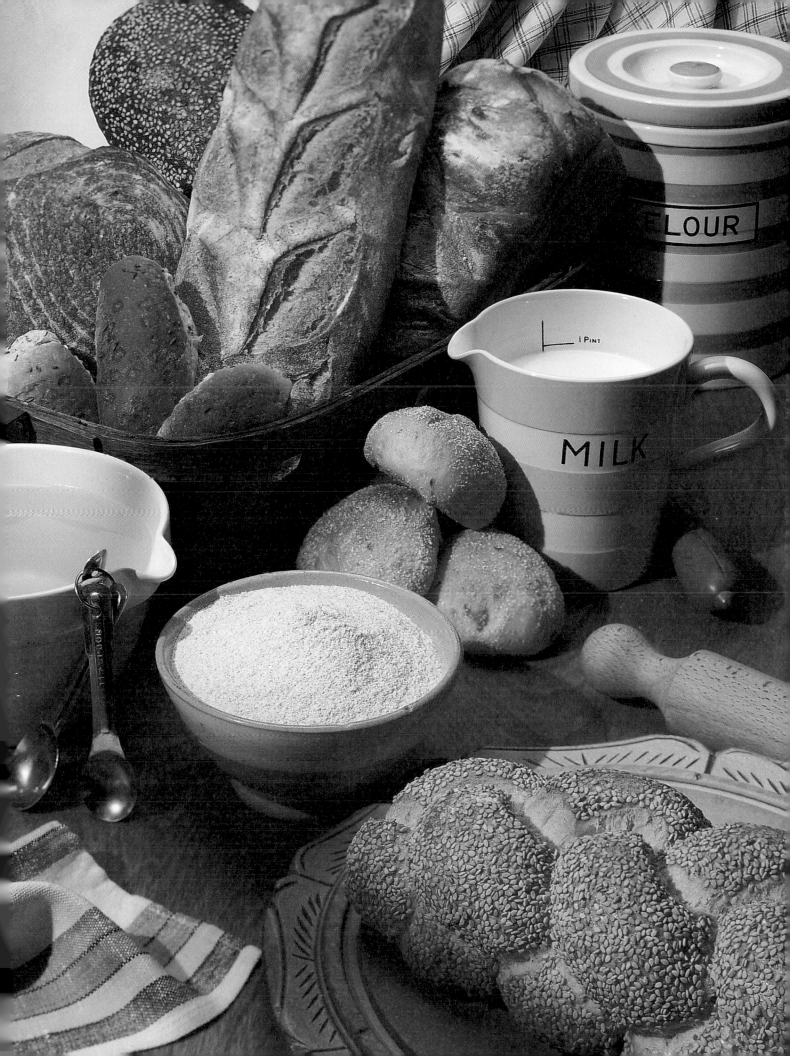

*M*agic Rye Bread *(a food-processor hit)*
~

YIELD: 1 LARGE LOAF; 27 LARGE ⅜-INCH SLICES

Easy to knead (thanks to the magic of the food processor), this plump, gorgeous loaf is as eye-filling as it is palate-pleasing. Savor the spongelike crumb (from a magic mix of buttermilk, gluten flour, and a little bit of baking powder). Watch it rise three times as if by magic. And in the finale of your breadcrafty act, bring down the house with 27 extra-large slices of slightly sourdough-tasting delight. There's no magic act like it.

About 2¾ cups unbleached flour

1 package dry yeast

¼ teaspoon sugar

¼ cup warm water (105°F to 115°F)

1¼ cups low-fat buttermilk (preferably without salt)

2 tablespoons Italian olive or canola oil, plus ½ teaspoon for bowl

1 tablespoon unsulfured molasses

3 tablespoons date sugar (see page 297 and Variations below)

1 tablespoon finely minced orange zest

1 cup light rye flour (see page 297)

½ cup gluten flour

½ teaspoon each ground cardamom and cinnamon

½ teaspoon baking powder

2 teaspoons caraway seeds

2 teaspoons well-crushed coriander seeds

½ teaspoon sweet soft corn oil margarine for pan

1½ teaspoons stone ground yellow cornmeal

1 egg white mixed with 2 teaspoons water (optional)

1. In a tall water glass, combine and blend 2 tablespoons flour, yeast, sugar, and water (a chopstick does a fine job here). Let stand until mixture foams and rises to the top of the glass (about 8 minutes).

2. In a small saucepan, combine buttermilk with 2 tablespoons oil, the molasses, date sugar, and orange zest. Over very low heat, stir and warm until date sugar dissolves. Remove from heat.

3. In workbowl of food processor fitted with steel blade, put 2¼ cups unbleached flour, the rye and gluten flours, spices, baking powder, 1½ teaspoons caraway seeds, and all the coriander seeds. Process for 10 seconds. With machine running, pour yeast through feed tube, scraping out glass; then gradually pour buttermilk mixture through feed tube. Process for 15 seconds. Stop machine and let dough rest for 2 minutes. Uncover workbowl. If dough has formed into cohesive ball(s), re-cover and process until one large ball forms and rotates around the bowl 20 times. If dough feels sticky to the touch, sprinkle with 1 to 2 tablespoons remaining flour, re-cover and process until a ball forms and rotates around the bowl 20 times. Stop machine and let dough rest for 2 minutes.

Per slice
Calories: 81
Carbohydrate: 15 g
Protein: 2 g
Fat: 1 g
Saturated fat: trace
Cholesterol: trace
Dietary fiber: 0.9 g
Sodium: 16 mg
Exchanges: 1 starch/bread

4. Remove and shape into a ball. If dough feels slightly sticky, lightly sprinkle work surface with flour and knead by hand until smooth and pliable. Shape into a ball. Drop into a lightly oiled fairly straight-sided bowl, turning to coat. Cover tightly with plastic wrap. Let rise at room temperature (70°F to 80°F) for 45 minutes. Punch down, briefly knead in bowl, reshape into a ball, re-cover and let rise until doubled (about 1½ hours). Punch down and knead out air bubbles (you'll hear them pop). Cover and let dough rest for 5 minutes.

5. Roll or stretch out into an 8" × 10" rectangle. Roll up tightly, pinching seams and sides. With hands, roll back and forth to smooth out.

6. Lightly margarine-grease a medium pan with sides (at least 7" × 9"). Sprinkle with cornmeal, shaking off excess. Place bread in pan. With a sharp serrated knife, cut 2 shallow diagonal slashes across loaf. Cover with plastic wrap (it won't stick when removed). Let rise until almost doubled (1 to 1¼ hours). Preheat oven to 400°F.

7. Brush bread with egg white mixture. Sprinkle with remaining ½ teaspoon caraway seeds, if desired. Bake in center section of oven for 20 minutes. Reduce heat to 375°F. Bake for 20 minutes longer, covering loosely with a sheet of aluminum foil if top of loaf browns too rapidly. Tap bottom of loaf with knuckles. A hollow sound indicates bread is done. If not, return to oven directly on rack and bake for 5 minutes. Cool completely on wire rack. Wrap in plastic for several hours for easy thin-slicing.

VARIATIONS:

1. Diet permitting, replace date sugar with 3 tablespoons firmly packed light brown sugar for a sweeter loaf.

2. Using Variation 1, convert this recipe into a raisin loaf by sprinkling ½ cup dark seedless raisins across dough before rolling up (step 5).

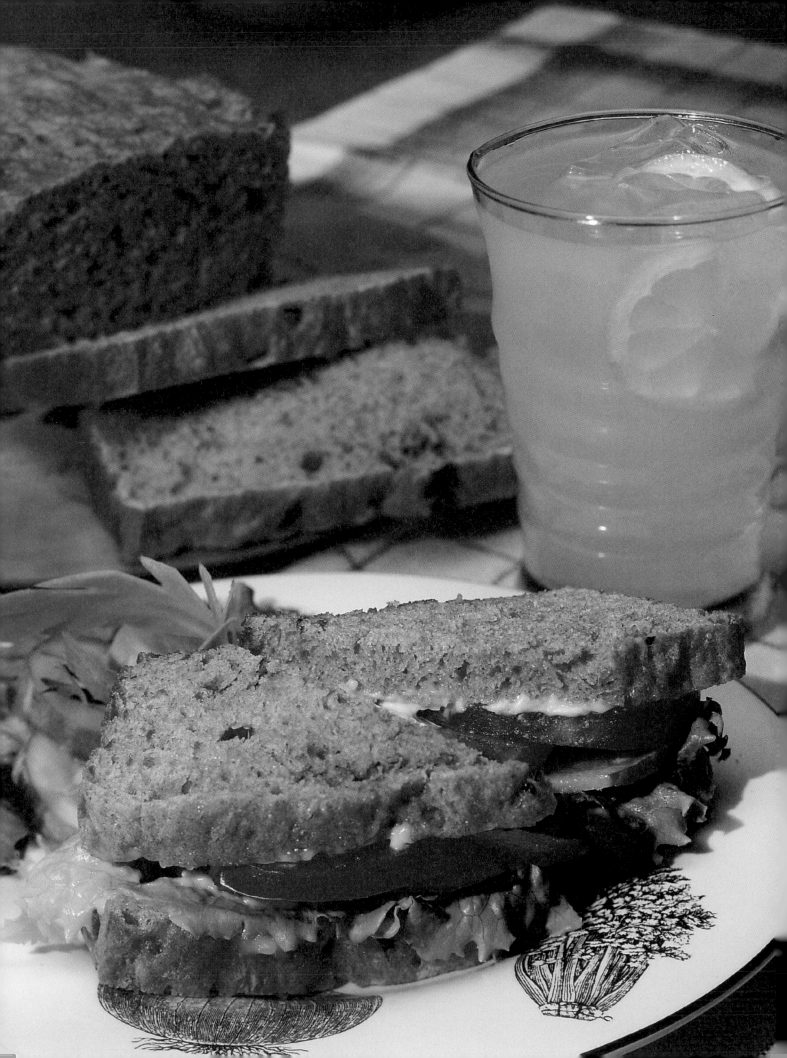

*N*o-Knead Barley Bread

YIELD: 1 LOAF (24 SLICES, ⅜ INCH EACH)

Can you beat a simple cake with an electric beater or a wooden spoon? Then you can prepare this bread just as easily. It's actually a three-flour bread, but it's the barley flour that sets it apart, adding a new, distinct texture. Barley flour is available in health-food stores.

Per slice
Calories: 72
Carbohydrate: 13 g
Protein: 2 g
Fat: 2 g
Saturated fat: trace
Cholesterol: 7 mg
Dietary fiber: 1.5 g
Sodium: 3 mg
Exchanges: 1 starch/bread

1½ cups unbleached flour

1 cup whole-wheat flour

1 package dry yeast

1 teaspoon granulated fructose (see page 297)

½ teaspoon ground cinnamon

1 teaspoon ground coriander

½ cup apple juice (no sugar added)

¾ cup water

2 tablespoons Italian olive oil or canola oil

1 teaspoon grated orange zest

1 egg, reserving 1 teaspoon egg white

¾ cup barley flour (see page 297)

¼ teaspoon sweet corn oil margarine for pan

2 teaspoons unshelled sesame seed or poppy seed (see page 297)

1. In large mixing bowl, combine all of unbleached flour, ½ cup whole-wheat flour, yeast, fructose, cinnamon, and coriander.

2. In saucepan, heat apple juice, water, oil, and orange zest until very warm (115°F to 120°F). Pour into dry mixture. Beat on medium speed of mixing machine or with wooden spoon for 15 seconds. Add egg. Beat with machine for 3 minutes, stopping machine and scraping down sides of bowl midway; or beat with wooden spoon until well blended.

3. Using wooden spoon, beat in balance of whole-wheat flour (½ cup) and all of barley flour, ¼ cup at a time. Mixture will be soft and sticky.

4. Lightly grease a 9½" × 6" × 2½" loaf pan with margarine. Spoon and spread batter into pan, making sure that all corners are filled. Smooth top with dampened fingers. Cover loosely with plastic wrap and let rise at room tempera-ture (70°F to 80°F) until doubled in bulk (about 1¼ hours). Preheat oven to 375°F.

5. Beat reserved egg white with 2 tea-spoons water. Gently brush over loaf. Sprinkle with sesame or poppy seed. Bake for 30 minutes. Cover loosely with aluminum foil and bake for additional 10 to 15 minutes. To test for doneness, insert a metal skewer into center of bread; skewer should come out dry. Place pan on rack and let cool for 10 minutes.

6. Gently remove bread from pan and let cool for 30 minutes. Delicious served slightly warm, at room tem-perature, or toasted.

NOTE: This bread freezes very well. Slice when completely cooled, then reassemble into loaf shape. Wrap securely in plastic wrap or waxed paper, then in aluminum foil, and freeze. Each slice when frozen can easily be flicked off for quick toasting.

Coriander Whole-Wheat Bread

YIELD: 3 LOAVES (20 SLICES, ⅜ INCH EACH, PER LOAF)

My happiest time in the kitchen is when I'm making bread. If you've never made bread before and want to share my bread-making joy, here's an easy recipe to start with. You'll get it right the first time, and puffed with pride you'll want to share your creation with everybody. Sweetened with fruit juices, cardamom, and other spices, here is a crisp, crunchy loaf with a delicate center. It's a perfect foil for chicken, meat, and cheese, and is excellent toasted or enjoyed as is (that's the way I like it).

2   packages dry yeast

⅓   cup nonfat dry milk

2   cups whole-wheat flour

3¼ cups unbleached flour

2   teaspoons ground coriander

1   teaspoon cinnamon

¼   teaspoon allspice

¾   cup apple juice (no sugar added)

1   tablespoon frozen orange juice concentrate

1   cup water

1   tablespoon Italian olive oil or canola oil, plus ¼ teaspoon for bowl

½   cup low-fat plain yogurt

1   tablespoon grated orange zest (preferably from navel orange)

½   teaspoon sweet soft corn oil margarine for baking pans and waxed paper

1. In large mixing bowl, combine yeast, milk, 1 cup each whole-wheat and unbleached flours, and spices. Combine apple juice, orange juice concentrate, water, and 1 tablespoon oil in saucepan. Heat until very warm (115°F to 120°F). Pour over dry ingredients. Beat with wooden spoon until well blended (about 1 minute). Cover and let stand for 10 minutes.

2. Stir in yogurt and orange zest.

3. Beat in balance of whole-wheat flour (1 cup). Add balance of unbleached flour, ½ cup at a time, beating with wooden spoon after each addition. When dough becomes too difficult to handle with wooden spoon, turn onto lightly floured board and knead, using additional flour if necessary, (up to ¼ cup) to make a smooth and elastic dough. When dough is fully kneaded, you'll find it delightfully pliant and soft to the touch. (If you have a dough hook attachment on your mixing machine, see Note.)

Per 2 slices

Calories: 86

Carbohydrate: 16 g

Protein: 3 g

Fat: 1 g

Saturated fat: trace

Cholesterol: 1 mg

Dietary fiber: 1.4 g

Sodium: 10 mg

Exchanges: 1 starch/bread

4. Shape dough into ball. Heat outside of fairly straight-sided bowl by placing it briefly under hot running water. Lightly oil inside of bowl. Drop dough into bowl. Cover tightly with plastic wrap, and let rise at room temperature (70°F to 80°F) until doubled in bulk (about 1½ hours).

5. Punch down. Transfer to board and knead briefly. The dough will be very easy to handle. Shape into loaf. Cut into 3 equal pieces. Shape into loaves. Place in 3 small margarine-greased loaf pans (7⅜" × 3⅝" × 2¼"). Cover loosely with waxed paper that has been lightly greased with margarine. Let rise until doubled in bulk (well above sides of pans, about 1½ hours). Preheat oven to 375°F.

6. Bake for 45 minutes. Loaves should be golden brown and crispy to the touch. Test doneness by removing loaves from pans and tapping bottoms of loaves with knuckles. Loaves are done when you hear a hollow sound. If not done, place back in oven directly on rack for 5 minutes.

7. Remove from oven and let cool completely on rack before slicing.

NOTE: When using a dough hook, start after dough becomes too difficult to handle with wooden spoon. Knead for 7 minutes after dough has cleaned sides of bowl and has clung to dough hook. Then knead briefly by hand to warm dough. Continue with recipe instructions.

Light and Spongy Loaf

YIELD: 2 LOAVES (EACH QUARTER LOAF MAKES 8 UNEVEN ½-INCH SLICES)

Probably the most fun I get in bread making is when I take two sets of similar ingredients and make entirely different kinds of breads from each of them. Case in point: You won't find much difference between the ingredients in this recipe and in the preceding one, but I've changed the proportions and the techniques—and what a difference in the results! Here are two round cakelike loaves that slice into a sandwich maker's delight. Or use one thick slice for my Pineapple French Toast (page 37)—and be amazed by the new taste sensation. Homemade bread is such fun to make, to use, and to savor bite by bite that once you get into bread making you'll never want to stock store-bought bread again.

2	packages dry yeast
2	teaspoons granulated fructose (see page 297)
5	cups unbleached flour
½	cup skim milk
1¾	cups water
1	tablespoon Italian olive oil or canola oil, plus ¼ teaspoon for bowl
1	cup whole-wheat flour
2	teaspoons anise seed, crushed
1	teaspoon ground coriander
1	tablespoon grated orange zest (preferably from navel orange)
½	teaspoon sweet soft corn oil margarine for baking sheet and waxed paper
1	tablespoon stone-ground cornmeal
1	egg white beaten with 1 tablespoon water
1	tablespoon unshelled sesame seed (see page 297)

1. The night before baking, combine 1 package yeast, fructose, and 2 cups unbleached flour in large mixing bowl. Heat milk and 1½ cups water until warmed to 105°F to 115°F. Pour over dry ingredients, stirring until well blended. Cover tightly with plastic wrap and let stand in draft-free warm spot overnight.

2. Next day, stir down mixture. Dissolve balance of yeast (1 package) in balance of water (¼ cup). Add to bowl and beat with wooden spoon until blended.

3. Stir in all of whole-wheat flour, anise seed, coriander, and orange zest. Add all but ¼ cup of balance of unbleached flour (2¾ cups), ½ cup at a time, beating with wooden spoon after each addition. When dough becomes too difficult to handle with spoon, scoop up, and turn onto lightly floured board and knead, adding balance of flour until dough is smooth and elastic. The mixture will be slightly sticky when you start kneading, but stickiness will disappear and dough will become resilient with delicate texture when fully kneaded.

Per 2 slices, ½ inch each, from quarter loaves or 2 slices, ⅜ inch each, from three loaves

Calories: 89

Carbohydrate: 17 g

Protein: 3 g

Fat: 1 g

Saturated fat: trace

Cholesterol: trace

Dietary fiber: 1.1 g

Sodium: 7 mg

Exchanges: 1 starch/bread

4. Shape dough into ball. Lightly oil fairly straight-sided bowl. Drop ball into bowl. Cover tightly with plastic wrap and let rise at room temperature (70°F to 80°F) until more than doubled in bulk (about 1¼ hours).

5. Punch dough down. Transfer to board and knead briefly. Shape into ball. Cut in half. Reshape into 2 balls. Grease an 11½" × 15½" jelly-roll pan with ¼ teaspoon margarine. Sprinkle with cornmeal, shaking out excess. Place loaves in opposite corners of pan. Grease a sheet of waxed paper with balance of margarine. Place over loaves, greased side down. Let rise until more than doubled. Preheat oven to 400°F.

6. Brush with egg-white mixture; sprinkle with sesame seed. Bake for 10 minutes. Reduce heat to 375°F and bake for 30 minutes or until done. Tap bottoms of loaves with knuckles. If you hear a hollow sound, your bread is done. If it is soft, return to the oven without the pan for 5 minutes.

VARIATION: In step 5, cut into 3 equal pieces. Shape into loaves. Place in 3 small margarine-greased loaf pans (7⅜" × 3⅝" × 2¼"). Let rise until more than doubled. Brush with egg-white mixture. Sprinkle with 1½ teaspoons each poppy seed and unshelled sesame seed. Bake in preheated 375°F oven for 45 minutes. Remove from pans and let cool completely on rack before slicing. Makes 3 loaves (20 slices, ⅜ inch each, per loaf).

24 Onion Rolls and One Loaf

~

YIELD: 24 ROLLS, 1 LOAF

Imagine—24 rolls and a substantial loaf for under one dollar. Eat the rolls as is for weeks after they emerge from the oven (they're wonderful freezers), or use them magically to lend sparkle to so-so fillings and panache to great ones. Bonus: They're such fun to make!

2   packages dry yeast

4½   cups unbleached flour

1   cup whole-wheat flour

4   dashes ground red (cayenne) pepper

2   teaspoons anise seed, crushed

½   cup each water and apple juice (no sugar added)

1   cup skim milk

1½   teaspoons granulated fructose (see page 297)

6   tablespoons minced dried onion

2   teaspoons prepared Dijon mustard

5   teaspoons Italian olive oil or canola oil, plus ¼ teaspoon for rising bowl

1   egg yolk

1   teaspoon sweet soft corn oil margarine

2   egg whites mixed with 2 teaspoons water

1   tablespoon poppy seed

⅓   cup water

1. In large mixing bowl, combine yeast, 1½ cups unbleached flour, all of whole-wheat flour, ground red pepper, and anise seed. Stir to combine.

2. In heavy-bottom saucepan, combine water, apple juice, milk, fructose, 3 tablespoons dried onion, mustard, and 5 teaspoons oil. Heat slowly until very warm (115°F to 120°F), stirring to dissolve fructose. Pour over dry mixture. Beat with wooden spoon or with electric beater until smooth. Cover bowl and let stand for 10 minutes.

3. Stir mixture down. Blend in egg yolk. Beat in balance of unbleached flour. When mixture becomes too difficult to handle with wooden spoon, use dough hook, or turn onto a lightly floured board. Knead until smooth and elastic, adding a little more flour if necessary to make a nonsticky dough. Shape into ball.

Per roll or slice (¹⁄₁₂ of loaf)
Calories: 75
Carbohydrate: 14 g
Protein: 2 g
Fat: 1 g
Saturated fat: trace
Cholesterol: 8 mg
Dietary fiber: 0.9 g
Sodium: 7 mg
Exchanges: 1 starch/bread

4. Drop into lightly greased, fairly straight-sided bowl. Cover tightly with plastic wrap. Let rise at room temperature (70°F to 80°F) until double in bulk (about 1 hour). Punch down. Transfer to board. Knead briefly, pressing out bubbles (you'll hear them pop). Divide into thirds. Cover with bowl and let rest for 5 minutes.

5. For the loaf, shape one-third of dough into a loaf. Place in small (7⅜" × 3⅝" × 2¼") loaf pan lightly greased with margarine. Brush with some egg-white mixture. Cover loosely with waxed paper. Let rise until doubled (about 1 hour). Preheat oven to 375°F. Brush again with some egg-white mixture. Sprinkle with some poppy seed. Bake for 40 to 45 minutes, or until crispy. Remove from pan. Let cool on rack before slicing.

6. For the rolls, cut each third of remaining dough in half. Then cut each half into 6 pieces. Shape pieces into balls. Flatten to 3-inch circles. Place on 3 margarine greased cookie sheets. Brush lightly with egg-white mixture. Cover loosely with waxed paper and let rise until double (30 to 40 minutes). Preheat oven to 375°F. Combine balance of minced onion (3 tablespoons) with ⅓ cup water. Let stand until softened. Lightly brush rolls again with egg-white mixture. Then sprinkle with equal amounts of softened onion. Sprinkle with balance of poppy seed. Bake for 20 to 25 minutes, or until lightly browned. Serve warm or at room temperature.

Food Processor Whole-Wheat Bran Loaf

~

YIELD: 2 MEDIUM LOAVES (20 SLICES, ⅜ INCH EACH, PER LOAF)

You'll scarcely need to touch this dough, but when you do, you'll find it ever so supple and easy to handle. You'll make a sweet loaf—crunchy, crusted, with a firm-textured yet tender center, and a novel kind of deliciousness. Prediction: Once the enticing baking aromas waft from your oven, you'll have a horde of drooling neighbors knocking at your door.

⅓ cup warm water (105°F to 115°F)

1 package dry yeast

½ teaspoon granulated fructose (see page 297)

2 tablespoons unbleached flour, plus 2¾ cups

1 cup whole-wheat flour

½ teaspoon baking powder

1 teaspoon ground coriander

½ teaspoon freshly grated nutmeg

2 teaspoons coarsely grated orange zest (preferably from navel orange)

2 tablespoons each oat bran and date sugar (see page 297)

¼ cup low-fat plain yogurt

1 cup apple juice (no sugar added)

1 tablespoon Italian olive oil or canola oil, plus ¼ teaspoon for bowl

½ teaspoon sweet soft corn oil margarine for pan and waxed paper

1. Combine water, dry yeast, fructose, and 2 tablespoons unbleached flour in mixing bowl. Stir to blend. Cover and let stand for 10 minutes. Mixture will puff up.

2. Fit food processor with steel blade. In processor bowl, combine 2½ cups unbleached flour, all of whole-wheat flour, baking powder, spices, orange zest, oat bran, and date powder. Turn processor on/off twice to blend. With machine on, pour risen yeast mixture through feed tube, scraping small bowl to remove every drop. Process for 15 seconds. Stop machine.

3. Pour yogurt through feed tube. Process for 5 seconds.

For 2 slices
Calories: 93
Carbohydrate: 18 g
Protein: 3 g
Fat: 1 g
Saturated fat: trace
Cholesterol: trace
Dietary fiber: 1.3 g
Sodium: 13 mg
Exchanges: 1 starch/bread

4. In a saucepan, heat apple juice and 1 tablespoon oil until warm (90°F). With machine running, pour through feed tube. Process until soft ball forms and rotates in processor 10 times, adding balance of flour (¼ cup) if dough sticks to sides of bowl and doesn't rotate freely. Remove to board and knead for 1 minute.

5. Shape dough into ball. Drop into large, fairly straight-sided, lightly oiled bowl, turning to coat. Cover tightly with plastic wrap and let rise at room temperature (70°F to 80°F) until doubled in bulk (about 1½ hours).

6. Punch dough down. Transfer to board and knead for 15 seconds. Shape into 2 loaves. Place in mar-garine-greased 9½" × 6" × 2½" loaf pans. Cover with waxed paper that has been lightly greased with margarine. Let rise until doubled (about 1 hour). Preheat oven to 375°F.

7. Bake in center section of oven for 40 minutes. Remove from pan. Finished loaves should be browned and bottom should be crisp to the touch. If not, place back in oven directly on rack and bake a few minutes more, taking care not to burn.

8. Let cool on rack for at least 30 minutes before slicing. Serve slightly warm, at room tempera-ture, or toasted—it's delicious all three ways.

Magnificent Rye Bread
~

YIELD: 2 LARGE LOAVES (EACH LOAF YIELDS 26 LARGE ⅜-INCH SLICES)

The true rye bread of my childhood is no more. But I've resurrected its magnificent flavor. The rye breads of the past, with their intense rye flavor, were made with sourdough starters, salt, and such sweeteners as molasses, honey, and brown sugar. My modern version derives its vigorous ryeness from dark rye flour, its slight sourness from a mixture of onions and selected seeds, and its balancing sweetness from apple juice, orange zest, milk, and date powder. An unusual combination? Not to the hundreds of thousands who have come to regard the unusual in my recipes—particularly my bread recipes—as the usual.

2 packages dry yeast

1½ cups dark rye flour (see Note)

5½ cups unbleached flour

2 tablespoons each oat bran and date sugar (see page 297)

⅓ cup nonfat dry milk

1 tablespoon grated orange zest (preferably from navel orange)

1 tablespoon each caraway seed and anise seed, partially crushed

1 teaspoon poppy seed

1 tablespoon minced dried onion

1 cup each water and apple juice (no sugar added)

1 tablespoon Italian olive oil or canola oil, plus ¼ teaspoon for rising bowl

¾ teaspoon sweet soft corn oil margarine

1 tablespoon stone-ground cornmeal

1 egg white mixed with 2 teaspoons water

1. In large mixing bowl, combine yeast, 1 cup rye flour, 2 cups unbleached flour, oat bran and date powder, dry milk, orange zest, seeds, and onion. Stir to combine.

2. Combine and heat water, apple juice, and 1 tablespoon oil until very warm (115°F to 120°F). Pour over flour mixture. Beat with wooden spoon until well blended. Cover bowl. Let stand for 10 minutes.

3. Stir mixture down. Add balance of rye flour (½ cup), and balance of unbleached flour, ½ cup at a time, beating with wooden spoon after each addition. When batter becomes too difficult to handle with spoon, use dough hook, or turn onto a lightly floured board. Knead, adding a little more flour if necessary to make a smooth and elastic dough. Mixture will be sticky at the start, but stickiness will diminish when dough is fully kneaded. Shape into ball.

Per slice

Calories: 68

Carbohydrate: 13 g

Protein: 2 g

Fat: 1 g

Saturated fat: trace

Cholesterol: trace

Dietary fiber: 1.0 g

Sodium: 5 mg

Exchanges: 1 starch/bread

4. Place outside of fairly straight-sided bowl under hot running water for a few seconds. Rub inside of bowl lightly with oil. Drop dough into bowl, turning to coat. Cover tightly with plastic wrap. Let rise at room temperature (70°F to 80°F) until more than doubled in bulk (about 1¼ hours). Dough will rise rapidly at the start, and will then continue to rise at a slower rate.

5. Punch down. Knead briefly on board. Cover with bowl, and let rest for 3 minutes. Shape each half into a 9-inch-long high loaf. Arrange loaves, well spaced, on a 11½" × 15½" baking sheet that has been greased with ½ teaspoon margarine and then sprinkled with cornmeal. Cover with large sheet of waxed paper that has been greased with balance of margarine. Let rise until doubled (about 1 hour). Preheat oven to 375°F.

6. Brush with egg-white mixture. Bake in center section of preheated 375°F oven for 10 minutes. Reduce heat to 350°F. Bake for 35 minutes. Finished bread should be chestnut brown and crispy. Place loaves on rack and let cool completely before slicing.

NOTE: Dark rye flour produces a more assertive rye flavor than medium rye flour. It is available in ethnic markets, grain stores, and health-food stores.

No-Fuss Cracked-Wheat Bread

YIELD: 3 LOAVES (20 SLICES, ⅜ INCH EACH, PER LOAF)

My version of this All-American favorite always gets <u>oohs</u> and <u>ahhs</u> whether it's served toasted or plain. It makes the best-ever toasted bread crumbs and French toast, too. Part of the secret is the subtle use of nutmeg, anise seed, and orange zest. Another part is a tested technique that's as easy to follow as it's fun to apply.

3½	cups unbleached flour
2	packages dry yeast
1	cup cracked-wheat cereal (see page 297)
2	teaspoons anise seed, crushed
½	teaspoon freshly grated nutmeg
1	teaspoon granulated fructose (see page 297)
1	cup apple juice (no sugar added)
¾	cup water

2	tablespoons Italian olive oil or canola oil, plus ¼ teaspoon for rising bowl
1	tablespoon grated orange zest (preferably from navel orange)
½	cup evaporated skim milk, plus 1 tablespoon
1	cup whole-wheat flour
½	teaspoon sweet soft corn oil margarine for pans and waxed paper

1. In large mixing bowl, combine 2 cups unbleached flour, yeast, cracked-wheat cereal, anise seed, and nutmeg.

2. In saucepan, combine fructose, apple juice, water, 2 tablespoons oil, and orange zest. Heat until very warm (115°F to 120°F). Pour over dry mixture. Beat with wooden spoon for 1 minute or until well blended. Cover and let stand for 15 minutes. Add ½ cup evaporated skim milk, beating to blend.

3. Add whole-wheat flour and 1 cup of unbleached flour, ½ cup at a time, beating with wooden spoon after each addition. When dough becomes too difficult to handle with wooden spoon, turn onto lightly floured board and knead, adding balance of flour (up to ½ cup) if necessary, to make a smooth and elastic dough.

Per 2 slices

Calories: 86

Carbohydrate: 16 g

Protein: 3 g

Fat: 1 g

Saturated fat: trace

Cholesterol: trace

Dietary fiber: 1.2 g

Sodium: 12 mg

Exchanges: 1 starch/bread

4. Shape dough into ball. Heat outside of a fairly straight-sided bowl by placing it briefly under hot running water. Lightly oil inside of bowl. Drop dough into bowl. Cover tightly with plastic wrap (you'll want to watch it rise), and let rise at room temperature (70°F to 80°F) until doubled in bulk (1¼ hours). Punch dough down. Knead briefly in bowl. Re-cover and let rise again until doubled. Preheat oven to 375°F.

5. Punch dough down. Transfer to board. Knead briefly. Cut into 3 equal pieces. Cover with waxed paper and let rest for 3 minutes. Shape into loaves. Place in 3 small margarine-greased loaf pans (7⅜" × 3⅝" × 2¼"). Let rise until doubled in bulk.

6. Bake for 40 minutes. Test for doneness by removing loaves from pans and tapping bottoms with knuckles. If you hear a hollow sound, your loaves are ready for the last step.

7. Mix balance of evaporated skim milk (1 tablespoon) with 1 teaspoon water. Brush tops of loaves with mixture. Let bread cool completely before slicing.

NOTE: Here's how to prepare bread crumbs: Preheat oven to 425°F. Cut sliced bread into cubes. Spread on cookie sheet and bake for 10 minutes, turning once midway with spatula. Let cool. Transfer to blender and blend on high speed for 1 minute.

Desserts

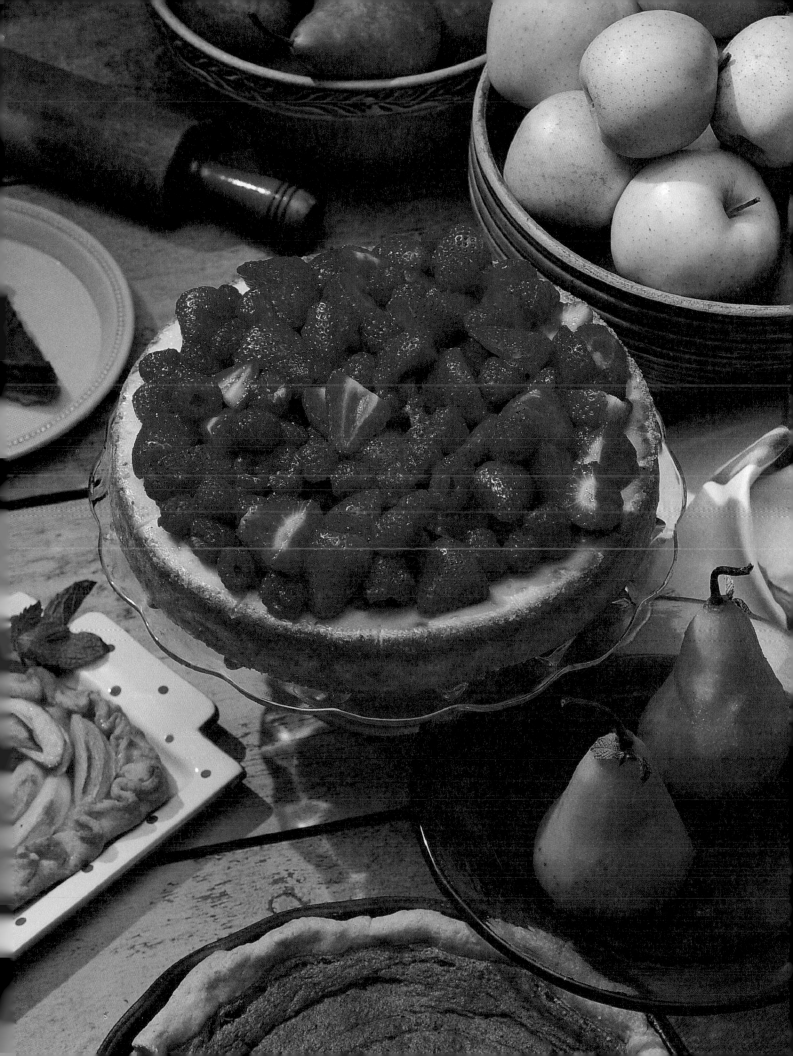

Fabulous Cheesecake I

~

YIELD: SERVES 14

For ages, humankind dreamed about flying to the moon. That's been done. And making luscious cheesecake that's low in fat, cholesterol, sugar, and salt and really tastes like cheesecake. Now even that's been done. You can do it yourself, either with this scrumptious version, its variation, or the recipe that follows.

FOR THE CAKE:

½   cup undiluted evaporated skim milk (see page 297)

½   cup each fresh orange juice and canned or frozen pineapple juice

2   envelopes plain gelatin

3   large eggs, separated

3   7½-ounce packages of farmer cheese (preferably without salt)

¼   teaspoon each freshly grated nutmeg and cinnamon

4   tablespoons granulated fructose (see page 297)

3   tablespoons fresh lemon juice

1   teaspoon minced lemon zest

1   teaspoon pure vanilla extract

2   tablespoons sugar

1   tablespoon finely minced orange zest, preferably from navel orange

2   teaspoons grated semisweet chocolate (optional)

FOR THE CRUST:

½   cup fine bread crumbs, preferably from Light and Spongy Loaf (page 226), or good-quality commercial white bread

3   tablespoons date sugar (see page 297)

½   teaspoon cinnamon

1   tablespoon sweet soft corn oil margarine, melted

Per serving
Calories: 132
Carbohydrate: 16 g
Protein: 12 g
Fat: 2 g
Saturated fat: 1 g
Cholesterol: 39 mg
Dietary fiber: 0.1 g
Sodium: 50 mg
Exchanges: 1 starch/bread
1 lean meat

This recipe contains a moderate amount of sugar and should be used only occasionally. It should be carefully worked into your individual meal plan.

1. Pour milk into a large mixing bowl. Place bowl and whipping utensil(s) in freezer. Chill until almost frozen (firm to the touch).

2. While milk is chilling, prepare the crust. Preheat oven to 400°F. In small bowl, combine and blend bread crumbs, date sugar, and cinnamon. Stir in margarine and blend. Sprinkle, then press onto bottom of a 9-inch springform pan. Bake until lightly brown (about 9 minutes), taking care not to burn. Cool.

3. To make the cake, first pour juices into top of double boiler. Then sprinkle with gelatin. Let soften for 3 minutes. Place over simmering water. Add the egg yolks. While whisking continuously, cook until slightly thickened and mixture coats spoon lightly (about 4 minutes). Remove from heat.

4. Place farmer cheese in a large bowl and mash, or beat with mixing machine, until smooth. Stir in heated mixture. Add spices, fructose, 2½ tablespoons lemon juice, lemon zest, and vanilla and blend. Place bowl in refrigerator and chill until mix is almost set (about 40–60 minutes), stirring occasionally.

5. Beat egg whites until soft peaks form. Sprinkle with sugar and beat until firm and glistening.

6. Beat almost-frozen milk with remaining ½ tablespoon lemon juice to the consistency of whipped cream. (See explicit whipping instructions under Frozen Chocolate Dessert, page 279.)

7. Fold beaten egg whites and beaten milk into cheese medley, half of each at a time. Spoon into prepared crust, smoothing out top. Sprinkle with orange zest and grated chocolate, if desired. Chill until firm (at least 6 hours or overnight).

8. Run a moistened blunt knife around sides of pan. Remove rim. Place cake (with bottom of pan) on doily-covered plate. Cut with a sharp moistened knife and serve chilled.

VARIATION: Substitute the crust from Enchanting Chocolate Chiffon Pie (page 244) for the bread crumb crust, pressing onto bottom and 1 inch up the sides of a 9-inch springform pan, and then baking until lightly brown (about 8 minutes), taking care not to burn. Cool.

Fabulous Cheesecake II

~

YIELD: SERVES 12

Per serving
Calories: 132
Carbohydrate: 14 g
Protein: 7 g
Fat: 4 g
Saturated fat: 2 g
Cholesterol: 39 mg
Dietary fiber: 0.2 g
Sodium: 78 mg
Exchanges: 1 medium-fat
meat
1 fruit

This recipe contains a moderate amount of sugar and should be used only occasionally. It should be carefully worked into your individual meal plan.

1   crust recipe from
Fabulous Cheesecake I

¾   cup drained canned pineapple
chunks (no sugar added) plus
⅓ cup juice from can

15 ounces part-skim ricotta cheese

½   cup low-fat plain yogurt

¾   cup pineapple juice
(no sugar added)

2   envelopes plain gelatin

4   tablespoons granulated fructose
(see page 297)

2   eggs, separated

3   tablespoons fresh lemon juice

2   teaspoons freshly grated lemon
zest

⅛   teaspoon each ground cinnamon
and freshly grated nutmeg

1   teaspoon pure vanilla extract

3   drops almond extract

1   tablespoon coarsely chopped
walnuts

1. Follow directions for bottom crust in preceding recipe, Fabulous Cheesecake Cake I, or use crust recipe from Enchanting Chocolate Chiffon Pie (page 244).

2. Place ½ cup pineapple chunks and ⅓ cup juice in food blender and puree until smooth. Pour into large bowl. Add cheese and yogurt. Beat with whisk or mixer until blended.

3. Pour ¾ cup pineapple juice into top of double boiler. Sprinkle with gelatin. Let soften for 3 minutes. Place over simmering water. Whisk in 3 tablespoons fructose and egg yolks. Whisk and cook until slightly thickened and mixture lightly coats spoon (about 4 minutes). Remove from heat. Cool.

4. Pour over cheese mixture. Add lemon juice, lemon zest, spices, and extracts. Blend. Chill until mixture begins to thicken (about 20 minutes). Do not let mixture set.

5. Beat egg whites until almost stiff. Sprinkle in balance of fructose (1 tablespoon) and beat until satiny. Fold into thickened mixture. Pour into prepared crust. Slice balance of pineapple chunks (¼ cup). Arrange in a decorative pattern on top of cake. Sprinkle walnuts around edges. Chill until completely set (5 hours or more).

6. Remove rim of pan. Place cake with bottom of pan on doily-covered serving plate. Cut with moistened knife.

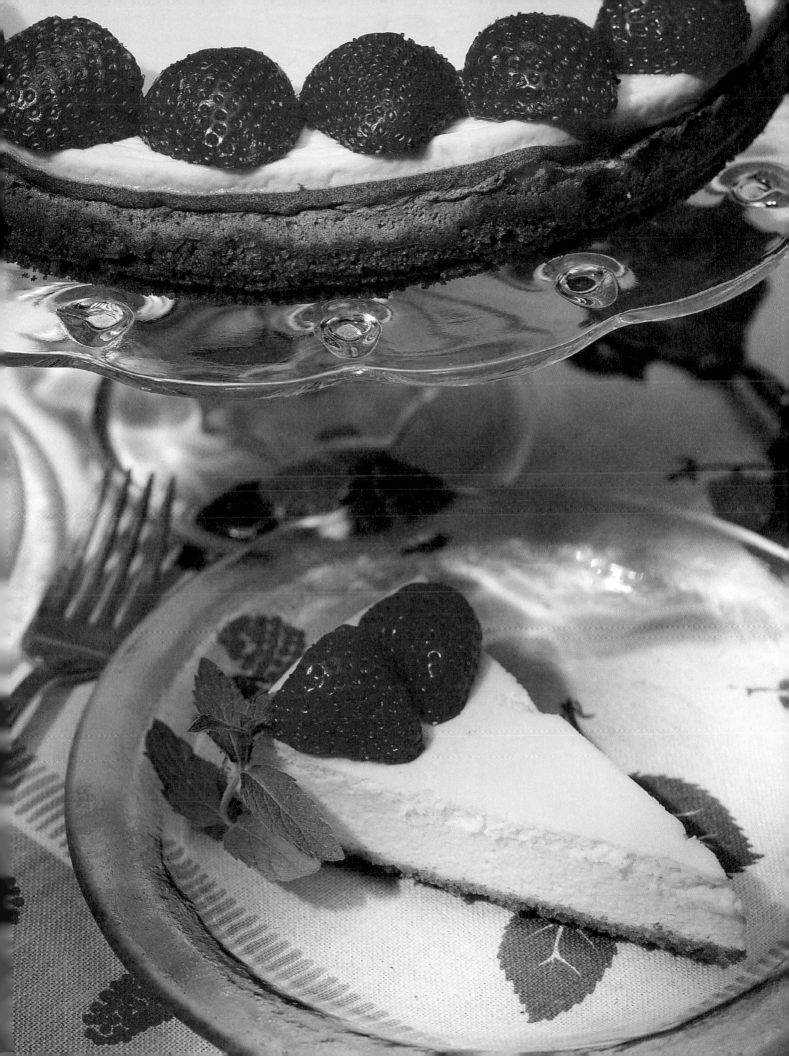

Chocolate Chestnut Mousse with Strawberry Sauce
~

YIELD: 12 SERVINGS

Roasted in its shell on a street vendor's brazier or gracing the sauce of a coupe marron, the chestnut is as sweet and as versatile as it is popular. It's one of my favorite ingredients because I can build a scrumptious dessert around it that can be devoured without a tinge of guilt. Extremely low in fat, the chestnut contributes less than ten calories per nut. Sample those virtues in this four-star confection, which you whisk up a day in advance of serving (yes, the whisk is a magical tool for creating that unforgettable texture). Both mousse and sauce retain their freshly made flavors for up to three days.

FOR THE MOUSSE:

¼ cup apple juice (no sugar added)

2 packets plain gelatin

1 15½-ounce can imported unsweetened whole peeled chestnuts packed in water

¾ cup undiluted evaporated skim milk

1 tablespoon honey

3 tablespoons frozen apple juice concentrate

¼ cup unsweetened cocoa

1 teaspoon finely minced orange zest

½ teaspoon each allspice and cinnamon

¼ teaspoon each ground cardamom and freshly grated nutmeg

3 large eggs (use 2 yolks and 3 whites)

1 teaspoon pure vanilla extract

½ teaspoon almond extract

¼ teaspoon cream of tartar

3 tablespoons granulated fructose (see page 297)

½ cup jarred or homemade applesauce (no sugar added)

FOR THE SAUCE:

1 20-ounce package frozen strawberries (no sugar added)

¼ teaspoon each freshly grated nutmeg and ground cardamom

½ teaspoon cinnamon

¼ teaspoon almond extract (optional)

1–2 tablespoons granulated fructose

1. Pour apple juice into a small bowl. Sprinkle with gelatin and let soften.

2. Drain chestnuts, reserving ¼ cup liquid. Pick out 4 whole chestnuts for garnish. Put half the remaining nuts into workbowl of food processor that has been fitted with steel blade (or use a food blender). Add reserved canned juices to the workbowl together with ¼ cup evaporated skim milk, honey and concentrate. Puree until smooth.

Pour into a large bowl, scraping out any residue.

3. Coarsely chop remaining chestnuts. Set aside.

4. Half-fill the bottom section of a double boiler with water. Bring to a boil. Reduce heat to simmering. Put remaining ½ cup milk, the cocoa, zest, and the spices into the top section. Combine pots and place over heat. While whisking, cook until cocoa dissolves.

Mousse
Per serving
Calories: 71
Carbohydrate: 11 g
Protein: 4 g
Fat: 1 g
Saturated fat: 1 g
Cholesterol: 46 mg
Dietary fiber: 3.0 g
Sodium: 40 mg
Exchanges: 1 starch/bread

Strawberry Sauce
Per serving
Calories: 18
Carbohydrate: 4 g
Protein: trace
Fat: 0
Saturated fat: 0
Cholesterol: 0
Dietary fiber: 1.0 g
Sodium: 1 mg
Exchanges: free
　(2 servings = ½ fruit)

This recipe contains a moderate amount of sugar and should be used only occasionally. It should be carefully worked into your individual meal plan.

5. Drop 2 egg yolks into a cup and the 3 egg whites into mixing machine bowl. To the cup, pour about 3 tablespoons warmed cocoa mix and blend with fork. Pour mixture back into the pot. Whisk constantly while cooking for 1 minute.

6. Add gelatin mix (it will have firmed up); whisk until mixture is smooth and lightly thickened. Pour into chestnut puree, blending well, scraping sides of pot with rubber spatula. Add extracts and blend. Place in refrigerator to chill until puree begins to thicken (20 to 25 minutes). Whisk until smooth.

7. Using whisk attachment of mixer, beat egg whites with cream of tartar on medium speed until foamy. Increase speed to high. Gradually add fructose while beating until soft peaks form, stopping machine once or twice to check that eggs don't become stiff.

8. Stir ½ cup into thickened chocolate puree. Fold in reserved chopped chestnuts; then fold in remaining beaten egg whites alternately with applesauce.

9. Turn into a 7- or 8-inch souffle dish and smooth out top. Split reserved whole chestnuts in half; arrange decoratively on top of mousse. Refrigerate until well chilled and set (about 3 hours).

10. To prepare sauce, put frozen berries into a wide heavy-bottom saucepan (do not add water). Cover and cook over very low heat until berries defrost. Stir in spices. Re-cover and simmer for 5 minutes. Pour into a large bowl and cool for 10 minutes. Stir in extract (if desired) and 1 tablespoon fructose. Taste. Add another tablespoon if sauce isn't sweet enough. Pour into a large jar and chill. Serve cold, spooned around individual servings of mousse.

Enchanting Chocolate Chiffon Pie

YIELD: SERVES 8

To enchant means to allure, enrapture, entice, enthrall, and wing you away from the commonplace. Can a dessert do that? Yes, when a sweet graham cracker shell nestles a cloudlike chocolate filling accented with confectionery spices and topped with toasted almond morsels. Enjoy a forkful and find the meaning of enchantment for yourself.

Per serving
Calories: 195
Carbohydrate: 24 g
Protein: 7 g
Fat: 7 g
Saturated fat: 3 g
Cholesterol: 69 mg
Dietary fiber: 1.6 g
Sodium: 157 mg
Exchanges: 1 starch/bread
            ½ milk
            1 fat

This recipe contains a moderate amount of sugar and should be used only occasionally. It should be carefully worked into your individual meal plan.

FOR THE CRUST:

12   honey graham crackers (2½-inch squares)

1   tablespoon regular wheat germ

½   teaspoon each ground nutmeg and cinnamon

2½ tablespoons sweet corn oil margarine, partially melted

FOR THE FILLING:

1   cup evaporated skim milk

1   package plus 1 teaspoon unflavored gelatin

1½ squares semisweet chocolate (1½ ounces)

3   large eggs (use 2 yolks and 3 whites)

¼   cup unsweetened apple juice

5   tablespoons unsweetened carob powder , sifted (see page 297)

3   tablespoons granulated fructose (see page 297)

¼   teaspoon ground nutmeg

1½ teaspoons pure vanilla extract

1   tablespoon coarsely chopped toasted almonds for garnish (optional)

1. Preheat oven to 375°F. Break crackers into workbowl of food processor that has been fitted with steel blade. Add wheat germ and spices. Process to fine crumbs. With machine running, pour the partially melted margarine through feed tube. Process until mixture appears moist. Turn into an 8-inch pie pan; press to sides and bottom. For a soft shell, chill for 1 hour before filling; for a crisp shell, bake until lightly browned (7 to 8 minutes). Cool before filling.

2. Put milk into a medium-size heavy-bottom saucepan. Sprinkle with gelatin. Let soften for 5 minutes. Place over very low heat and cook, while whisking, until warm (do not boil). Remove from heat.

3. In another medium-size heavy-bottom saucepan, melt chocolate over very low heat. Set aside.

4. Drop 2 yolks into a cup and 3 whites into large mixing bowl. To yolks, add apple juice, beating with fork to blend. Pour into milk mixture. Place saucepan again over very low heat and while whisking, cook until liquid returns to warm temperature.

5. Add carob, one tablespoon at a time, whisking after each addition. Continue to cook and whisk until carob is completely dissolved. Wisk in melted chocolate. Cool for two minutes. Then whisk in two tablespoons fructose, the nutmeg, and the vanilla.

6. Pour into a large bowl. Chill until thickened but not set, stirring from time to time.

7. Beat the egg whites on medium speed until soft peaks form. Sprinkle in remaining tablespoon fructose and beat on high speed until just firm, taking care that dry peaks do not form. Whisk one-third into thickened chocolate mixture; fold in remainder.

8. Spoon into prepared shell. Sprinkle with nuts. Chill until set (about 3 hours).

NOTE: Pie may be prepared a day ahead. In that event, bake the shell.

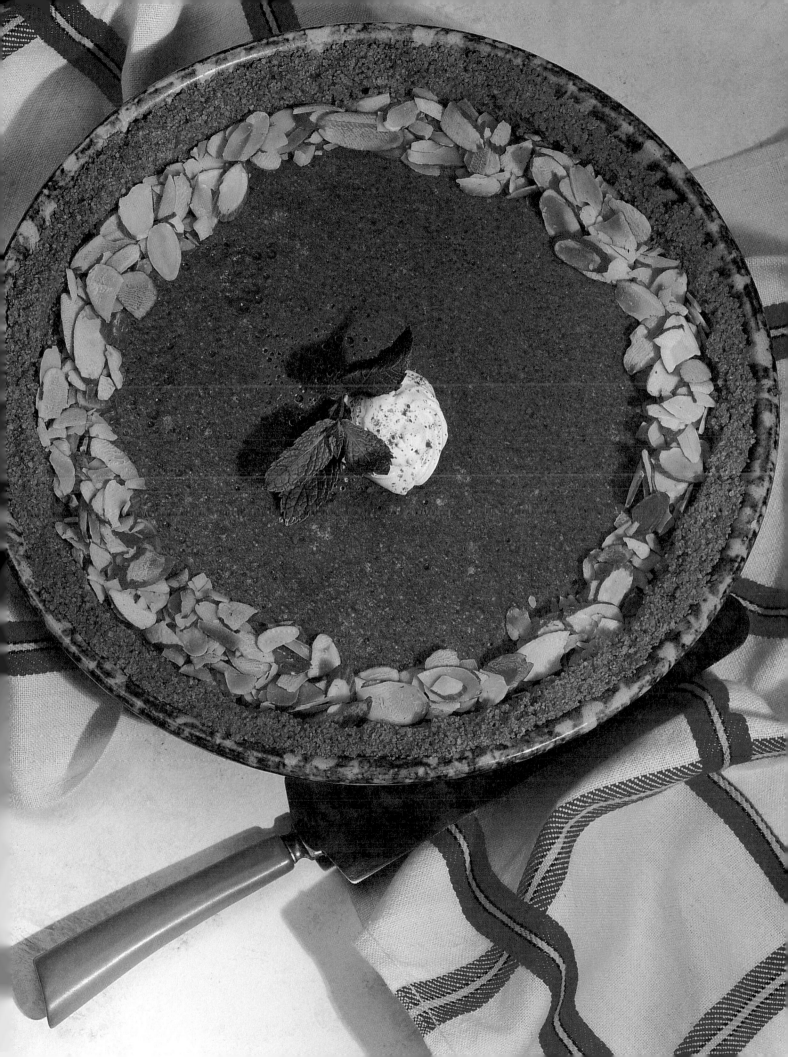

Picture-Perfect Chocolate Pear Pie

YIELD: SERVES 10

For your next gourmet dessert, picture a crispy pie shell with a pudding-like chocolate filling topped with an extravagance of cranberry-poached pears. Picture perfect!

FOR THE PIE:

1 recipe Pretty Poached Pears in Cranberry Juice (page 252)

1 pastry recipe from Chocolate Pumpkin Pie (page 255)

1½ squares unsweetened chocolate

2 tablespoons reduced-fat cream cheese (Neufchâtel)

1 envelope plain gelatin

2 tablespoons granulated fructose (see page 297)

FOR THE GARNISH:

½ cup Pretty Poached Pears

1½ tablespoons reduced-fat cream cheese (Neufchâtel)

1½ tablespoons reduced-fat sour cream

¼ teaspoon almond extract

1. Prepare the poached pears a day ahead. Preheat oven to 425°F. Make the pastry following directions from Chocolate Pumpkin Pie through step 3. Then roll out to an 11-inch circle to fit a 9-inch metal pie pan. Cut away ragged edges, leaving a ½-inch overhang (crust shrinks after baking). To keep the unfilled crust from puffing up while baking, cut an 11-inch circle of aluminum foil and fit over the dough, pressing lightly against sides of pan. Fill to the rim with dried beans. Bake until lightly browned (about 15 minutes). Lift out foil with beans (store them in a jar for future use). Reduce oven heat to 400°F. Return pan to oven and bake until bottom of shell is lightly browned (8 to 10 minutes). Stand pan on a wire rack and cool completely. Cover with plastic wrap.

Per serving
Calories: 181
Carbohydrate: 31 g
Protein: 2 g
Fat: 5 g
Saturated fat: 2 g
Cholesterol: 4 mg
Dietary fiber: 3.6 g
Sodium: 64 mg
Exchanges: 1 starch/bread
1 fruit
1 fat

2. With slotted spoon, transfer chilled pears to a bowl. Pour ¼ cup of the juices into a small heavy-bottom saucepan. Add chocolate and melt over low heat, stirring often. Remove from heat. Cool for 5 minutes. Then whisk in cheese. Transfer to a medium-size bowl and set aside. Rinse out saucepan.

3. Pour remaining juices into the saucepan. Sprinkle with gelatin. Let soften for 3 minutes. Stir over low heat until gelatin dissolves. Whisk into the chocolate mixture. Chill until it mounds slightly when dropped from a spoon (about 30 minutes). Whisk and return to refrigerator for 5 minutes. Pour into prepared pie crust. Chill for 15 minutes.

4. Thinly slice pears lengthwise. Measure out ½ cup and reserve for garnish. Arrange remaining slices in a decorative pattern over filling, starting close to the edge of pie and continuing in a circle until filling is completely covered.

5. To prepare the garnish, put the ½ cup reserved pears in the workbowl of food processor that has been fitted with steel blade. Add cheese, sour cream, and extract; process until smooth. Put a ½ teaspoon at a time in a circle between the crust and pears. Drop a rounded teaspoon in the center of the pie. Chill for at least 3 hours before cutting.

Sumptuous Chocolate Cake

~

YIELD: SERVES 12

Revel in the luxurious texture and real chocolate flavor of this sumptuous confection. It's totally satisfying with or without frosting. If your meal plan allows, a creamy chocolate frosting follows this recipe.

Per serving
Calories: 148
Carbohydrate: 22 g
Protein: 4 g
Fat: 5 g
Saturated fat: 2 g
Cholesterol: 9 mg
Dietary fiber: 1.1 g
Sodium: 212 mg
Exchanges: 1½ starch/bread
　　　　　　1 fat

This recipe contains a moderate amount of sugar and should be used only occasionally. It should be carefully worked into your individual meal plan.

3　tablespoons unsweetened cocoa (preferably Dutch process)

1　ounce (1 square) semisweet chocolate

2　teaspoons freeze-dried coffee granules (regular or decaffeinated)

2½　tablespoons frozen apple juice concentrate

1　teaspoon pure vanilla extract

1½　cups sifted unbleached flour, plus 1 teaspoon for pan

1　teaspoon baking soda

¼　teaspoon baking powder

½　teaspoon salt

3　tablespoons each granulated fructose (see page 297) and sugar

¼　cup cold margarine, cut into small pieces, plus ½ teaspoon for pan

1　large egg

¾　cup cold evaporated skim milk

1. Preheat oven to 350°F. Combine first 4 ingredients in a small heavy-bottom saucepan. Place pan over very low heat and, while stirring, warm until ingredients dissolve. Remove from heat and cool. Then stir in vanilla. Mixture will be very thick.

2. Resift the 1½ cups flour, baking soda, baking powder, and salt into large mixing bowl. Stir in fructose and sugar. Strew the cut-up butter over all. Beat on low speed until shortening is absorbed (about 1 minute).

3. In a cup, combine egg with ½ cup milk, beating with fork to blend. Increase speed of mixer to medium and, while beating, gradually pour mixture into batter.

4. Add chocolate mixture a tablespoon at a time, scraping down sides of bowl once or twice. Dribble in remaining ¼ cup milk and blend (do not overbeat).

5. Lightly grease an 8-inch loose-bottom layer pan with shortening; sprinkle with flour and shake out the excess. Spoon batter into pan, and smooth out the top with a spatula. Bake in center section of oven for 30 to 35 minutes; test for doneness after 30 minutes (cake is fully baked when a toothpick inserted in center comes out clean). Cake may crack slightly. Place pan on a wire rack and cool for 5 minutes. Remove rim and let cake cool completely before removing bottom section.

Creamy Chocolate Frosting
~

YIELD: ENOUGH FOR AN 8- OR 9-INCH CAKE

Light, silky, smooth. A once-in-a-while treat and the perfect frosting for Sumptuous Chocolate Cake.

Per serving
Calories: 61
Carbohydrate: 6 g
Protein: 4 g
Fat: 2 g
Saturated fat: 1 g
Cholesterol: 4 mg
Dietary fiber: 0.7 g
Sodium: 60 mg
Exchanges: ½ starch/bread
½ lean meat

½ pound tofu, cut and drained on paper toweling

½ cup low-fat cottage cheese (1% milkfat) drained

3 tablespoons reduced-fat cream cheese (Neufchâtel), (see Note)

2 tablespoons granulated fructose

3 tablespoons unsweetened cocoa

2 teaspoons freeze-dried coffee granules (regular or decaffeinated)

2 tablespoons frozen apple juice concentrate

1 teaspoon pure vanilla extract

1 teaspoon finely minced orange zest (optional)

1. Put tofu into workbowl of food processor fitted with steel blade (or use a blender). Process to the consistency of sour cream. Measure out ½ cup; discard remainder. Return puree to workbowl.

2. Add cottage cheese, cream cheese, and fructose to workbowl. Process until very smooth. Place bowl in refrigerator and chill for at least 30 minutes. (Mixture may be prepared a day ahead.)

3. Put cocoa, coffee granules, and concentrate in a small heavy-bottom saucepan. Place pan over low heat and, while stirring, warm until ingredients dissolve. Cool. Stir in vanilla and orange zest if desired.

4. Place workbowl of processor or blender on stand. Add cocoa mixture and process until combined. (Chilled cheese mix can also be scraped into a bowl; the cocoa mélange can then be stirred into puree.) Refrigerate until ready to spread on cake.

NOTE: Philly Light (a brand of Neufchâtel), with one third less fat than cream cheese, works well in this recipe.

Chocolate Pudding the Way You Like It

~

YIELD: SERVES 6

*H*ow can chocolate pudding be creamy without cream or even whole milk? Easy. Just use fresh skim milk and canned evaporated skim milk, and follow the explicit instructions in the recipe.

How can you make it sweet when you don't use sugar? To begin with, evaporated skim milk adds its own sweetness. So does pureed canned unsweetened pineapple. Even more sweetness is contributed by vanilla extract, sweet spices, fruit juices, and just a hint of fructose. Sweet enough? Yes!

Creamy, sweet, and with no no-nos: chocolate pudding just the way you like it.

Per serving
Calories: 118
Carbohydrate: 20 g
Protein: 7 g
Fat: 1 g
Saturated fat: trace
Cholesterol: 1 mg
Dietary fiber: 1.5 g
Sodium: 63 mg
Exchanges: ½ fruit
         1 milk

½ cup evaporated skim milk

2 teaspoons plain gelatin

1¾ cups skim milk

3 tablespoons unsweetened cocoa

3 tablespoons cornstarch

1 cup drained and pureed unsweetened canned pineapple

2 tablespoons frozen pineapple juice concentrate

¼ teaspoon each allspice and ground cardamom

½ teaspoon cinnamon

1½ tablespoons granulated fructose (see page 297)

1 teaspoon pure vanilla extract

1. Pour evaporated skim milk into a measuring cup. Sprinkle with gelatin and let soften.

2. Put 1½ cups skim milk and cocoa into the top of a double boiler. Half-fill bottom section with water and bring to a boil. Assemble pots and cook mixture, while stirring, until cocoa dissolves and milk begins to scald. (For smooth results, use a wire whisk.)

3. Put cornstarch into a cup. While stirring, gradually add remaining ¼ cup skim milk (mixture should be smooth with all of the cornstarch dissolved). Pour into hot liquid and cook while whisking until blended and thickened (4 to 5 minutes).

4. Whisk in softened gelatin and cook for 2 minutes. Remove from heat. Whisk in ½ cup of the pineapple puree, the concentrate, and spices. Cool for 5 minutes. Then whisk in fructose and vanilla.

5. Immediately pour into 6 dessert dishes, allowing a little more than ½ cup for each serving. Chill until set (about 2 hours). Top each serving with 1 tablespoon of the remaining pineapple puree. Cover any leftovers with plastic film to lock in freshness for up to 3 days.

Frozen Mixed Fruit Mousse

~

YIELD: SERVES 10

Smooth, creamy, luxurious, superspecial, and guilt-free. Doesn't that describe a perfect dessert?

Per serving
Calories: 71
Carbohydrate: 14 g
Protein: 3 g
Fat: trace
Saturated fat: 0 g
Cholesterol: trace
Dietary fiber: 0.6 g
Sodium: 41 mg
Exchanges: 1 fruit

⅔ cup evaporated skim milk (see page 297)

1 20-ounce can pineapple chunks packed in pineapple juice (no sugar added)

¼ teaspoon ground cloves

2 teaspoons finely grated orange zest (preferably from navel orange)

1 tablespoon cognac or kirsch

⅓ cup pineapple juice from chunk pineapple

1 envelope plain gelatin

1 cup sliced ripe bananas

½ teaspoon ground cinnamon

2 tablespoons granulated fructose (see page 297) (optional)

3 egg whites (see Note 1)

¼ teaspoon cream of tartar

1. Pour milk into mixing bowl. Place bowl and beater(s) in freezer compartment of your refrigerator. Chill until almost frozen.

2. Meanwhile, drain pineapple chunks. Place pineapples in food processor. Set aside. Measure out ⅓ cup pineapple juice. Pour into saucepan. Sprinkle with gelatin. Let soften for 3 minutes. Heat, stirring until dissolved. Cool. Pour into a large bowl.

3. Add banana, spices, orange zest, and liqueur to food processor. Puree for 15 seconds. Pour into gelatin mixture.

4. Beat almost-frozen evaporated skim milk until as thick as whipped cream. Taste. Add fructose if desired and blend. Fold into pureed fruit mixture. Wash off beaters.

5. Beat egg whites with cream of tartar until stiff but not until dry peaks form. Then fold into dessert.

6. Turn into 1-quart freezeproof bowl. Freeze for 3 hours (see Note 3). Spoon into individual dessert dishes and serve.

NOTES:
1. When eggs are uncooked, I recommend using organic eggs.

2. If your diet does not permit uncooked alcohol, substitute 1 teaspoon pure vanilla extract or ½ teaspoon almond extract.

3. The efficiency of your freezer will determine length of freezing time. Check mixture after 2½ hours. Finished dessert should be the consistency of spoonable sherbet.

*P*retty Poached Pears in Cranberry Juice

~

YIELD: SERVES 8

*F*resh luscious pears, cranberry-tinted to a fuchsia hue, make a light and satisfying dessert after a full meal. For a very special presentation, top with Hot-Pink Sherbet (page 278).

Per serving
Calories: 106
Carbohydrate: 25 g
Protein: trace
Fat: trace
Saturated fat: trace
Cholesterol: 0 mg
Dietary fiber: 3.3 g
Sodium: 3 mg
Exchanges: 2 fruit

This recipe contains a moderate amount of sugar and should be used only occasionally. It should be carefully worked into your individual meal plan.

1½ cups fresh cranberries, rinsed and picked over

2 cups apple juice (no sugar added)

1 tablespoon honey

4 large, firm, almost-ripe Bartlett or d'Anjou pears (about 2 pounds), halved, cored, and peeled

¼ teaspoon cinnamon

⅛ teaspoon ground cardamom or nutmeg

2 tablespoons granulated fructose (see page 297)

¼ teaspoon almond extract

1. Put cranberries and apple juice in a 3-quart heavy-bottom saucepan. Bring to a boil. Reduce heat to simmering. Cover and cook until all the berries pop (about 7 minutes). Stain into a bowl, pressing out juices with a large spoon. Stir honey into juices. Discard solids.

2. Arrange pears in layers in saucepan, rounded sides down. Cover with cranberry liquid. Bring to a boil. Reduce heat to simmering. Cover and simmer until firm-tender (about 10 minutes). Sprinkle with spices. Gently spoon liquid over pears. Uncover and let stand for 10 minutes.

3. With slotted spoon, transfer pears to a 3-quart covered bowl. Add fructose to juices, stirring until dissolved. Then pour over fruit. Cover and refrigerate several hours (or overnight) to permit flavors to develop fully.

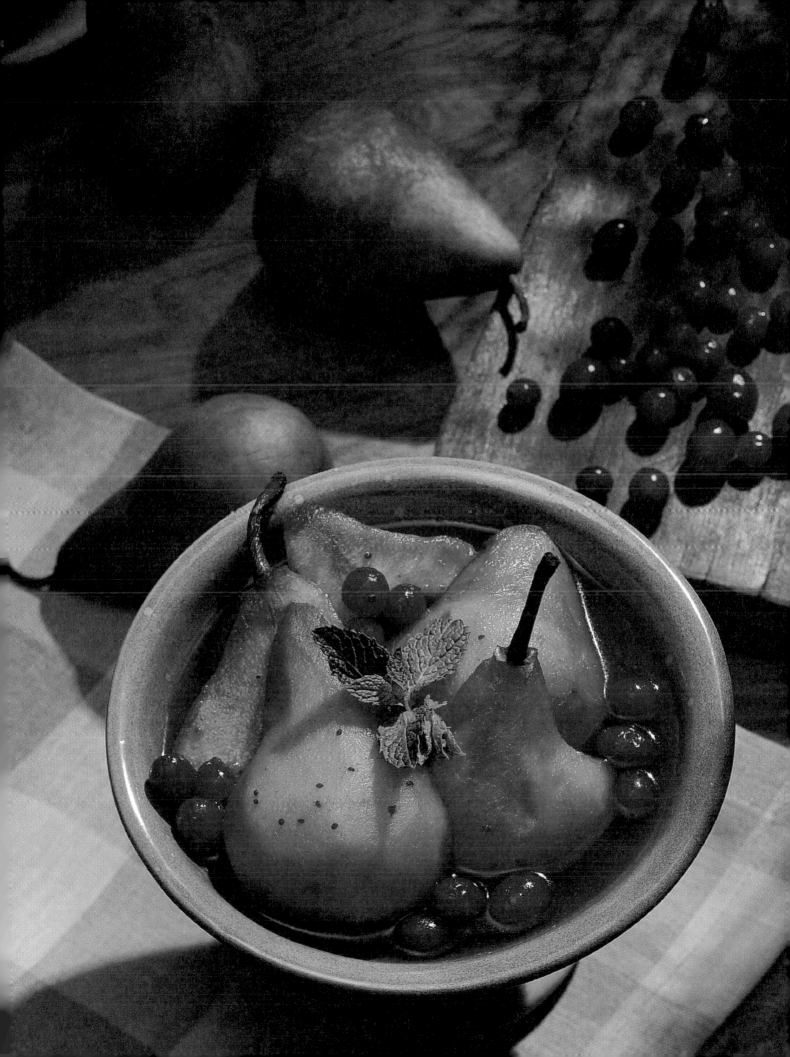

Crunchy Cookies

~

YIELD: ABOUT 40 COOKIES

*D*o you like cookies?
Do you like granola?
Here's a crunchy granola-
like cookie just bursting
with nutrition and
unusual flavors (run down
the list of ingredients, and
you'll see why).

Per cookie
Calories: 44
Carbohydrate: 7 g
Protein: 1 g
Fat: 1 g
Saturated fat: trace
Cholesterol: trace
Dietary fiber: 0.7 g
Sodium: 2 mg
Exchanges: ½ starch/bread

¼	cup bulgur
¾	cup apple juice (no sugar added)
3	tablespoons dark seedless raisins
¼	cup water
3	tablespoons canola oil
⅓	cup buttermilk (preferably without salt)
1	cup whole-wheat flour
⅓	cup brown rice flour (see page 297)

⅓	cup date sugar (see page 297)
¼	cup unsweetened carob powder (see page 297)
¼	cup chopped walnuts
½	teaspoon each ground ginger and cinnamon
¼	teaspoon ground cardamom
½	teaspoon sweet soft corn oil margarine for cookie sheet

1. Preheat oven to 370°F. Combine first 4 ingredients in saucepan. Bring to boil. Reduce heat to simmering point. Simmer uncovered for exactly 8 minutes. Some of the liquid will remain. Remove from heat. Add oil and buttermilk, stirring to blend. Set aside.

2. Place flours, date sugar, carob, nuts, and spices in mixing bowl. Stir to blend. Add bulgur mixture to dry mixture and stir with wooden spoon until well blended.

3. Lightly grease 2 cookies sheets with margarine. Drop by spoonfuls onto sheets, pressing with moist fork, to ⅛-inch thickness. Bake in center section of preheated oven for 15 to 18 minutes until browned. Cool on rack.

NOTES:
1. Unbleached flour may be substituted for brown rice flour (cookies will be less sweet).

2. Cookies may be recrisped next day by baking in 350°F oven for 8 minutes.

Chocolate Pumpkin Pie
~

YIELD: SERVES 12

The pastry for this luscious dessert is paper-thin, easy to roll and gently spiced. Failure-proof, it's also the crust for New Classic Apple Tart (page 260), and Picture Perfect Chocolate Pear Pie (page 246). Here it's filled with an amalgam of unsweetened chocolate, canned pumpkin (available year-round), and sweet spices. Don't wait for a holiday to enjoy it.

FOR THE PASTRY:

⅔   cup unbleached flour

3   tablespoons 1-minute quick oats

1   tablespoon date sugar (see page 297) or regular wheat germ

¼   teaspoon baking powder

¼   teaspoon each cinnamon and freshly grated nutmeg

3   tablespoons cold, sweet, soft corn oil margarine

3   tablespoons ice water

FOR THE FILLING:

¼   cup apple juice (no sugar added)

2   tablespoons honey

1   square unsweetened chocolate (1 ounce)

1   16-ounce can solid pack pumpkin (1¾ cup)

1   teaspoon cinnamon

½   teaspoon ground ginger

¼   teaspoon each freshly grated nutmeg and allspice

⅛   teaspoon ground cloves

2   tablespoons granulated fructose (see page 297)

2   large eggs, separated

1   cup undiluted evaporated skim milk

½   cup skim milk

1. Using a ⅓-cup measure, spoon ⅓ cup flour into cup and level it off with a knife. Turn into workbowl of food processor that has been fitted with steel blade. Repeat measuring and leveling off ⅓ cup more flour, and turning into workbowl. (This measuring tactic assures you of a perfect crust every time.)

2. Add oats, date sugar (or alternative), baking powder, and spices. Process for 15 seconds. Remove cover. Drop margarine in 3 separate spots over dry mixture. Cover and process until mixture is crumbly (about 6 seconds). With machine running, pour water through feed tube. Process until a mass forms (about 10 seconds). Stop machine. Tear off a large

Per serving

Calories: 131

Carbohydrate: 17 g

Protein: 5 g

Fat: 5 g

Saturated fat: 2 g

Cholesterol: 29 mg

Dietary fiber: 1.6 g

Sodium: 74 mg

Exchanges: 1 starch/bread
1 fat

sheet of waxed paper and lay on work surface. Lift out dough and place on waxed paper. Scrape bowl for any residue. Knead briefly into a cohesive ball. Press into a 9-inch circle. Cover with another sheet of waxed paper. Place on a flat plate and chill for 30 minutes.

3. Moisten rolling surface, then put a large sheet of waxed paper on the surface. Remove top sheet of waxed paper from pastry. Invert dough onto paper-covered work surface. Gently roll dough between the two sheets of waxed paper to an 11- to 12-inch circle (pastry will be very thin), changing sheets of waxed paper if they tear. Carefully peel off top sheet. Lift up bottom sheet with dough; invert and ease into a 9- or 10-inch pie pan. Pull off paper by tearing down center first, then peeling each half outwards to edge of pan. Flute edges of dough. Preheat oven to 375°F.

4. To prepare filling, put apple juice, honey, and chocolate into a small heavy-bottom saucepan. Cook

over very low heat until chocolate melts. Stir to combine. Cool.

5. Put pumpkin, spices, and fructose into large mixing bowl. Beat on medium speed until well blended. Add egg yolks and beat to blend. Reduce speed to low and add milks a little at a time. Blend in chocolate mixture.

6. In another bowl, beat egg whites until firm but not until dry peaks form. Stir one-quarter of the beaten egg white into batter; fold in remainder. Pour into pastry and smooth out the top. Bake in center section of oven until set (45 to 50 minutes). Cool pan on rack. Serve at room temperature or chilled.

SERVING SUGGESTION: Top with Creamy Vanilla Sauce (page 208), Frozen Chocolate Dessert (page 279), or Chocolate-Raspberry Sauce (page 264).

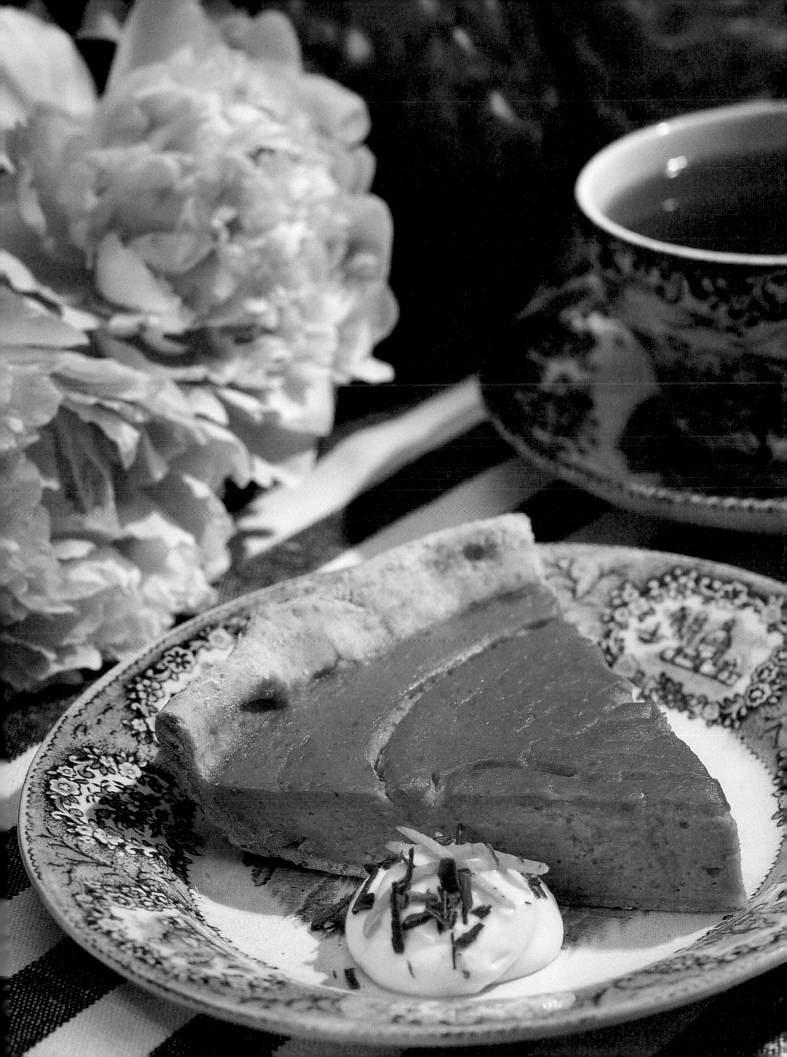

Warm Apple Crunch

YIELD: SERVES 5

Per serving

Calories: 142

Carbohydrate: 22 g

Protein: 3 g

Fat: 5 g

Saturated fat: 1 g

Cholesterol: 3 mg

Dietary fiber: 3.0 g

Sodium: 59 mg

Exchanges: ½ starch/bread
        1 fruit
        1 fat

This recipe contains a moderate amount of sugar and should be used only occasionally. It should be carefully worked into your individual meal plan.

1   tablespoon fresh lemon juice

2   tablespoons frozen orange juice concentrate

3   dashes ground cloves

½   teaspoon ground cinnamon

3   crisp sweet apples (1¼ pounds), peeled, cored, and cut lengthwise into thick slices

1   tablespoon sweet soft corn oil margarine, plus ½ teaspoon for pan

3   tablespoons part-skim ricotta cheese

1   slice Food Processor Whole-Wheat Bran Loaf (page 230), or good-quality commercial whole-wheat bread

2   tablespoons date sugar (see page 297)

¼   teaspoon freshly grated nutmeg

2   tablespoons coarsely chopped walnuts

1. In small bowl, combine lemon juice, orange juice concentrate, cloves, and ¼ teaspoon ground cinnamon. Mash with fork to dissolve concentrate; then beat with fork to blend.

2. Drop sliced apples into mixture, turning well to coat. Set aside.

3. Prepare topping by combining and blending in a cup 1 tablespoon margarine with ricotta cheese (a pastry blender does a good job here).

4. Tear bread into small pieces and bake in a 400°F oven until lightly toasted. (A tabletop toaster-oven does this job speedily.) Then crumble pieces with fingers and toast again for 1 minute. Transfer to a cup.

5. Add balance of cinnamon (¼ teaspoon), 1 tablespoon date sugar, nutmeg, and walnuts to cup. Mix thoroughly. Preheat oven to 375°F.

6. Drain apples, reserving juices. Arrange in a neat pattern in a lightly greased 9-inch-square pan. Sprinkle with topping (it will be clumpy to handle). Sprinkle with balance of date sugar. Pour reserved juices evenly over mixture.

7. Bake until apples are tender but not oversoft (about 30 minutes). Serve immediately.

NOTE: Reheat any leftover portion in covered ovenproof crock in preheated 400°F oven for about 10 minutes. It will taste just-baked.

Chocolate-Carrot Biscotti

~

YIELD: SERVES 18

Biscotti is the Italian word for cookies. But biscotti are not traditional American cookies with a foreign name. They are not the roll-out or the drop-onto-a-cookie-sheet kind of cookies familiar to American kitchens. Rather, a moist sweet batter is shaped into logs and baked; then the warm cake is cut into narrow slices which are arranged flat on a cookie sheet and returned to the oven until almost dry. While the technique comes from Italy, the ingredients for these one-of-a-kind biscotti spin from an American culinary imagination

These biscotti are just the thing to enjoy with your tea (or coffee).

For 2 biscotti
Calories: 126
Carbohydrate: 18 g
Protein: 3 g
Fat: 5 g
Saturated fat: 2 g
Cholesterol: 10 mg
Dietary fiber: 1.5 g
Sodium: 76 mg
Exchanges: 1 starch/bread
1 fat

2 ounces semisweet chocolate

½ cup pineapple juice (no sugar added)

2½ cups unbleached flour, plus 2 tablespoons for board

½ teaspoon baking soda

1½ teaspoons baking powder

1 teaspoon cinnamon

½ teaspoon each ground allspice, cardamom, and ginger

2 tablespoons sweet soft corn oil margarine

½ cup Ambrosia (page 267)

1½ tablespoons each sugar and granulated fructose (see page 297)

1 large egg

1 cup firmly packed, finely grated carrot

½ cup finely chopped, shelled whole almonds

2 teaspoons pure vanilla extract

½ teaspoon almond extract

1. Preheat oven to 350°F. Put chocolate and pineapple juice into a small heavy-bottom saucepan. Cook over very low heat until chocolate melts. Stir and set aside to cool.

2. Sift 2½ cups flour, baking soda, baking powder, and spices into a bowl.

3. Using large mixing bowl, combine margarine, Ambrosia, fructose, and sugar. Beat on medium speed until fluffy. Add egg and beat on high speed to blend.

4. With machine on low, add carrots and nuts. When well incorporated, pour in chocolate mixture. Beat in flour mix, a little at a time.

5. Increase speed of mixer to medium and blend in extracts. Dough will be thick and somewhat sticky.

6. Sprinkle remaining 2 tablespoons flour across a board. Scrape batter onto the board. Gently knead, turning and folding dough over

until it is no longer sticky. Cut into 2 equal pieces. Shape into logs 1½ inches high and 7 inches long with squared-off ends.

7. Line a cookie sheet with parchment paper. Transfer logs to paper. Bake in center section of oven until center of cake when pierced with a toothpick comes out clean (30 to 35 minutes). Logs expand and may crack on the sides; not to worry. Let cool for 5 minutes. Raise oven heat to 400°F.

8. With a spatula, lift up and transfer logs to a cutting board. Using a sharp serrated knife, cut into ⅜-inch slices. Arrange slices (in two batches) flat and close together back onto the parchment. Bake until toasted (10 to 12 minutes). Cool on wire rack (do not cover). To preserve flavor and crispness, store in tightly closed container and freeze. Cookies thaw out rapidly at room temperature.

New Classic Apple Tart

YIELD: SERVES 8

To most of us, the "classic apple tart" means a buttery pie crust, a cream filling, a topping of fruit slathered in butter, and an excessive amount of sugar. My New Classic Apple Tart is based on the concept that if the crust is multitextured and crisp, the filling is all fruit, and the total confection is just sweet enough—you'll never miss the butter, the cream, and the superfluous sugar. And it's so easy to make. Serve warm as is, or follow the serving suggestions for Chocolate Pumpkin Pie (page 255).

Per serving
Calories: 148
Carbohydrate: 26 g
Protein: 1 g
Fat: 4 g
Saturated fat: 1 g
Cholesterol: 0 mg
Dietary fiber: 2.5 g
Sodium: 49 mg
Exchanges: 1 starch/bread
½ fruit
1 fat

This recipe contains a moderate amount of sugar and should be used only occasionally. It should be carefully worked into your individual meal plan.

1 recipe pastry from Chocolate Pumpkin Pie (page 255)

½ cup well drained crushed pineapples (no sugar added)

2 teaspoons fresh lemon juice

1½ pounds Golden Delicious apples (4 medium apples)

½ teaspoon each ground cardamom, allspice, cinnamon, and nutmeg

2 tablepoons unbleached flour

2 tablespoons sugar

1 tablespoon granulated fructose (see page 297)

1. To prepare pastry, follow directions through step 3 on page 256. Roll pastry to a 12-inch circle and invert onto a cookie sheet lined with parchment paper. Preheat oven to 400°F.

2. Combine pineapples and lemon juice in a large bowl. Peel, core, quarter, and thin-slice apples, adding them to the bowl as they're sliced. Sprinkle with spices, gently tossing several times to coat evenly.

3. In a cup, combine flour with 1 tablespoon sugar. Leaving a 2-inch circular margin, sprinkle mixture evenly over pastry. Arrange apples around flour, round sides out; then fill the flour-covered pastry with the remaining fruit in a decorative pattern. Fold up uncovered margin of pastry, pleating to hold. Sprinkle apples with remaining 1 tablespoon sugar.

4. Bake in center section of oven until pastry is lightly brown (40 to 45 minutes). Transfer paper with tart to a wire rack. Cool for 10 minutes. Sprinkle with fructose. With the aid of 2 spatulas, transfer to a large serving plate. Serve warm.

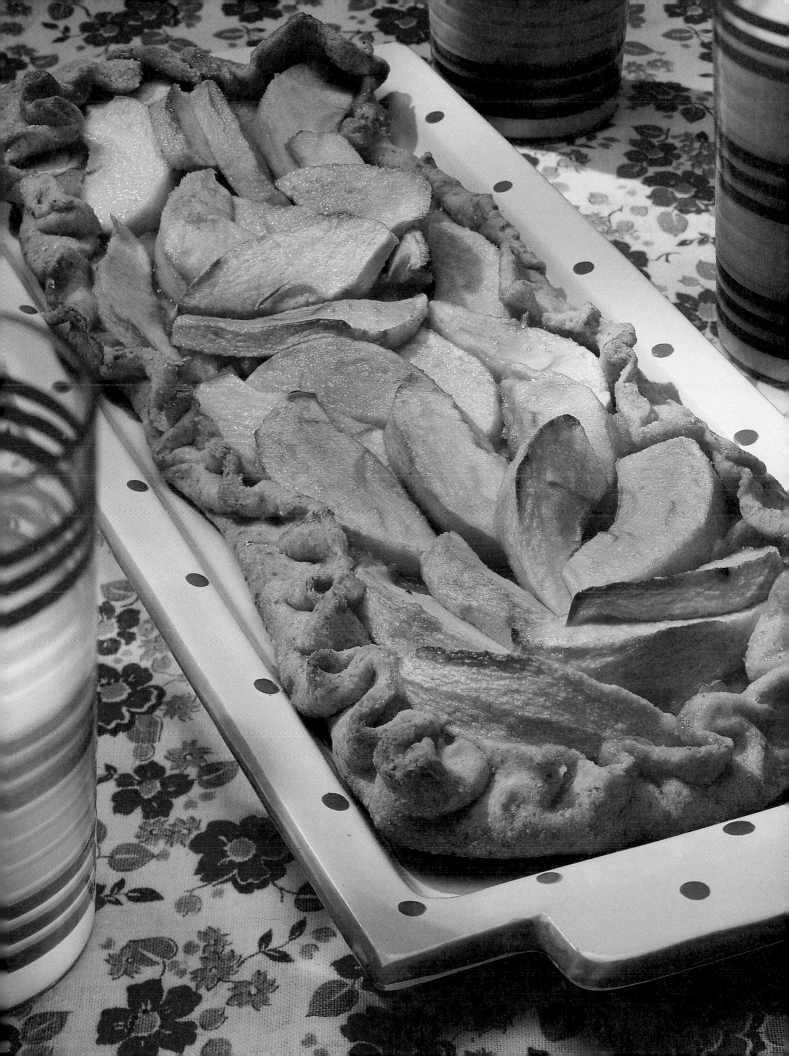

Chocolate Swirl Coffee Cake

YIELD: SERVES 12

*High on any choco-
late-lover's wish list,
this dream cake—moist,
tender and chocolatey,
chocolatey—comes with an
overture: a tantalizing
baking aroma that height-
ens the taste sensation of
that first bite. You'll want
to keep one cake frozen for
drop-in guests to dramatize
that anybody can enjoy
great desserts as much as we
can.*

FOR THE SWIRL:

2	tablespoons unsweetened cocoa
2	teaspoons freeze-dried coffee granules (preferably decaffeinated)
3½	tablespoons undiluted evaporated skim milk
1	tablespoon frozen pineapple juice concentrate
2	tablespoons honey
½	teaspoon cinnamon
½	teaspoon each freshly grated nutmeg and ground cardamom (or 1 teaspoon cinnamon)
2½	tablespoons date sugar (see page 297)

FOR THE CAKE:

2	cups unbleached flour
¾	teaspoon baking soda
2	teaspoons baking powder
½	teaspoon cinnamon
⅓	cup sweet soft corn oil margarine, plus ¾ teaspoon for pan
3	tablespoons granulated fructose (see page 297)
½	cup (plus 1 tablespoon) date sugar
1½	teaspoons pure vanilla extract
3	eggs (use 2 yolks and 3 whites)
1	cup plain low-fat yogurt

Per serving
Calories: 215
Carbohydrate: 33 g
Protein: 5 g
Fat: 7 g
Saturated fat: 2 g
Cholesterol: 47 mg
Dietary fiber: 0.7 g
Sodium: 197 mg
Exchanges: 2 starch/bread
                1 fat

This recipe contains a moderate amount of sugar and should be used only occasionally. It should be carefully worked into your individual meal plan.

1. Preheat oven to 350°F. Prepare swirl first. Put first four ingredients in a small heavy-bottom saucepan. Over very low heat, while stirring, cook until cocoa dissolves (2 to 3 minutes). Remove from heat. Stir in honey. Let cool. In cup, combine and blend spices with date sugar. Set aside.

2. Sift flour, baking soda, baking powder, and cinnamon into a bowl.

3. In large mixing bowl, combine ⅓ cup margarine, fructose, all of the date sugar, and vanilla. Beat on medium speed until well blended, scraping down sides of bowl once. Beat in eggs, then yogurt.

4. With machine running at low speed, add dry ingredients to batter, a ¼ cup at a time. Then increase speed to medium and beat for 10 seconds. Batter will be thick.

5. Grease an 8- or 9-inch loose-bottom tube pan with remaining ¾ teaspoon shortening. Spoon batter into pan, distributing evenly. Drizzle chocolate swirl mix over batter; then sprinkle with spice mixture. With blunt knife or large spoon, fold bottom batter over toppings in a down and then upward motion in 5 places (do not mix). Smooth out top.

6. Bake in center section of oven for 30 to 35 minutes. Check doneness after 30 minutes. Cake is done when toothpick inserted comes out clean. Place pan on a rack and cool for 10 minutes. Run a blunt knife around the sides of pan and lift out tube with cake. Cook completely on rack. Run a spatula under cake to loosen from bottom of pan. Then, with both hands, lift (do not invert) onto a serving plate. Freeze leftovers.

*S*piced Chocolate Banana Cake with Chocolate-Raspberry Sauce

~

YIELD: SERVES 10

*I*f you like pound cake, you'll love this spiced banana cake, which resembles pound cake without the "pounds" of sugar and butter. The banana is used as a natural sweetener not as the dominant flavor, so be sure the banana you choose is fully ripe so you can glean all of its sweetness. This cake is equally delicious with or without the cocoa (see Variation); and the sauce can be served atop Griddle Cakes, Blintzes, and New Classic Apple Tart (pages 36, 276, and 260, respectively) as well as on other confections in this book.

FOR THE CAKE:

2 cups unbleached flour

1½ teaspoons baking powder

½ teaspoon baking soda

2 tablespoons unsweetened cocoa

½ teaspoon each ground cardamom, ground coriander, and cinnamon

¼ teaspoon ground ginger

¼ cup sweet soft corn oil margarine, plus ½ teaspoon for pan

5 tablespoons granulated fructose (see page 297)

2 tablespoons sugar

1 tablespoon frozen pineapple or apple juice concentrate

½ cup mashed ripe banana (1 medium banana)

2 large eggs

1½ teaspoons pure vanilla extract

¼ teaspoon almond extract

1 cup low-fat buttermilk (preferably without salt)

FOR THE SAUCE:

1 12-ounce bag frozen raspberries (no sugar added)

2½ tablespoons granulated fructose

1 square unsweetened chocolate (1 ounce)

3 tablespoons frozen apple juice concentrate

4 tablespoons undiluted evaporated skim milk

¼ teaspoon cinnamon

½ teaspoon pure vanilla extract

Per serving

Calories: 222

Carbohydrate: 31 g

Protein: 5 g

Fat: 9 g

Saturated fat: 3 g

Cholesterol: 35 mg

Dietary fiber: 1.0 g

Sodium: 167 mg

Exchanges: 2 starch/bread
2 fat

Chocolate Raspberry Sauce

Per serving

Calories: 34

Carbohydrate: 7 g

Protein: 1 g

Fat: trace

Saturated fat: 0

Cholesterol: trace

Dietary fiber: 1.7 g

Sodium: 6 mg

Exchanges: ½ fruit

This recipe contains a moderate amount of sugar and should be used only occasionally. It should be carefully worked into your individual meal plan.

1. Preheat oven to 350°F. Sift first 6 ingredients into a bowl. Set aside.

2. In mixing bowl, combine ¼ cup margarine with fructose, sugar, and concentrate. Beat on medium speed until blended. Scrape down sides of bowl.

3. Beat in banana, then eggs and extracts. Scrape down sides of bowl once more.

4. Add buttermilk alternately with dry ingredients and beat until smooth.

5. Pour into a lightly greased 8-inch loaf pan and smooth out the top. Bake in center section of oven for 45 minutes. Insert a toothpick into center of cake. If it comes out moist, return pan to oven for 5 minutes and test again for doneness. When fully baked, set pan on a wire rack for 15 minutes. Run a blunt knife around the sides and invert cake onto the rack. Let cool for 1 hour before slicing.

6. To prepare the sauce, put frozen berries into a 1½- to 2-quart heavy-bottom saucepan. Cover and place over very low heat stirring from time to time, until berries give up their liquid. With bowl underneath, puree through a food mill (not a blender). Stir in fructose.

7. Rinse out saucepan. Put chocolate and concentrate into pan. Cook over very low heat, uncovered, until chocolate melts. Stir in 3 tablespoons milk and cinnamon. Remove from heat and cool for 5 minutes. Whisk into puree; then whisk in vanilla. Taste for sweetness, adding remaining tablespoon of milk, if desired. Serve chilled.

VARIATION: Cake is also delicious without cocoa. Just reduce fructose measurement to 4 tablespoons, proceed with recipe, and bake for 40 minutes before testing for doneness.

NOTE: To preserve the texture of uneaten portions of cake, wrap in plastic film, then in aluminum foil, and freeze.

Chocolate Chip Oatmeal Cookies with Ambrosia Topping

YIELD: 45 COOKIES

During a guest appearance on a radio program, I couldn't resist belting out the following parody of "Sugar in the Morning": "Don't have that/ Sugar in the morning,/ Sugar in the evening,/ Sugar at suppertime./ Cutting down on sugar/ Can make your life sublime!"

Heeding the advice of my theme song, I created these confections with only about ⅛ teaspoon of sugar per cookie—an all-time low.

Bonus: Oatmeal gives you that satisfied feeling after just one cookie (maybe two).

Per cookie
Calories: 62
Carbohydrate: 8 g
Protein: 1 g
Fat: 3 g
Saturated fat: 1 g
Cholesterol: 4 mg
Dietary fiber: 1.0 g
Sodium: 25 mg
Exchanges: ½ starch/bread
  ½ fat

1½ cups unbleached flour

½ teaspoon each baking powder and baking soda

1½ teaspoons cinnamon

¼ teaspoon each allspice and nutmeg

¼ cup sweet soft corn oil margarine

2 tablespoons sugar

1 cup Ambrosia (page 267)

2 tablespoons frozen apple juice concentrate

2 teaspoons pure vanilla extract

1 large egg

¾ cup 1-minute Quick Oats

2 tablespoons undiluted evaporated skim milk

½ cup coarsely chopped walnuts

½ cup semisweet chocolate chips

1. Preheat oven to 375°F. Sift first 4 ingredients into a bowl. Set aside.

2. Put margarine, sugar, ½ cup Ambrosia, and concentrate into large mixing bowl. Blend on medium speed. Scrape down sides of bowl. Beat in egg and vanilla. Scrape down sides of bowl once more.

3. With machine running on low speed, add oats a ¼ cup at a time; then add milk, nuts, and chocolate chips. Turn speed up to medium and beat for 15 seconds. Batter will be thick.

4. Line 1 or 2 cookie sheets with parchment paper. Drop batter by the teaspoonful onto paper, arranging 16 cookies on each baking sheet. With a moistened fork, flatten dough to a ¼-inch thickness (cookies will be about 2¾ inches in diameter).

5. Bake in center section of oven for 8 minutes (or bake one batch at a time if both sheets don't fit on your oven rack). Remove from oven. Immediately spoon ¾ teaspoon Ambrosia atop each cookie; then spread it across the cookie almost to the edge. Return baking sheet(s) to the oven until the cookies are lightly browned (6 to 7 minutes). Repeat procedure with remaining batter (parchment may be reused each time). Cool on wire racks. Serve slightly warm or at room temperature.

NOTE: To preserve freshness of cookies after bake day, pack loosely in tightly sealed container(s) and store in freezer. Cookies thaw out at room temperature in 10 minutes.

Ambrosia
(mixed dried fruit puree)
~

YIELD: 2 CUPS

Ambrosia, the sweetest of sweets, was created, legends inform us, for the delectation of the ancient Greek gods and goddesses. My ambrosia is a puree of dried figs, dates, apricots, and seedless dark raisins aided and abetted by the sweet scents of vanilla, mint, cinnamon, and apple juice. Enjoy it to satisfy that need for a sweet pick-me-up (without added sugar). Try it, too, as a sweetener in Chocolate-Carrot Biscotti (page 259) and as a sugar substitute and topping in Chocolate Chip Oatmeal Cookies (page 266).

6	ounces dried figs (about 12 medium-size)	¼	cup dark seedless raisins
6	ounces dried apricots (about 34 halves), preferably unsulfured, well rinsed	½	vanilla bean
		1	cup apple juice (no sugar added)
4	ounces dried, pitted dates (about 12), each date cut in half	1¼	cups brewed mint herb tea
		1	teaspoon cinnamon

1. Put all ingredients in a 2-quart heavy-bottom saucepan. Bring to a boil. Reduce heat to simmering. Cover and cook for 20 minutes, stirring from time to time. Remove from heat and let stand, covered, until cooled. (Most of liquid will be absorbed.)

2. Turn into a food mill (not a blender) and puree. Store in tightly closed container for up to 2 weeks.

Per tablespoon
Calories: 37
Carbohydrate: 9 g
Protein: trace
Fat: trace
Saturated fat: 0 g
Cholesterol: 0 mg
Dietary fiber: 1.3 g
Sodium: 1 mg
Exchanges: ½ fruit

Light Pineapple Tapioca

YIELD: SERVES 6

"Tapioca is a farinaceous food derived from the roots of a tropical food plant called manioc"—and that description is admittedly a turn-off. But several years back a major Manhattan restaurant featured a tapioca dessert that was as brilliantly conceived and executed as any sweet we've ever savored. No, this is not the recipe for that wonder ("We are very sorry, madame, but it is a secret of the proprietor"), but it is a recipe that's creamy and sweet, and ever so different—and that's pretty wonderful, too.

Per serving
Calories: 87
Carbohydrate: 16 g
Protein: 4 g
Fat: 1 g
Saturated fat: trace
Cholesterol: 29 mg
Dietary fiber: 0.2 g
Sodium: 48 mg
Exchanges: ½ fruit
         ½ milk

3 tablespoons quick-cooking tapioca

1¼ cups skim milk

¼ cup evaporated skim milk

1 egg, separated

¼ cup pineapple juice (drain it from the pineapple tidbits used below)

2 tablespoons frozen apple juice concentrate

2 tablespoons granulated fructose (see page 297)

¼ teaspoon each ground allspice and freshly grated nutmeg

2 dashes ground cloves

½ teaspoon pure vanilla extract

⅛ teaspoon almond extract

½ cup well-drained canned pineapple tidbits (no sugar added)

1. Place tapioca, milks, egg yolk, and juices in heavy-bottom saucepan. Mix well. Let stand for 5 minutes.

2. Beat egg white until foamy. Then sprinkle with fructose and beat until soft peaks form. Set aside.

3. Bring tapioca mixture to boil. Reduce heat to slow boil and cook, stirring constantly, for 6 minutes. Stir in spices. Slowly dribble mixture into beaten egg whites, stirring only until just blended.

4. Stir in extracts. Let cool for 20 minutes. Gently fold in pineapple. Spoon into 6 decorative dessert dishes. Serve warm or chilled.

Carob Loaf
~

YIELD: 12 SLICES

Slightly spicy, slightly fruity, deliciously moist, and finely textured, this mahogany-hued loaf, with just a hint of chocolate flavor, is enriched with only healthful ingredients. A breeze to make!

Per slice
Calories: 125
Carbohydrate: 17 g
Protein: 4 g
Fat: 5 g
Saturated fat: 1 g
Cholesterol: 28 mg
Dietary fiber: 0.9 mg
Sodium: 97 mg
Exchanges: 1 starch/bread
1 fat

1¼ cups unbleached flour

2 teaspoons baking powder

½ teaspoon each ground coriander and cinnamon

3 tablespoons sweet soft corn oil margarine, plus ½ teaspoon for pan

3 tablespoons granulated fructose (see page 297)

1 teaspoon pure vanilla extract

2 eggs

2 tablespoons each orange juice concentrate and water

1 tablespoon coffee substitute or decaffeinated coffee

¼ cup unsweetened carob powder (see page 297)

¼ cup each evaporated skim milk and low-fat plain yogurt

¼ cup coarsely chopped walnuts

1. Preheat oven to 350°F. Sift flour, baking powder, and spices 3 times into bowl. Set aside.

2. Beat 3 tablespoons margarine with fructose and vanilla until fluffy. Add eggs and beat until blended.

3. In small heavy-bottom saucepan or enamel pot, over low heat, combine and heat orange juice concentrate, water, coffee substitute, and carob, stirring constantly, until carob is dissolved. (Carob powder sometimes tends to lump up in box.) Let cool. Pour in evaporated milk, stirring to blend. Add to egg mixture. Beat only until blended.

4. Add half of flour mixture to mixing bowl and beat briefly. Add yogurt. Blend. Then add balance of flour mixture. Beat or stir until flour is absorbed.

5. Spoon into small margarine-greased loaf pan (7⅜" × 3⅝" × 2¼"). Sprinkle with nuts. Swirl nuts through cake with knife. Bake for 45 minutes. Cake is done when toothpick inserted into center comes out clean. Let pan cool on rack for 10 minutes. Loosen around sides with blunt knife. Remove loaf from pan and let cool thoroughly on rack before slicing.

SERVING SUGGESTION: Serve with Creamy Vanilla Sauce (page 208).

Apricot-Pineapple Pie with Crunchy Crust

YIELD: SERVES 12

Want to create a local sensation? Offer wedges of this pie to your neighbors and wait for their exclamations of delight.

Per serving
Calories: 214
Carbohydrate: 37 g
Protein: 5 g
Fat: 5 g
Saturated fat: 1 g
Cholesterol: trace
Dietary fiber: 3.5 g
Sodium: 24 mg
Exchanges: 1 starch/bread
1½ fruit
1 fat

This recipe contains a moderate amount of sugar and should be used only occasionally. It should be carefully worked into your individual meal plan.

FOR THE CRUST:

½ cup whole-wheat flour

½ cup old-fashioned rolled oats

½ cup date sugar (see page 297)

½ cup buckwheat flour (see page 297)

½ cup unbleached flour

½ teaspoon ground cinnamon

¼ cup Italian olive oil or canola oil

FOR THE FILLING:

1 recipe (1 cup) Stewed Apricots (page 38)

½ cup drained canned pineapple chunks (no sugar added)

½ cup evaporated skim milk

2 tablespoons low-fat cottage cheese (no salt added), drained

2 teaspoons granulated fructose (see page 297)

¼ teaspoon freshly grated nutmeg

⅔ cup pineapple juice from pineapple chunks

2 envelopes plain gelatin

2 egg whites, stiffly beaten (see Note 1, page 251)

1. Preheat oven to 350°F. Prepare crust first. If you have a food processor, fit with steel blade. In processor bowl, combine and process all ingredients except water, turning machine on/off 4 times. Then turn machine on and slowly pour ice water through feed tube. Dough will form into ball.

2. If you don't have a food processor, combine all dry ingredients in medium-size bowl. Add oil a little at a time and blend with fork. Finally, dribble ice water into mixture, using only enough water to hold mixture together. Knead briefly.

3. Turn into a 10-inch metal pie pan. Press to bottom and sides of pan. Bake for 20 minutes. Crust is fully baked when it starts to come away from sides of pan. Place on rack and let cool.

4. Now prepare filling. Place first 6 ingredients and ⅓ cup pineapple juice in bowl of food processor or blender. Process until smooth.

5. Pour balance of pineapple juice (⅓ cup) into saucepan. Sprinkle with gelatin. Let soften for 3 minutes. Heat and stir until gelatin dissolves. Add to processor bowl. Process on/off twice. Pour into bowl and chill until mixture begins to thicken (about 25 minutes). Do not let mixture set.

6. Whisk one-third of beaten egg whites into thickened mixture. Fold in balance.

7. Pour filling into pie shell. Refrigerate until set (about 2 hours).

VARIATION: The filling alone makes a delicious and eye-appealing dessert. Pour mixture (step 7) into 8 decorative dessert dishes. Sprinkle with nuts. Refrigerate until set.

*A*pricot Delight
~

YIELD: SERVES 9

Satiny smooth, sinfully delicious, sweet and tart, and simple to make. Use it as a pie filling, too.

Per serving
Calories: 124
Carbohydrate: 26 g
Protein: 4 g
Fat: 1 g
Saturated fat: 0 g
Cholesterol: 1 mg
Dietary fiber: 2.7 g
Sodium: 42 mg
Exchanges: 2 fruit

Apricot Pie
Per serving
Calories: 334
Carbohydrate: 59 g
Protein: 8 g
Fat: 8 g
Saturated fat: 1 g
Cholesterol: 1 mg
Dietary fiber: 5.4 g
Sodium: 47 mg
Exchanges: 1½ starch/bread
         2 fruit
         1 fat

This recipe contains a moderate amount of sugar and should be used only occasionally. It should be carefully worked into your individual meal plan.

1	recipe Stewed Apricots, including syrup (page 38)
¾	cup cold evaporated skim milk
1	tablespoon granulated fructose (see page 297)
¾	cup pineapple juice (no sugar added)
¼	cup fresh orange juice
1	envelope plain gelatin
1	teaspoon finely grated orange zest (preferably from navel orange)
¼	teaspoon freshly grated nutmeg
2	large egg whites (see Note 1, page 251)
1	tablespoon coarsely chopped walnuts (optional)

1. Place apricots, skim milk, and fructose in food processor that has been fitted with steel blade. Blend until smooth (about 30 seconds). Turn into large bowl.

2. Pour pineapple and orange juices into small heavy-bottom saucepan. Sprinkle with gelatin. Let gelatin soften for 3 minutes. Add orange zest and nutmeg. Warm mixture over low heat, stirring until gelatin dissolves.

3. Whisk into apricot puree until smooth. Chill until mixture begins to thicken (about 30 minutes).

4. Whisk in one-third of egg whites. Fold in balance of egg whites.

5. Spoon into decorative dessert dishes. Sprinkle with nuts. Chill until set (about 2 hours).

VARIATION: Use as a pie filling. Prepare pie shell for Apricot-Pineapple Pie with Crunchy Crust (page 270). Pour thickened mixture into shell and chill until set. Serves 8.

Apricot Spice Cake

YIELD: 18 SLICES

For dessert or a snack. For breakfast. For anytime you want something spicy and delicious.

Per slice
Calories: 113
Carbohydrate: 15 g
Protein: 3 g
Fat: 5 g
Saturated fat: 1 g
Cholesterol: 10 mg
Dietary fiber: 1.2 g
Sodium: 68 mg
Exchanges: 1 starch/bread
           1 fat

⅓ cup chopped dried apricots (unsulfured preferred, see page 297)

½ cup pineapple or apple juice (no sugar added)

¾ cup whole-wheat flour

1½ cups unbleached flour

3 teaspoons baking powder

3 tablespoons date sugar (see page 297)

1 teaspoon each ground ginger, coriander, and cinnamon

2 tablespoons each Italian olive oil or canola oil and sweet soft corn oil margarine, plus ¼ teaspoon for pan

1 whole egg

¾ cup buttermilk (preferably without salt)

¼ cup chopped walnuts or almonds

1. Preheat oven to 350°F. Place apricots in small bowl. In a saucepan, bring juice to simmering point. Pour over apricots and stir to separate. Set aside.

2. Sift flours and baking powder into mixing bowl. Add date sugar and spices, stirring to blend.

3. In medium-size bowl, whisk oil and margarine until well blended. Add egg and beat until smooth. Add buttermilk, blending briefly with whisk. Pour in apricot mixture.

4. Gradually add liquid mixture to dry ingredients, beating with wooden spoon until blended. Stir in nuts.

5. Pour batter into a lightly greased 9" × 5" loaf pan. Bake for 50 minutes. When done, toothpick inserted into center of cake should come out clean.

6. Place pan on rack and let cool for 5 minutes. Loosen around sides with blunt knife. Remove cake from pan. Place on rack and let cool completely before slicing.

VARIATION: Diet permitting, add 1 tablespoon Grand Marnier or cognac in step 4.

$\mathcal{S}$*peedy Spice Cake*

YIELD: 12 SLICES, ⅔ INCH EACH

All you need to prepare this delicious textured cake is 5 minutes, a large mixing bowl, a whisk, and a spoon. Why not prepare a double recipe, and keep a frozen loaf available for slicing off a snack any time of day (diet permitting).

Per slice
Calories: 136
Carbohydrate: 17 g
Protein: 3 g
Fat: 6 g
Saturated fat: 1 g
Cholesterol: 14 mg
Dietary fiber: 0.8 g
Sodium: 67 mg
Exchanges: 1 starch/bread
          1 fat

1⅓ cups unbleached flour

1 teaspoon each ground coriander and cinnamon

¼ teaspoon each ground ginger and freshly grated nutmeg

2 teaspoons baking powder

2 tablespoons each oat bran and date sugar (see page 297)

2 tablespoons each canola oil and sweet soft corn oil margarine, plus ½ teaspoon for pan

1 whole egg (room temperature)

1 tablespoon granulated fructose (see page 297)

⅓ cup each evaporated skim milk and apple juice (no sugar added)

1 teaspoon finely grated orange zest

¼ cup raisins

2 tablespoons coarsely chopped walnuts

1. Preheat oven to 350°F. Sift flour, spices, and baking powder into large mixing bowl. Stir in oat bran and date powder.

2. In small bowl, whisk oil and margarine until blended. Add egg and fructose, whisk until smooth.

3. Combine skim milk, apple juice, and orange zest. Add to mixture. Stir. Pour over dry ingredients, a little at a time, and stir with wooden spoon (do not beat) until all flour is absorbed. Stir in raisins.

4. Pour into small loaf pan (7⅜" × 3⅝" × 2¼"). Sprinkle with walnuts. Bake for 40 to 45 minutes. Test for doneness: Toothpick inserted into center of cake should come out dry.

5. Place pan on rack for 5 minutes. Loosen around sides of pan with blunt knife. Remove loaf from pan. Let cool on rack. Delicious served warm or at room temperature.

*S*pecial Treat Coffee Cake

~

YIELD: 16 SQUARES

*R*eserve this special treat for whenever (diet permitting) that irresistible urge for something sweet consumes you. But don't worry about overconsumption; just a few bites and you'll glow with that satisfied feeling. It keeps well in your freezer.

FOR THE STREUSEL:

3   tablespoons date sugar (see page 297)

⅓   cup toasted pine nuts or coarsely chopped walnuts (see Note 1)

1   tablespoon sweet soft corn oil margarine or butter

1   tablespoon whole-wheat flour

3   tablespoons raisins

FOR THE CAKE:

¼   cup sweet soft corn oil margarine, plus ½ teaspoon for pan

5   tablespoons granulated fructose (see page 297)

3   eggs, separated (use 2 egg yolks, 3 egg whites)

1   cup low-fat plain yogurt

1   teaspoon grated orange zest (preferably from navel orange)

1   tablespoon frozen pineapple juice concentrate

1   teaspoon pure vanilla extract

2¼ cups unbleached flour

2¼ teaspoons baking powder

1. Prepare streusel first by combining all ingredients in small bowl and blending. (Your fingers will do the best job here.) Set aside.

2. Preheat oven to 350°F. Have all cake ingredients at room temperature. In large bowl, combine ¼ cup margarine and fructose. Beat until well blended, stopping beaters and scraping down sides of bowl. Add 2 egg yolks and beat until smooth.

3. Add yogurt, orange zest, and orange juice concentrate to bowl. Beat only until combined. Beat in vanilla.

Per square
Calories: 156
Carbohydrate: 22 g
Protein: 4 g
Fat: 6 g
Saturated fat: 1 g
Cholesterol: 35 mg
Dietary fiber: 1.0 g
Sodium: 114 mg
Exchanges: 1½ starch/bread
1 fat

This recipe contains a moderate amount of sugar and should be used only occasionally. It should be carefully worked into your individual meal plan.

4. Sift flour and baking powder. With beater going, add flour mixture ½ cup at a time.

5. In a separate bowl, beat 3 egg whites until stiff. Fold into batter.

6. Lightly grease an 8- or 9-inch-square metal baking pan. Spoon and spread half of mixture into pan. Sprinkle with half of streusel mixture. Cover with balance of thick batter. (It's easiest to drop spoonfuls in various spots and then spread evenly with spatula into corners of pan.) Sprinkle balance of streusel over cake, pressing into batter with spoon.

7. Bake for 45 to 50 minutes. Top of cake should be golden brown and cake should start to come away from sides. Place pan on rack to cool. Cut into 16 squares. Serve slightly warm.

NOTES:
1. To toast pine nuts, place in preheated skillet and toast over medium heat, shaking skillet from time to time until nuts are lightly toasted (3 to 4 minutes). Take care not to burn.

2. This cake freezes magnificently. Wrap each portion in waxed paper, then place in aluminum foil. Seal tightly in plastic bag. To serve, unwrap; lay on baking sheet. Cover with aluminum foil, and bake in preheated 350°F oven for about 12 minutes, or until cake is heated through. Serve warm.

Blintzes: Traditional Style and a Chocolate-Cheese Variation

~

YIELD: 16 BLINTZES

Paper-thin wrappers (as svelte as crepes) deserve this elegant filling of low-fat cheeses, fresh tangerine juice, and spices. For the variation, speckle the filling with chocolate bits which, when cooked, melt to just the right consistency. Both blintzes are just as lovely to look at as they are to taste, particularly when they're spooned with my colorful Strawberry Sauce (see page 242).

FOR THE FILLING:

1	7½-ounce package farmer cheese, without salt
2	tablespoons reduced-fat cream cheese (Neufchâtel)
¼	cup tangerine juice
2	teaspoons fresh lemon juice
¼	cup mashed ripe banana (½ medium banana)
1	large egg
2	teaspoons sugar
½	teaspoon pure vanilla extract
3	tablespoons unbleached flour
¼	teaspoon each cinnamon and allspice (or ground cardamom)
2	teaspoons sweet soft margarine for sautéing
1½	teaspoons granulated fructose (see page 297)

FOR THE WRAPPERS:

1	large egg, plus reserved egg from filling
½	cup each skim milk and undiluted evaporated skim milk
¾	cup sifted unbleached flour
¼	teaspoon each cinnamon and freshly grated nutmeg (or ground cardamom)
1	tablespoon sweet soft corn oil margarine, melted
⅛	teaspoon almond extract
2	teaspoons Italian olive oil (or canola oil) for sautéing

1. To prepare the filling, put the farmer cheese and cream cheese into a medium bowl and mash. Add juices and stir to blend. Then stir in banana.

2. Put egg into a cup and beat with a fork until well blended. Measure out 2 tablespoons and add to the cheese mixture (reserve the remainder for the wrappers).

3. Stir in sugar and vanilla extract. Sift flour and spices over filling; fold in. Cover and refrigerate for 30 minutes.

4. To prepare the wrappers, put reserved egg from filling and 1 whole egg in a medium-size bowl. Whisk in the milks. While whisking, gradually add flour, then the spices. Stir in the melted margarine and almond extract. Let stand for 10 minutes.

For 2 blintzes
Calories: 157
Carbohydrate: 17 g
Protein: 10 g
Fat: 5 g
Saturated fat: 2 g
Cholesterol: 47 mg
Dietary fiber: 0.5 g
Sodium: 88 mg
Exchanges: 1 starch/bread
           1 lean meat
           ½ fat

5. Lightly brush two 7-inch nonstick skillets with oil. Place over medium heat. When drops of water bounce off the cooking surface of pans, they're hot enough for the batter. Half-fill a ¼-cup measure with batter and pour into each pan. Immediately tilt pans to distribute batter evenly; patch any holes with a bit more batter. Cook until edges begin to curl and tops of pancakes are dry to the touch (1 to 1½ minutes). Lift up sides with spatula, turn, and cook for 10 seconds. Transfer to a plate. Repeat procedure with remaining batter, regulating heat when necessary to assure even cooking. Stack wrappers, second side up, as they're made.

6. To assemble blintzes, spoon a heaping teaspoon of filling in the center of each blintz. Then flip over the edges to make a rectangle; first fold over two opposite sides, then the remaining open sides. Place seam down on a plate as they're assembled.

7. Heat 1 or 2 large nonstick skillets, using 1 teaspoon shortening for each skillet. Place bundles, seam side down, in pans and cook over moderate heat until they're lightly browned. Turn carefully. Cover and cook for 1 minute. Uncover, and cook until browned.

8. Slide onto a hot serving platter. Sprinkle with fructose and serve immediately.

VARIATION: Put 4 semisweet chocolate bits on top of filling in step 6 before flipping over the edges to make a package. For a serving size of 2 blintzes, this adds 15 calories.

SERVING SUGGESTION: Try this with Strawberry Sauce (page 242), on the side in a sauceboat.

NOTES:
1. A 7-inch pan assures rounded edges for the wrappers. If you already own an 8-inch nonstick pan, it can be used. You may need a little practice in using a circular motion when tilting it so that all the batter doesn't run to one side.

2. These blintzes are just as delicious served the next day. Store your leftovers in a tightly closed container large enough to hold the blintzes without crushing them. Reheat, covered, over moderate heat in a nonstick skillet (do not add any fat), turning once.

Hot-Pink Sherbet

YIELD: SERVES 8

Bright red cranberry juices mingle with the soft yellows of pineapples and bananas to give this delicious dessert a hot-pink hue. The title reads "hot" but the taste is cool, cool. Your whole family will love it.

1 cup fresh cranberries, rinsed and picked over

2 tablespoons frozen pineapple juice concentrate

2 medium-size ripe bananas

1 20-ounce can pineapple chunks (no sugar added)

2 tablespoons honey

4 teaspoons granulated fructose (see page 297)

¼ cup low-fat buttermilk, preferably without salt

Per serving
Calories: 96
Carbohydrate: 22 g
Protein: 1 g
Fat: trace
Saturated fat: trace
Cholesterol: trace
Dietary fiber: 1.4 g
Sodium: 5 mg
Exchanges: 1½ fruit

This recipe contains a moderate amount of sugar and should be used only occasionally. It should be carefully worked into your individual meal plan.

1. Put cranberries and concentrate in a small saucepan. Place over very low heat. Cover and cook until berries pop, stirring twice (about 5 minutes). Cool. Spoon into an ice-cube tray, half-filling sections. Freeze.

2. Peel and cut bananas into ⅜-inch slices. Arrange flat on a cookie sheet. Drain pineapples, reserving juices. Cut each chunk into thirds. Place on the cookie sheet in one layer and freeze about 2½ hours. (Frozen fruit may be transferred to a plastic bag and kept in freezer for up to 2 days.)

3. Remove fruit from freezer and let stand for 10 minutes to slightly soften. Using a food processor fitted with a steel blade, put half each of cranberries, bananas, and pineapples into workbowl. Add 1 tablespoon of the reserved pineapple juice and half each of honey, fructose, and buttermilk. Process until smooth. Scrape into a chilled bowl. Repeat procedure with remaining fruit, 1 tablespoon pineapple juice, and balance of honey, fructose, and buttermilk. Combine with first batch. Mixture will resemble the soft consistency of Italian water ices.

4. Cover and place in freezer. Sherbet will firm up in about 2 hours. Scoop servings into chilled parfait glasses.

NOTE: Dessert maintains its distinctive flavor for 2 days. To enjoy the next day, soften by transferring to refrigerator for 30 minutes before serving.

$\mathcal{F}$rozen Chocolate Dessert

~

YIELD: SERVES 8

Don't you sometimes dream that some-where over the rainbow there's a land of happy food lovers consuming globs of luscious chocolate ice cream made without cream or even whole milk? Stop dreaming; that land is as near as your mixing machine. You don't have to be the Wizard of Oz to mix this smooth, creamy, and, above all, chocolatey confection. It's amazing that carob mixed with apple juice concentrate and the smallest amount of real chocolate can produce such a true chocolate taste.

Per serving
Calories. 97
Carbohydrate: 19 g
Protein: 2 g
Fat: 1 g
Saturated fat: 1 g
Cholesterol: 1 mg
Dietary fiber: 0.6 g
Sodium: 35 mg
Exchanges: 1 fruit
½ milk

This recipe contains a moderate amount of sugar and should be used only occasionally. It should be carefully worked into your individual meal plan.

¾ cup evaporated skim milk (see page 299)

4 ounces frozen apple juice concentrate

1 tablespoon freeze-dried decaffeinated coffee granules

3 tablespoons unsweetened carob powder (see page 299)

½ square (½ ounce) semisweet chocolate

¼ teaspoon each cinnamon and ground cardamom

½ teaspoon pure vanilla extract

1 teaspoon fresh lemon juice

2½ tablespoons granulated fructose (see page 299)

1. Pour milk into a large metal mix-ing bowl. Place bowl and whipping utensil(s) in freezer. Chill until firm to the touch (about 2 hours).

2. Combine half the apple juice concentrate, the coffee, carob, chocolate, and spices in a heavy-bottom saucepan; place over low heat. Cook while stirring until mixture is smooth and chocolate has completely melted. Remove from heat, and cool for 5 minutes.

3. Whisk in remaining apple juice concentrate and vanilla. Pour into a small covered bowl (or plastic container) and place in freezer until mixture is thick and almost frozen. (If it freezes completely before milk is ready to beat, let it stand at room temperature for a few minutes, then cut it into chunks.)

4. Attach cold beating utensil(s) to mixing machine. Sprinkle lemon juice over milk and beat on medium speed until milk begins to congeal. Turn up to highest speed and beat until milk reaches the consistency of whipped cream (it will take several minutes).

5. With machine running, spoon in cold coffee mixture and beat until well blended. Sprinkle in fructose, a little at a time, and continue beating for 2 minutes.

6. Spoon (do not compress) into a large freezer tray that has been rinsed in cold water. Cover tray loosely with plastic wrap or wax paper and place in freezer. Freezing time is 1 to 1½ hours for the consistency of frozen custard; 4 to 5 hours for the consistency of ice cream. (Freezing time will vary with size of tray and efficiency of your freezer.) Dessert maintains its smooth texture and flavor in your freezer for 2 days. Keep dessert in freezer until ready to serve.

Spiced Applesauce
~

YIELD: SERVES 8

2   pounds crisp, sweet apples (such as Washington State), unpeeled, cored, and thickly sliced

1   slice orange, including skin

1   cup apple juice (no sugar added)

½   teaspoon each ground coriander and cardamom

1   teaspoon cinnamon

6   whole cloves

Yes, you can enjoy sweet-tasting applesauce without sugar or artificial sweeteners. Just add a bright orange slice, sweet spices, and naturally sweet apple juice. A sugar-free sweet can be that simple.

Per serving
Calories: 70
Carbohydrate: 17 g
Protein: trace
Fat: trace
Saturated fat: trace
Cholesterol: 0 mg
Dietary fiber: 2.8 g
Sodium: 1 mg
Exchanges: 1 fruit

1. Combine all ingredients in heavy-bottom saucepan. Bring to simmering point. Cover and simmer for 10 minutes, stirring twice. Uncover partially and let cool in pot. Discard orange slice.

2. Pour into food mill and puree.

NOTE: Combine the Cortland and Delicious and/or Winesap apples for excellent flavor and texture.

Frosty Yogurt Milk Shake
~

YIELD: SERVES 2

6   canned apricot halves, packed in water (no sugar added), drained (see Note)

2   teaspoons frozen orange juice concentrate

½   cup each skim milk and low-fat plain yogurt, or nonfat plain yogurt

½   teaspoon each ground coriander and cinnamon

1   dash ground cloves

3   crushed ice cubes

½   teaspoon pure vanilla extract (optional)

This is the answer to high-caloric jumbo shakes. It's a smooth, bubbly refresher—apricot, pineapple, or banana flavored.

Per serving
Calories: 94
Carbohydrate: 15 g
Protein: 6 g
Fat: 1 g
Saturated fat: 1 g
Cholesterol: 5 mg
Dietary fiber: 1.1 g
Sodium: 73 mg
Exchanges: ½ fruit
            ½ milk

1. Combine all ingredients in blender and puree until smooth and bubbly.

2. Pour into 2 chilled glasses. Serve immediately.

NOTE: For a different flavor with roughly the same nutrition and calories, substitute 1 banana or 2 slices of canned pineapple.

APPENDIX
EXCHANGE LISTS FOR MEAL PLANNING

Exchange Lists for Meal Planning is a widely used meal-planning system for people with diabetes and anyone interested in weight loss or healthy diets. Exchange lists help people to eat a nutritionally balanced diet from a wide variety of foods without having to count calories.

The exchanges are based on the grams of carbohydrate, protein, fat, and calories in foods. Each exchange, or serving of food, has a similar amount of nutrients as other foods on the same list. Therefore, one food in the serving size listed can be exchanged for any other food in the same list while providing a similar amount of carbohydrate, protein, fat, and calories. Exchange Lists for Meal Planning groups foods into six lists: starch/bread, meat, vegetable, fruit, milk, and fat.

People with diabetes often have a meal plan that outlines the number of exchanges from each food list to eat at meals and snacks. A meal plan must be individualized to take into account factors such as age, weight, medications, activity level, and other lifestyle considerations. A meal plan serves as a guide to what—and when—food should be eaten during the day.

If you don't have an individualized meal plan, it would be a good idea to contact a registered dietitian; your physician or nurse educator can help you find one in your area. A registered dietitian can assess your current eating habits, recommend changes to help you achieve your nutritional goals, and develop a meal plan appropriate for you.

The following Exchange Lists (© 1989 American Diabetes Association, The American Dietetic Association) are reprinted with the permission of the American Diabetes Association and the American Dietetic Association. The Exchange Lists are the basis of a meal planning system designed by a committee of the American Diabetes Association and The American Dietetic Association. While designed primarily for people with diabetes and others who must follow special diets, the Exchange Lists are based on principles of good nutrition that apply to everyone.

STARCH/BREAD LIST

Each item in this list contains approximately 15 grams of carbohydrate, 3 grams of protein, a trace of fat, and 80 calories. Whole grain products average about 2 grams of fiber per exchange. Some foods are higher in fiber. Those foods that contain 3 or more grams of fiber per exchange are identified with the fiber symbol ▨.

You can choose your starch exchanges from any of the items on this list. If you want to eat a starch food that is not on this list, the general rule is as follows:

- ½ cup of cereal, grain, or pasta is one exchange

- 1 ounce of a bread product is one exchange

Your dietitian can help you be more exact.

CEREALS/GRAINS/PASTA

Bran cereals, concentrated (such as Bran Buds ®, All Bran®) ▨	⅓ cup
Bran cereals, flaked ▨	½ cup
Bulgur (cooked)	½ cup
Cooked cereals	½ cup
Cornmeal (dry)	2½ tbsp
Grape-Nuts	3 tbsp
Grits (cooked)	½ cup

Other ready-to-eat unsweetened cereals	¾ cup
Pasta (cooked)	½ cup
Puffed cereal	1½ cups
Rice, white or brown (cooked)	⅓ cup
Shredded wheat	½ cup
Wheat germ ▨	3 tbsp

DRIED BEANS/PEAS/LENTILS

Beans and peas (cooked) (such as kidney, white, split, blackeye) ▨	⅓ cup
Lentils (cooked) ▨	⅓ cup
Baked beans ▨	¼ cup

STARCHY VEGETABLES

Corn ▨	½ cup
Corn on cob, 6 in. long ▨	1
Lima beans ▨	½ cup
Peas, green (canned or frozen) ▨	½ cup
Plantain ▨	½ cup
Potato, baked (small)	1 (3 oz)
Potato, mashed	½ cup
Squash, winter (acorn, butternut) ▨	1 cup
Yam, sweet potato, plain	⅓ cup

▨ *3 grams or more of fiber per exchange*

BREAD

Bagel . . . . ½ (1 oz)
Bread sticks, crisp, ... 2 (⅔ oz)
    4 in. long × ½ in.
Croutons, low-fat . . . . 1 cup
English muffin . . . . ½
Frankfurter or . . . . ½ (1 oz)
    hamburger bun
Pita, 6 in. across . . . . ½
Plain roll, small . . . . 1 (1 oz)
Raisin, unfrosted . . . . 1 slice (1 oz)
Rye, pumpernickel . . . . 1 slice (1 oz)
Tortilla, 6 in. across 1
White (including . . . . 1 slice
    French, Italian)   (1 oz)
Whole wheat . . . . 1 slice (1 oz)

CRACKERS/SNACKS

Animal crackers 8
Graham crackers, 2½ in. square 3
Matzoh . . . . ¾ oz
Melba toast . . . . 5 slices
Oyster crackers 24
Popcorn . . . . 3 cups
    (popped, no fat added)
Pretzels . . . . ¾ oz
Rye crisp, 2 in. × 3½ in. 4
Saltine-type crackers 6
Whole-wheat crackers, ... 2–4 slices
    no fat added   (¾ oz)
    (crisp breads, such as
    Finn®, Kavli®, Wasa®) 🌾

STARCH FOODS PREPARED WITH FAT

(Count as 1 starch/bread exchange, plus 1 fat exchange)

Biscuit, 2½ in. across 1
Chow mein noodles . . . . ½ cup
Corn bread, 2 in. cube . . . . 1 (2 oz)
Cracker, round butter type 6
French fried potatoes, ... 10
    2 in. to 3½ in. long   (1½ oz)
Muffin, plain, small 1
Pancake, 4 in. across 2
Stuffing, bread (prepared) . . . . ¼ cup
Taco shell, 6 in. across 2
Waffle, 4½ in. square 1
Whole-wheat crackers, ... 4–6
    fat added   (1 oz)
    (such as Triscuit®) 🌾

MEAT LIST

E ach serving of meat and substitutes on this list contains about 7 grams of protein. The amount of fat and number of calories varies, depending on what kind of meat or substitute you choose. The list is divided into three parts based on the amount of fat and calories: lean meat, medium-fat meat, and high-fat meat. One ounce (one meat exchange) of each of these includes the following:

	Carbohydrates (grams)	Protein (grams)	Fat (grams)	Calories
Lean	0	7	3	55
Medium-Fat	0	7	5	75
High-Fat	0	7	8	100

You are encouraged to use more lean and medium-fat meat, poultry, and fish in your meal plan. This will help decrease your fat intake, which may help decrease your risk for heart disease. The items from the high-fat group are high in saturated fat, cholesterol, and calories. You should limit your choices from the high-fat group to three (3) times per week. Meat and substitutes do not contribute any fiber to your meal plan.

ꙮ Meats and meat substitutes that have 400 milligrams or more of sodium per exchange are indicated with this symbol.

★ Meats and meat substitutes that have 400 mg or more of sodium if two or more exchanges are eaten are indicated with this symbol.

TIPS

1. Bake, roast, broil, grill, or boil these foods rather than frying them with added fat.

2. Use a nonstick pan spray or a nonstick pan to brown or fry these foods.

3. Trim off visible fat before and after cooking.

4. Do not add flour, bread crumbs, coating mixes, or fat to these foods when preparing them.

5. Weigh meat after removing bones and fat, and after cooking. Three ounces of cooked meat is about equal to 4 ounces of raw meat. Some examples of meat portions are:
   2 oz meat (2 meat exchanges)=
     1 small chicken leg or thigh,
     ½ cup cottage cheese
     or tuna
   3 oz meat (3 meat exchanges)=
     1 medium pork chop,
     1 small hamburger,
     ½ of a whole chicken breast,
     1 unbreaded fish fillet,
     cooked meat the size of a
       deck of cards

6. Restaurants usually serve prime cuts of meat, which are high in fat and calories.

LEAN MEAT AND SUBSTITUTES
(One exchange is equal to any one of the following items)

Beef:	USDA Select Choice grades of lean beef, such as round, sirloin, and flank steak; tenderloin; and chipped beef 🖐	1 oz
Pork:	Lean pork, such as fresh ham; canned, cured or boiled ham 🖐 ; Canadian bacon 🖐 ; tenderloin	1 oz
Veal:	All cuts are lean except for veal cutlets (ground or cubed). Examples of lean veal are chops and roasts.	1 oz
Poultry:	Chicken, turkey, Cornish hen (without skin)	1 oz
Fish:	All fresh and frozen fish	1 oz
	Crab, lobster, scallops, shrimp, clams (fresh or canned in water)	2 oz
	Oysters	6 medium
	Tuna ⭐ (canned in water)	¼ cup
	Herring ⭐ (uncreamed or smoked)	1 oz
	Sardines (canned)	2 medium
Wild Game:	Venison, rabbit, squirrel	1 oz
	Pheasant, duck, goose (without skin)	1 oz
Cheese:	Any cottage cheese ⭐	¼ cup
	Grated Parmesan	2 tbsp
	Diet cheeses 🖐 (with less than 55 calories per ounce)	1 oz
Other:	95% fat-free luncheon meat 🖐	1½ oz
	Egg whites	3 whites
	Egg substitutes (with less than 55 calories per ½ cup)	½ cup

🖐 *400 mg or more of sodium per exchange*

⭐ *400 mg or more of sodium if two or more exchanges are eaten*

MEDIUM-FAT MEAT AND SUBSTITUTES
(One exchange is equal to any one of the following items)

Beef:	Most beef products fall into this category.	1 oz
	Examples are: all ground beef,	
	roast (rib, chuck, rump),	
	steak (cubed, Porterhouse, T-bone),	
	and meat loaf.	
Pork:	Most pork products fall into this category.	1 oz
	Examples are: chops, loin roast,	
	Boston butt, cutlets.	
Lamb:	Most lamb products fall into this category.	1 oz
	Examples are: chops, leg, and roast.	
Veal:	Cutlet (ground or cubed, unbreaded)	1 oz
Poultry:	Chicken (with skin), domestic duck or goose	1 oz
	(well drained of fat), ground turkey	
Fish:	Tuna ☆ (canned in oil and drained)	¼ cup
	Salmon ☆ (canned)	¼ cup
Cheese:	Skim or part-skim cheeses, such as:	
	Ricotta	¼ cup
	Mozzarella	1 oz
	Diet cheeses ✍ (with 56–80 calories per ounce)	1 oz
Other:	86% fat-free luncheon meat ☆	1 oz
	Egg (high in cholesterol, limit to 3 per week)	1
	Egg substitutes (with 56–80 calories per ¼ cup)	¼ cup
	Tofu (2½ in. × 2¾ in. × 1 in.)	4 oz
	Liver, heart, kidney, sweetbreads	1 oz
	(high in cholesterol)	

✍ *400 mg or more of sodium per exchange*

☆ *400 mg or more of sodium if two or more exchanges are eaten*

HIGH-FAT MEAT AND SUBSTITUTES
(One exchange is equal to any one of the following items)

Remember, these items are high in saturated fat, cholesterol, and calories, and should be used only three (3) times per week.

Beef: Most USDA prime cuts of beef, ... 1 oz
                        such as ribs, corned beef

Pork: Spareribs, ground pork, pork sausage 🖐 . . . . 1 oz
                        (patty or link)

Lamb: Patties (ground lamb) . . . . 1 oz

Fish: Any fried fish product . . . . 1 oz

Cheese: All regular cheeses, such as American 🖐 , Blue 🖐 , ... 1 oz
                        Cheddar ⭐ , Monterey Jack ⭐ , Swiss

Other: Luncheon meat, such as bologna, salami, ... 1 oz
                        pimento loaf

            Sausage 🖐 , such as Polish, Italian smoked . . . . 1 oz

            Knockwurst . . . . 1 oz

            Bratwurst ⭐ . . . . 1 oz

            Frankfurter 🖐 (turkey or chicken) . . . . 1 frank
                                                  (10/lb)

            Frankfurter 🖐 (beef, pork, or combination) . . . . 1 frank
                    Count as one high-fat meat plus one fat exchange   (10/lb)

            Peanut butter (contains unsaturated fat) . . . . 1 tbsp

🖐 *400 mg or more of sodium per exchange*
⭐ *400 mg or more of sodium if two or more exchanges are eaten*

VEGETABLE LIST

Each vegetable serving on this list contains about 5 grams of carbohydrate, 2 grams of protein, and 25 calories. Vegetables contain 2–3 grams of dietary fiber. Vegetables which contain 400 mg or more of sodium per exchange are identified with a ❧ symbol.

Vegetables are a good source of vitamins and minerals. Fresh and frozen vegetables have more vitamins and less added salt. Rinsing canned vegetables will remove much of the salt.

Unless otherwise noted, the serving size for vegetables (one vegetable exchange) is as follows:

- ½ cup of cooked vegetables or vegetable juice

- 1 cup of raw vegetables

Artichoke (½ medium)
Asparagus
Beans (green, wax, Italian)
Bean sprouts
Beets
Broccoli
Brussels sprouts

Cabbage, cooked
Carrots
Cauliflower
Eggplant
Greens (collard, mustard, turnip)
Kohlrabi
Leeks
Mushrooms, cooked
Okra
Onions
Pea pods
Peppers (green)
Rutabaga
Sauerkraut ❧
Spinach, cooked
Summer squash (crookneck)
Tomato (one large)
Tomato/vegetable juice ❧
Turnips
Water chestnuts
Zucchini, cooked

Starchy vegetables such as corn, peas, and potatoes are found on the Starch/Bread list. For free vegetables, see Free Food List on page 293.

FRUIT LIST

Each item on this list contains about 15 grams of carbohydrate and 60 calories. Fresh, frozen, and dried fruits have about 2 grams of fiber per exchange. Fruits that have 3 or more grams of fiber per exchange have a 🌿 symbol. Fruit juices contain very little dietary fiber.

The carbohydrate and calorie content for a fruit exchange are based on the usual serving of the most commonly eaten fruits. Use fresh fruits or fruits frozen or canned without sugar added. Whole fruit is more filling than fruit juice and may be a better choice for those who are trying to lose weight. Unless otherwise noted, the serving size for one fruit exchange is as follows:

~ ½ cup of fresh fruit or fruit juice

~ ¼ cup of dried fruit

FRESH, FROZEN, AND UNSWEETENED CANNED FRUIT

Apple (raw, 2 in. across). 1
Applesauce (unsweetened). . . . . ½ cup
Apricots (medium, raw). 4
Apricots (canned). . . . . ½ cup or
4 halves
Banana (9 in. long) . . . . ½
Blackberries (raw) 🌿 . . . . ¾ cup
Blueberries (raw) 🌿 . . . . ¾ cup
Cantaloupe (5 in. across) . . . . ⅓
(cubes) . . . . 1 cup
Cherries (large, raw). 12
Cherries (canned) . . . . ½ cup
Figs (raw, 2 in. across) 2
Fruit cocktail (canned). . . . . ½ cup
Grapefruit (medium) . . . . ½
Grapefruit (segments) . . . . ¾ cup
Grapes (small). 15
Honeydew melon (medium) . . . . ⅛
(cubes) . . . . 1 cup
Kiwi (large) 1

Mandarin oranges . . . . ¾ cup
Mango (small) . . . . ½
Nectarine (2½ in. across) 🌾 1
Orange (2½ in. across) 1
Papaya. . . . . 1 cup
Peach (2¾ in. across). . . . . 1 or ¾ cup
Peaches (canned) . . . . ½ cup or 2 halves
Pear (small) . . . . 1 or ½ large
Pears (canned). . . . . ½ cup or 2 halves
Persimmon 2
    (medium, native)
Pineapple (raw) . . . . ¾ cup
Pineapple (canned) . . . . ⅓ cup
Plum (raw, 2 in. across) 2
Pomegranate 🌾 . . . . ½
Raspberries (raw) 🌾 . . . . 1 cup
Strawberries . . . . 1¼ cup
    (raw, whole) 🌾
Tangerine 2
    (2½ in. across) 🌾
Watermelon (cubes) . . . . 1¼ cup

DRIED FRUIT

Apples 🌾 . . . . 4 rings
Apricots 🌾 . . . . 7 halves
Dates (medium) 2½
Figs 🌾 1½
Prunes (medium) 🌾 3
Raisins . . . . 2 tbsp

FRUIT JUICE

Apple juice/cider . . . . ½ cup
Cranberry juice cocktail . . . . ⅓ cup
Grapefruit juice . . . . ½ cup
Grape juice . . . . ⅓ cup
Orange juice. . . . . ½ cup
Pineapple juice. . . . . ½ cup
Prune juice . . . . ⅓ cup

MILK LIST

E ach serving of milk or milk products on this list contains about 12 grams of carbohydrate and 8 grams of protein. The amount of fat in milk is measured in percent (%) of butter-fat. The calories vary, depending on what kind of milk you choose. The list is divided into three parts based on the amount of fat and calories: skim/very-low-fat milk, low-fat milk, and whole milk. One serving (one milk exchange) of each of these includes the following:

	Carbohydrate (grams)	Protein (grams)	Fat (grams)	Calories
Skim/Very-Low-Fat	12	8	trace	90
Low-Fat	12	8	5	120
Whole	12	8	8	150

Milk is the body's main source of calcium, the mineral needed for growth and repair of bones. Yogurt is also a good source of calcium. Yogurt and many dry or powdered milk products have different amounts of fat. If you have questions about a particular item, read the label to find out the fat and calorie content.

Milk is good to drink, but it can also be added to cereal, and to other foods. Many tasty dishes such as sugar-free pudding are made with milk (see the Combination Foods list). Add life to plain yogurt by adding one of your fruit exchanges to it.

SKIM AND VERY-LOW-FAT MILK
Skim milk . . . . 1 cup
½% milk . . . . 1 cup
1% milk . . . . 1 cup
Low-fat buttermilk . . . . 1 cup
Evaporated skim milk . . . . ½ cup
Dry nonfat milk . . . . ⅓ cup
Plain nonfat yogurt . . . . 8 oz

LOW-FAT MILK
2% milk . . . . 1 cup
Plain low-fat yogurt . . . . 8 oz
  (with added nonfat milk solids)

WHOLE MILK
The whole milk group has much more fat per serving than the skim and low-fat groups. Whole milk has more than 3¼% butterfat. Try to limit your choices from the whole milk group as much as possible.

Whole milk . . . . 1 cup
Whole plain yogurt . . . . 8 oz
Evaporated whole milk . . . . ½ cup

FAT LIST

Each serving on the fat list contains about 5 grams of fat and 45 calories.

The foods on the fat list contain mostly fat, although some items may also contain a small amount of protein. All fats are high in calories and should be carefully measured. Everyone should modify fat intake by eating unsaturated fats instead of saturated fats. The sodium content of these foods varies widely. Check the label for sodium information.

UNSATURATED FATS

Avocado (medium) . . . . ⅛
Margarine . . . . 1 tsp
Margarine, diet ☆ . . . . 1 tbsp
Mayonnaise . . . . 1 tsp
Mayonnaise, ... 1 tbsp
   reduced-calorie ☆
Nuts and Seeds:
   Almonds, dry roasted . . . . 6 whole
   Cashews, dry roasted . . . . 1 tbsp
   Pecans . . . . 2 whole
   Peanuts . . . . 20 small or 10 large
   Walnuts . . . . 2 whole
   Other nuts . . . . 1 tbsp
   Seeds, pine nuts, sunflower . . . . 2 tsp
     (without shells)
   Pumpkin seeds . . . . 2 tsp

Oil (corn, cottonseed, ... 1 tsp
   safflower, soybean,
   sunflower, olive, peanut)
Olives ☆ . . . . 10 small or 5 large
Salad dressing, ... 2 tsp
   mayonnaise-type
Salad dressing, ... 1 tbsp
   mayonnaise-type,
   low-calorie
Salad dressing . . . . 1 tbsp
   (oil varieties) ☆
Salad dressing, ... 2 tbsp*
   low-calorie 🖐

* Two tablespoons of low-calorie salad dressing is a free food.

SATURATED FATS

Butter . . . . 1 tsp
Bacon ☆ . . . . 1 slice
Chitterlings . . . . ½ oz
Coconut, shredded . . . . 2 tbsp
Coffee whitener, liquid . . . . 2 tbsp
Coffee whitener powder . . . . 4 tsp
Cream (light, coffee, table) . . . . 2 tbsp
Cream, sour . . . . 2 tbsp
Cream (heavy, whipping) . . . . 1 tbsp
Salt pork ☆ . . . . ¼ oz

🖐 *400 mg or more of sodium per exchange*

☆ *400 mg or more of sodium if two or more exchanges are eaten*

FREE FOODS

A free food is any food or drink that contains less than 20 calories per serving. You can eat as much as you want of those items that have no serving size specified. You may eat two or three servings per day of those items that have a specific serving size. Be sure to spread them out through the day.

Fruit: (½ cup)
Cranberries, unsweetened
Rhubarb, unsweetened

Condiments:
Catsup (1 tbsp)
Horseradish
Mustard
Pickles 🐚, dill, unsweetened
Salad dressing, low-calorie (2 tbsp)
Taco sauce (3 tbsp)
Vinegar

Salad Greens:
Endive
Escarole
Lettuce
Romaine
Spinach

Drinks:
Bouillon 🐚 or broth without fat
Bouillon, low-sodium
Carbonated drinks, sugar-free
Carbonated water
Club soda
Cocoa powder, unsweetened (1 tbsp)
Coffee/Tea
Drink mixes, sugar-free
Tonic water, sugar-free

Sweet Substitutes:
Candy, hard, sugar-free
Gelatin, sugar-free
Gum, sugar-free
Jam/Jelly, sugar-free (less than 20 cal/2 tsp)
Pancake syrup, sugar-free (1–2 tbsp)
Sugar substitutes (saccharin, aspartame)
Whipped topping (2 tbsp)

Vegetables: (raw, 1 cup)
Cabbage
Celery
Chinese cabbage 🌾
Cucumber
Green onion
Hot peppers
Mushrooms
Radishes
Zucchini 🌾

Nonstick Pan Spray

Seasonings
Seasonings can be very helpful in making food taste better. Be careful of how much sodium you use. Read the label, and choose those seasonings that do not contain sodium or salt.

Basil (fresh)
Celery seeds
Chili powder
Chives
Cinnamon
Curry
Dill
Flavoring extracts
    (vanilla, almond, walnut,
    peppermint,butter,
    lemon, etc.)

Garlic
Garlic powder
Herbs
Hot pepper sauce
Lemon
Lemon juice
Lemon pepper
Lime
Lime juice
Mint
Onion powder
Oregano
Paprika
Pepper
Pimiento
Spices
Soy sauce 🥢
Soy sauce, low-sodium ("lite") 🥢
Wine, used in cooking (¼ cup)
Worcestershire sauce

🌾 *3 grams or more of fiber per exchange*

🥢 *400 mg or more of sodium per exchange*

COMBINATION FOODS

Much of the food we eat is mixed together in various combinations. These combination foods do not fit into only one exchange list. It can be quite hard to tell what is in a certain casserole dish or baked food item. This is a list of average values for some typical combination foods. This list will help you fit these foods into your meal plan. Ask your dietitian for information about any other foods you'd like to eat. *The American Diabetes Association/American Dietetic Association Family Cookbooks* and the *American Diabetes Association Holiday Cookbook* have many recipes and further information about many foods, including combination foods. Check your library or local bookstore.

FOOD	AMOUNT	EXCHANGES
Casseroles, homemade	1 cup (8 oz)	2 starch, 2 medium-fat meat, 1 fat
Cheese pizza 🌢 thin crust	¼ of 15 oz or ¼ of 10 in.	2 starch, 1 medium-fat meat, 1 fat
Chili with beans 🌢 (commercial)	1 cup (8 oz)	2 starch, 2 medium-fat meat, 2 fat
Chow mein 🌢 (without noodles or rice)	2 cups (16 oz)	1 starch, 2 vegetable, 2 lean meat
Macaroni and cheese 🌢	1 cup (8 oz)	2 starch, 1 medium-fat meat, 2 fat

Soup:

FOOD	AMOUNT	EXCHANGES
Bean 🗲 🌢	1 cup (8 oz)	1 starch, 1 vegetable, 1 lean meat
Chunky, all varieties 🌢	10¾ oz can	1 starch, 1 vegetable, 1 medium-fat meat
Cream 🌢 (made with water)	1 cup (8 oz)	1 starch, 1 fat
Vegetable 🌢 or broth-type 🌢	1 cup (8 oz)	1 starch
Spaghetti and meatballs 🌢 (canned)	1 cup (8 oz)	2 starch, 1 medium-fat meat, 1 fat
Sugar-free pudding (made with skim milk)	½ cup	1 starch

If beans are used as a meat substitute:

FOOD	AMOUNT	EXCHANGES
Dried beans 🗲, peas 🗲, lentils 🗲	1 cup (cooked)	2 starch, 1 lean meat

🗲 *3 grams or more of fiber per exchange*

🌢 *400 mg or more of sodium per exchange*

FOODS FOR OCCASIONAL USE

Moderate amounts of some foods can be used in your meal plan, in spite of their sugar or fat content, as long as you can maintain blood-glucose control. The following list includes average exchange values for some of these foods. Because they are concentrated sources of carbohydrate, you will notice that the portion sizes are very small. Check with your dietitian for advice on how often and when you can eat them.

FOOD	AMOUNT	EXCHANGES
Angel food cake	¹⁄₁₂ cake	2 starch
Cake, no icing	¹⁄₁₂ cake, or a 3 in. square	2 starch, 2 fat
Cookies, small (1¾ in. across)	2	1 starch, 1 fat
Frozen fruit yogurt	⅓ cup	1 starch
Gingersnaps	3	1 starch
Granola	¼ cup	1 starch, 1 fat
Granola bars, small	1	1 starch, 1 fat
Ice cream, any flavor	½ cup	1 starch, 2 fat
Ice milk, any flavor	½ cup	1 starch, 1 fat
Sherbet, any flavor	¼ cup	1 starch
Snack chips ★ all varieties	1 oz	1 starch, 2 fat
Vanilla wafers, small	6	1 starch

★ *400 mg or more of sodium if two or more exchanges are eaten*

SOURCES OF SOME FAVORED INGREDIENTS

1. The following ingredients, which have been specified in a number of recipes in this cookbook, are readily available in health-food stores: granulated fructose, cracked-wheat flour, light and dark rye flours, buckwheat flour, brown rice flour, carob powder, non-aluminum baking powder, natural dried fruits (unsulfured), unshelled sesame seed, date sugar (also available from Sunshine Valley, P.O. Box 5517, Sherman Oaks, CA 91413), smoked yeast (Bakon-Yeast; also available from Bakon-Yeast, Inc., P.O. Box 651, Rhinelander, WI 54501).

2. Wherever instructions indicate whipping evaporated skim milk, I suggest Pet Light, manufactured by Pet, Inc. It's generally available in supermarkets and is the only brand I know of that whips to the consistency of whipped cream and retains its shape while combining with other ingredients. For best results, use the large whisk attachment of your mixing machine, and use a mixer on a stand rather than a hand-held mixer.

INDEX